Understanding Mechanical Ventilation

Ashfaq Hasan

Understanding Mechanical Ventilation

A Practical Handbook

Second Edition

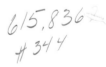

Springer

Ashfaq Hasan
1 Maruthi Heights Road No.
Banjara Hills
Hyderabad-500034
Flat 1-E
India
ashfaqhasanmd@gmail.com

ISBN: 978-1-84882-868-1 e-ISBN: 978-1-84882-869-8

DOI: 10.1007/978-1-84882-869-8

Springer Dordrecht Heidelberg London New York

Library of Congress Control Number: 2010920240

Cover design: eStudio Calamar, Figueres/Berlin

Printed on acid-free paper

Springer is part of Springer Science+Business Media (www.springer.com)

'To my parents'

Preface to the Second Edition

Simplify, simplify!

Henry David Thoreau

For writers of technical books, there can be no better piece of advice.

Around the time of writing the first edition – about a decade ago – there were very few monographs on this subject: today, there are possibly no less than 20.

Based on critical inputs, this edition stands thoroughly revamped. New chapters on ventilator waveforms, airway humidification, and aerosol therapy in the ICU now find a place. Novel software-based modes of ventilation have been included. Ventilator-associated pneumonia has been separated into a new chapter. Many new diagrams and algorithms have been added.

As in the previous edition, considerable energy has been spent in presenting the material in a reader-friendly, conversational style. And as before, the book remains firmly rooted in physiology.

My thanks are due to Madhu Reddy, Director of Universities Press – formerly a professional associate and now a friend, P. Sudhir, my tireless Pulmonary Function Lab technician who found the time to type the bits and pieces of this manuscript in between patients, A. Sobha for superbly organizing my time, Grant Weston and Cate Rogers at Springer, London, Balasaraswathi Jayakumar at Spi, India for her tremendous support, and to Dr. C. Eshwar Prasad, who, for his words of advice, I should have thanked years ago.

Above all, I thank my wife and daughters, for understanding.

Hyderabad, India Ashfaq Hasan

Preface to the First Edition

In spite of technological advancements, it is generally agreed upon that mechanical ventilation is as yet not an exact science: therefore, it must still be something of an art. The science behind the art of ventilation, however, has undergone a revolution of sorts, with major conceptual shifts having occurred in the last couple of decades.

The care of patients with multiple life-threatening problems is nothing short of a monumental challenge and only an envied few are equal to it. Burgeoning information has deluged the generalist and placed increasing reliance on the specialist, sometimes with loss of focus in a clinical situation. Predictably, this has led to the evolution of a team approach, but, for the novice in critical care, beginning the journey at the confluence of the various streams of medicine makes for a tempestuous voyage. Compounding the problem is the fact that monographs on specialized areas such as mechanical ventilation are often hard to come by. The beginner has often to sail, as it were, "an uncharted sea," going mostly by what he hears and sees around him.

It is the intent of this book to familiarize not only physicians, but also nurses and respiratory technologists with the concepts that underlie mechanical ventilation. A conscious attempt has been made to stay in touch with medical physiology throughout this book, in order to specifically address the hows and whys of mechanical ventilation. At the same time, this book incorporates currently accepted strategies for the mechanical ventilation of patients with specific disorders; this should be of some value to specialists practicing in their respective ICUs. The graphs presented in this book are representative and are not drawn to scale.

This book began where the writing of another was suspended. What was intended to be a short chapter in a handbook of respiratory diseases outgrew its confines and expanded to the proportions of a book.

No enterprise, however modest, can be successful without the support of friends and well wishers, who in this case are too numerous to mention individually. I thank my wife for her unflinching support and patience and my daughters for showing maturity and understanding beyond their years; in many respects, I have taken a long time to write this book. I also acknowledge Mr. Samuel Alfred for his excellent secretarial assistance and my colleagues, residents, and respiratory therapists for striving tirelessly, selflessly, and sometimes thanklessly to mitigate the suffering of others.

Ashfaq Hasan, 2003

Contents

Chapter 1
Historical Aspects of Mechanical Ventilation

As early as in the fifth century BC, Hippocrates, described a technique for the prevention of asphyxiation. In his work, "Treatise on Air," Hippocrates stated, "One should introduce a cannula into the trachea along the jawbone so that air can be drawn into the lungs." Hippocrates thus provided the first description of endotracheal intubation (ET).[4,10]

The first form of mechanical ventilator can probably be credited to Paracelsus, who in 1530 used fire-bellows fitted with a tube to pump air into the patient's mouth. In 1653, Andreas Vesalius recognized that artificial respiration could be administered by tracheotomising a dog.[24] In his classic, "De Humani Corporis Fabricia," Vesalius stated, "But that life may … be restored to the animal, an opening must be attempted in the trunk of the trachea, in which a tube of reed or cane should be put; you will then blow into this so that the lung may rise again and the animal take in air… And also as I do this, and take care that the lung is inflated in intervals, the motion of the heart and arteries does not stop…."

A hundred years later, Robert Hooke duplicated Vesalius' experiments on a thoracotomised dog, and while insufflating air into an opening made into the animal's trachea, observed that "the dog… capable of being kept alive by the reciprocal blowing up of his lungs with Bellows, and they suffered to subside, for the space of an hour or more, after his Thorax had been so displayed, and his Aspera arteria cut off just below the Epiglottis and bound upon the nose of the Bellows."[11] Hooke also made the important observation that it was not merely

A. Hasan, *Understanding Mechanical Ventilation*,
DOI: 10.1007/978-1-84882-869-8_1,

the regular movement of the thorax that prevented asphyxia, but the maintenance of phasic airflow into the lungs. What was possibly the first successful instance of human resuscitation by mouth-to-mouth breathing was described in 1744 by John Fothergill in England.

The use of bellows to resuscitate victims of near-drowning was described by the Royal Humane Society in the eighteenth century.[20] The society, also known as the "Society for the Rescue of Drowned Persons" was constituted in 1767, but the development of fatal pneumothoraces produced by vigorous attempts at resuscitation led to subsequent abandonment of such techniques. John Hunter's innovative double-bellows system (one bellow for blowing in fresh air, and another for drawing out the contaminated air) was adapted by the Society in 1782, and introduced a new concept into ventilatory care.

In 1880, the endotracheal route was used, possibly for the first time, for cannulation of the trachea, and emerged as a realistic alternative to tracheotomy.[14] Appreciation of the fact that life could be sustained by supporting the function of the lungs (and indeed the circulation) by external means led to the development of machines devised for this purpose. In 1838, Scottish physician John Dalziez described the first tank ventilator. In 1864 a body-tank ventilator was developed by Alfred Jones of Kentucky.[9] The patient was seated inside an air-tight box which enclosed his body, neck downwards. Negative pressure generated within the apparatus produced inspiration, and expiration was aided by the cyclical generation of positive pressure at the end of each inspiratory breath. Jones took out a patent on his device which claimed that it could cure not only paralysis, neuralgia, asthma and bronchitis, but also rheumatism, dyspepsia, seminal weakness and deafness. Woillez's hand-cranked "spirophore" (1876) and Egon Braun's small wooden tank for the resuscitation of asphyxiated children followed. The former, the doctor operated by cranking a handle; the latter needed the treating physician to vigorously suck and blow into a tube attached to the box that enclosed the patient. In respect of Wilhelm Shwake's pneumatic chamber, the patient himself could lend a hand by pulling and pushing against the bellows.

In 1929, Philip Drinker, Louis Shaw, and Charles McKhann at the Department of Ventilation, Illumination, and Physiology, of the Harvard Medical School introduced what they termed "an apparatus for the prolonged administration of artificial respiration."[9] This team which included an engineer (Drinker), a physiologist (Shaw), and a physician (McKhann) saw the development of what was dubbed "the iron lung." Drinker's ventilator relied on the application of negative pressure to expand the chest, in a manner similar to Alfred Jones' ventilator. The subject (at first a paralyzed cat, and then usually a patient of poliomyelitis) was laid within an air-tight iron tank. A padded collar around the patient's neck provided a seal, and the pressure within the tank was rhythmically lowered by pumps or bellows. Access to the patient for nursing was understandably limited, though ports were provided for auscultation and monitoring.* Emerson, in 1931 in a variation upon this theme incorporated an apparatus with which it was possible to additionally deliver positive pressure breaths at the mouth; this made nursing easier. The patient could now be supported on positive pressure breaths alone, while the tank was opened periodically for nursing and examination.

Toward the end of the nineteenth century, a ventilator functioning on a similar principle as the iron tank was independently developed by Ignaz von Hauke of Austria, Rudolf Eisenmenger of Vienna, and Alexander Graham Bell of the USA. Named so because of its similarity to the fifteenth century body armor, the "Cuirass" consisted of a breast plate and a back plate secured together to form an air-tight seal. Again, negative pressure generated by means of bellows (and during subsequent years, by a motor from a vacuum cleaner) provided the negative pressure to repetitively expand the thoracic cage and so move air in and out of the lungs. The Cuirass, by leaving the patient's arms unencumbered, and by

*A rich American financier's son who developed poliomyelitis during a visit to China was transported back home in a Drinker-tank by a dozen caregivers which included seven Chinese nurses. He used the iron lung for more than two decades during which he married and fathered three children.

causing less circulatory embarrassment, offered certain advantages over the tank respirator; in fact, Eisenmenger's Cuirass was as much used for circulatory assistance during resuscitation as it was for artificial ventilation. Despite its advantages, the Cuirass proved to be somewhat less efficient than the tank respirator in providing mechanical assistance to breathing.

During the earliest years of the twentieth century, advances in the field of thoracic surgery saw the design of a surgical chamber by Ferdinand Sauerbruch in 1904. This chamber functioned much on the same lines as the tank respirator except that the chamber included not only the patient's torso, but the surgeon himself.[4] Brauer reversed Sauerbruch's principle of ventilation by enclosing only the patient's head within a much smaller chamber which provided a positive pressure. In 1911, Drager designed his "Pulmotor," a resuscitation unit which provided positive pressure inflation to the patient by means of a mask held upon the face. A tilted head position along with cricoid pressure (to prevent gastric insufflation of air) aided ventilation. The unit was powered by a compressed gas cylinder, and used by the fire and police departments for the resuscitation of victims.[18]

Negative pressure ventilators were extensively used during the polio epidemic that ravaged Los Angeles in 1948 and Scandinavia in 1952. During the Scandinavian epidemic, nearly three thousand polio-affected patients were treated in the Community Diseases Hospital of Copenhagen over a period of less than 6 months.[16] The catastrophic mortality during the early days of the epidemic saw the use of the cuffed tracheostomy tube for the first time, in patients outside operating theaters. The polio epidemics in USA and Denmark saw the development and refinement of many of the principles of positive pressure ventilation.

In 1950, responding to a need for better ventilators, Ray Bennet and colleagues developed an accessory attachment with which it became possible to intermittently administer positive pressure breaths in synchrony with the negative pressure breaths, delivered by a tank ventilator.[3] The supplementation of negative pressure ventilation with intermittent positive pressure breaths did result in a substantial reduction in mortality.[9,12,13] Bennet's valve had originally been designed to enable pilots to breathe comfortably at high altitudes. The end of the Second World War saw the adaptation of the Bennet valve to regulate the flow of gases within mechanical ventilators.[17] Likewise, Forrest Bird's aviation experiences led to the design of the Bird Mark seven ventilator.

Around this time, interest predictably focused on the physiological effects of mechanical ventilation. Courmand and then Maloney and Whittenberger made important observations on the hemodynamic effects of mechanical ventilation.[15,17] By the mid 1950s, the concept of controlled mechanical ventilation had emerged. Engstrom's paper, published in 1963, expostulated upon the clinical effects of prolonged controlled ventilation.[7] In this landmark report, Engstrom stressed on the "complete substitution of the spontaneous ventilation of the patient by taking over both the ventilatory work and the control of the adequacy of ventilation" and so brought into definition, the concept of CMV. Engstrom developed ventilator models in which the minute volume requirements of the patient could be set. Setting the respiratory rate within a given minute ventilation determined the backup tidal volumes, and the overall effect was remarkably similar to the IMV mode in vogue today.

Improvements in the design of the Bennet ventilators saw the emergence of the familiar Puritan-Bennet machines. The popularity of the Bennet and Bird ventilators in USA (both of which were pressure cycled) soon came to be rivaled by the development of volume-cycled piston-driven ventilators. These volume preset Emerson ventilators better guaranteed tidal volumes, and became recognized as potential anesthesia machines, as well as respiratory devices for long-term ventilatory support.

Toward the end of the 1960s, with increasing challenges being presented during the treatment of critically ill patients on artificial ventilation, there arose a need for specialized areas for superior supportive care. During this period, a new disease entity came to be recognized, the Adult Respiratory Distress Syndrome, or the acute respiratory distress syndrome

(ARDS) as it is known today. Physicians were confronted with rising demands for the supportive care of patients with this condition. The Respiratory Intensive Care Unit emerged as an important area for the treatment of critically ill patients requiring intensive monitoring. The use of positive end-expiratory pressure (PEEP) for the management of ARDS patients came into vogue, principally through Ashbaugh and Petty's revival of Poulton and Barach's concepts of the 1930s. A number of investigators staked claim to the development of the concept of PEEP, but controversy did not preclude its useful application.[19,21]

In 1971, Gregory et al applied continuous positive pressure to the care of neonates with the neonatal respiratory distress syndrome (NRDS) and showed that pediatric mechanical ventilation was possible. Several departures from the original theme of positive pressure ventilation followed, including the development of heroic measures for artificial support.[1,5,8]

Today's ventilators have evolved from simple mechanical devices into highly complex microprocessor controlled systems which make for smoother patient-ventilator interaction. Such sophistication has, however, shifted the appreciation of the ventilator's operational intricacies into the sphere of a new and now indispensable specialist – the biomedical engineer.

Of late, resurgence in the popularity of noninvasive positive pressure breathing and the advent of high frequency positive pressure ventilation have further invigorated the area of mechanical ventilation; it also remains to be seen whether the promise of certain as yet unconventional modes of ventilation will be borne out in the near future.

References

1. Anderson HL, Steimle C, Shapiro M, et al Extracorporeal life support for adult cardiorespoiratory failure. *Surgery*. 1993; 114:161
2. Ashbaugh DG, Bigelow DB, Petty TL, et al Acute respiratory distress in adults. *Lancet*. 1967;2:319–323

3. Bennet VR, Bower AE, Dillon JB, Axelrod B. Investigation on care and treatment of poliomyelitis patients. *Ann West Med Surg*. 1950;4:561–582
4. Comroe JH. *Retrospectorscope: Insights into Medical Discovery*. Menlo park, CA: Von Gehr; 1977
5. Downs JB, Stock MC. Airway pressure release ventilation: a new concept in ventilatory support. *Crit Care Med*. 1987;15:459
6. Drinker P, Shaw LA. An apparatus for the prolonged administration of artificial respiration. 1. A design for adults and children. *J Clin Invest*. 1929;7:229–247
7. Engstrom CG. The clinical application of prolonged controlled ventilation. *Acta Anasthesiol Scand [Suppl]*. 1963;13: 1–52
8. Fort PF, Farmer C, Westerman J, et al High-frequency oscillatory ventilation for adult respiratory distress syndrome. *Crit Care Med*. 1997;25:937
9. Grenvik A, Eross B, Powner D. Historical survey of mechanical ventilation. *Int Anesthesiol Clin*. 1980;18:1–9
10. Heironimus TW. Mechanical Artificial Ventilation, Springfield, III, Charles C. Thomas; 1971
11. Hooke M. Of preserving animals alive by blowing through their lungs with bellows. *Philo Trans R Soc*. 1667;2:539–540
12. Ibsen B. The anesthetist's view point on treatment of respiratory complications in polio during epidemic in Copenhagen. *Proc R Soc Med*. 1954;47:72–74
13. Laurie G. Ventilator users, home care and independent living: An historical perspective. In: Kutscher AH, Gilgoff I (eds). The Ventilator: Psychosocial and Medical aspects. New York Foundation of Thanatology, 2001; p147–151.
14. Macewen W. Clinical observations on the introduction of tracheal tubes by the mouth instead of performing tracheotomy or laryngotomy. *Br Med J*. 1880;2(122–124):163–165
15. Maloney JV, Whittenberger JL. Clinical implications of pressures used in the body respiration. *Am J Med Sci*. 1951;221: 425–430
16. Meyers RA. Mechanical support of respiration. *Surg Clin North Am*. 1974;54:1115
17. Motley HL, Cournand A, Werko L, et al Studies of intermittent positive pressure breathing as a means of administering artificial respiration in a man. *JAMA*. 1948;137:370–387
18. Mushin WI, et al *Automatic Ventilation of the Lungs*. 2nd ed. Oxford, England: Blackwell Scientific; 1979

19. Petty TL, Nett LM, Ashbaugh DG. Improvement in oxygenation in the adult respiratory distress syndrome by positive end expiratory pressure (PEEP). *Respir Care*. 1971;16:173–176
20. Randel-Baker L. History of thoracic anesthesia. In: Mushin WW, ed. *Thoracic anesthesia*. Philadelphia: FA Davis; 1963:598–661
21. Springer PR, Stevens PM. The influence of PEEP on survival of patients in respiratory failure. *Am J Med*. 1979;66:196–200
22. Standiford TJ, Morganroth ML. High-frequency ventilation. *Chest*. 1989;96:1380
23. Stock MC, Downs JB, Frolicher DA. Airway pressure release ventilation. *Crit Care Med*. 1987;15:462
24. Vesalius A. De humani corporis fabrica, Lib VII, cap. XIX De vivorum sectione nonulla, Basle, Operinus, 1543;658

Chapter 2
The Indications for Mechanical Ventilation

Apart from its supportive role in patients undergoing operative procedures, mechanical ventilatory support is indicated when spontaneous ventilation is inadequate for the sustenance of life.

The word *support* bears emphasis, for mechanical ventilation is not a cure for the disease for which it is instituted: it is at best a form of support, offering time and rest to the patient until the underlying disease processes are resolved. Results with mechanical ventilation are consistently better when mechanical ventilatory support is initiated early and electively rather than in a crash situation.

The indications for mechanical ventilation may be viewed as falling under several broad categories (Fig. 2.1).

2.1 Hypoxia

Mechanical ventilation is often electively instituted when it is not possible to maintain an adequate oxygen saturation of hemoglobin. While optimization of tissue oxygenation is the goal, it is rarely possible to reliably assess the extent of *tissue* hypoxia. Instead, indices of *blood* oxygenation may rather need to be relied upon. Increasing the fraction of inspired oxygen (FIO_2) indiscriminately in an attempt to improve oxygenation may unnecessarily subject the patient to the danger of oxygen toxicity (these concepts will be addressed at a later stage). Mechanical ventilation enables better control

A. Hasan, *Understanding Mechanical Ventilation*,
DOI: 10.1007/978-1-84882-869-8_2,

Indications for intubation	Indications for ventilation
• Need to secure airway • Depressed sensorium • Depressed airway reflexes • Upper airway instability after trauma • Decreased airway patency • Need for sedation in the setting of poor airway control • Imaging (CT, MRT) and transportation of an unstable patient	• Hypoxia: acute hypoxemic respiratory failure • Hypoventilation • Unacceptably high work of breathing • Hemodynamic compromise • Cardiorespiratory arrest • Refractory shock • Raised intracranial pressure • Flail chest

FIGURE 2.1. Indications for intubation & ventilation.

of hypoxemia with relatively low inspired O_2 concentrations, thereby diminishing the risk of oxygen toxicity.

2.2 Hypoventilation

A major indication for mechanical ventilation is when the alveolar ventilation falls short of the patient's requirements. Conditions that depress the respiratory center produce a decline in alveolar ventilation with a rise in arterial CO_2 tension. A rising $PaCO_2$ can also result from the hypoventilation that results when fatiguing respiratory muscles are unable to sustain ventilation, as in a patient who is expending considerable effort in moving air into stiffened or obstructed lungs. Under such circumstances, mechanical ventilation may be used to support gas exchange until the patient's respiratory drive has been restored, or tired respiratory muscles rejuvenated, and the inciting pathology significantly resolved (Fig. 2.2).

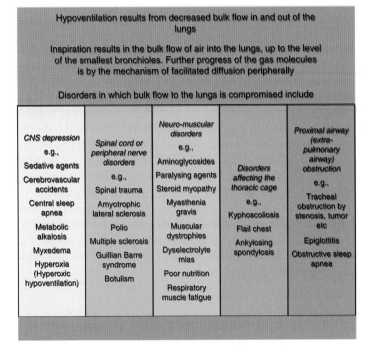

Hypoventilation results from decreased bulk flow in and out of the lungs

Inspiration results in the bulk flow of air into the lungs, up to the level of the smallest bronchioles. Further progress of the gas molecules is by the mechanism of facilitated diffusion peripherally

Disorders in which bulk flow to the lungs is compromised include

CNS depression	*Spinal cord or peripheral nerve disorders*	*Neuro-muscular disorders*	*Disorders affecting the thoracic cage*	*Proximal airway (extra-pulmonary airway) obstruction*
e.g.,	e.g.,	e.g.,	e.g.,	e.g.,
Sedative agents Cerebrovascular accidents Central sleep apnea Metabolic alkalosis Myxedema Hyperoxia (Hyperoxic hypoventilation)	Spinal trauma Amyotrophic lateral sclerosis Polio Multiple sclerosis Guillian Barre syndrome Botulism	Aminoglycosides Paralysing agents Steroid myopathy Myasthenia gravis Muscular dystrophies Dyselectrolytemias Poor nutrition Respiratory muscle fatigue	Kyphoscoliosis Flail chest Ankylosing spondylosis	Tracheal obstruction by stenosis, tumor etc Epiglottitis Obstructive sleep apnea

FIGURE 2.2. Causes of Hypoventilation.

2.3 Increased Work of Breathing

Another major category where assisted ventilation is used is in those situations in which excessive work of breathing results in hemodynamic compromise. Here, even though gas exchange may not be actually impaired, the increased work of breathing because of either high airway resistance or poor lung compliance may impose a substantial burden on, for example, a compromised myocardium.

When oxygen delivery to the tissues is compromised on account of impaired myocardial function, mechanical ventilation by resting the respiratory muscles can reduce the work of breathing. This reduces the oxygen consumption of the respiratory muscles and results in better perfusion of the myocardium itself.

2.4 Other Indications

In addition to these major indications, mechanical ventilation may be of value in certain specific conditions. The vasoconstriction produced by deliberate hyperventilation can reduce the volume of the cerebral vascular compartment, helping to reduce raised intracranial pressures. In flail chest, mechanical ventilation can be used to provide internal stabilization of the thorax when multiple rib fractures compromise the integrity of the chest wall; in such cases, mechanical ventilation using positive end-expiratory pressure (PEEP) normalizes thoracic and lung mechanics, so that adequate gas exchange becomes possible.

Where postoperative pain or neuromuscular disease limits lung expansion, mechanical ventilation can be employed to preserve a reasonable functional residual capacity within the lungs and prevent atelectasis. These issues have been specifically addressed in Chap. 9.

2.5 Criteria for Intubation and Ventilation

While the prevailing criteria for defining the need for intubation and ventilation of a patient in respiratory failure have met general acceptance, these are largely intuitive and based upon the subjective assessment of a patient's condition (Fig. 2.3 and Table 2.1). *See also Chap. 12* .

Objective criteria that are in current use are a forced expiratory volume in the first second (FEV_1) of less than 10 mL/kg body weight and a forced vital capacity (FVC) of less than 15 mL/kg body weight, both of which indicate a poor ventilatory capability.

Similarly, a respiratory rate higher than 35 breaths/min would mean an unacceptably high work of breathing and a substantial degree of respiratory distress, and is recognized as one of the criteria for intubation and ventilation. A $PaCO_2$ in excess of 55 mmHg (especially if rising, and in the presence of acidemia) would likewise imply the onset of respiratory muscle fatigue. Except in habitual CO_2 retainers, a $PaCO_2$ of

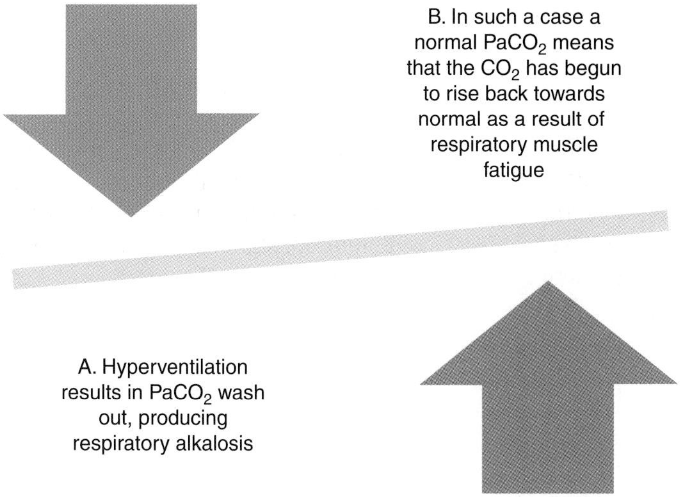
B. In such a case a normal $PaCO_2$ means that the CO_2 has begun to rise back towards normal as a result of respiratory muscle fatigue
A. Hyperventilation results in $PaCO_2$ wash out, producing respiratory alkalosis

FIGURE 2.3. $PaCO_2$ in status asthmaticus.

55 mmHg and over would normally reflect severe respiratory muscle dysfunction.

Documented $PaCO_2$ from an earlier stage of the patient's present illness may have considerable bearing on the interpretation of subsequent $PaCO_2$ levels (Fig. 2.3). For example, in an asthmatic patient in acute severe exacerbation, bronchospasm-induced hyperventilation can be expected to "wash out" the CO_2 from the blood, producing respiratory alkalosis. If in such a patient, the blood gas analysis were to show a normal $PaCO_2$ level, this would imply that the hypoventilation produced by respiratory muscle fatigue has allowed the $PaCO_2$ to rise back to normal. It is important to realize here, that although the $PaCO_2$ is now in the normal range, it is actually on its way up, and if this is not appreciated, neither the $PaCO_2$ nor the patient will stay normal for very long. A supranormal $PaCO_2$ in status asthmaticus should certainly be a cause of alarm and reinforce the need for mechanical ventilatory support.

A PaO_2 of less than 55–60 mmHg on 0.5 FIO_2 or a widened A-a DO_2 gradient (of 450 mmHg and beyond on 100% O_2)

TABLE 2.1. Criteria for ventilation.

Criteria value	Normal range	Critical level	Comment
Respiratory muscle performance			
Maximum inspiratory pressure (MIP)	−50 to −100 cm H_2O	More positive than −20 cm H_2O	Useful in neuromuscular patients. Can be measured by a Bourdon manometer interfaced to the patient by a mask, mouthpiece, or ET adaptor. Ideally, MIP measurements should be made after maximal exhalation
Maximum expiratory pressure (MEP)	+100 cm H_2O	Less than 40 cm H_2O	
Vital capacity (VC)	65–75 mL/kg	<15 mL/kg	Measured at the bedside with a pneumotachometer or a hand-held spirometer
Tidal volume (V1)	5–8 mL/kg	<5 mL/kg	Measured at the bedside with a pneumotachometer or a hand-held spirometer
Respiratory frequency (f)	12–20 breaths/min	>35 breaths/min	A high respiratory frequency indicates increased work of breathing, and may be indicative of impending respiratory muscle exhaustion
Forced expired volume at 1 s (FEV_1)	50–60 mL/kg	<10 mL/kg	Important in evaluating the degree of airway obstruction in COPD/asthma. May be difficult or exhausting for the severely obstructed patient
Peak expiratory flow	350–600 L/min	<100 L/min	Important in evaluating the degree of airway obstruction in COPD/asthma. May be difficult or exhausting for the severely obstructed patient
Ventilation			
pH	7.35–7.45	<7.25	A falling pH from respiratory acidosis is a late feature of respiratory muscle fatigue

Criteria value	Normal range	Critical level	Comment
$PaCO_2$	35–45 mmHg	>55 mmHg, and rising	A rising $PaCO_2$ from respiratory acidosis is a late feature of respiratory muscle fatigue
VD/VT	0.3–0.4	>0.6	Dead-space ventilation can be easily calculated at the bedside using capnometry and blood gas analysis (see Chap. 3)
Oxygenation (low values indicate the need for oxygen therapy or PEEP/CPAP; mechanical ventilation may be required if hypoxemia is nonresponsive to the above support, or is very severe)			
PaO_2	80–100 mmHg	<60 mmHg (on FIO_2 0.5)	A PaO_2 of 60 mmHg represents the approximate point where the slope of the oxy-hemoglobin dissociation curve abruptly changes. As the PaO_2 drops further below 60 mmHg, the SpO_2 can be expected to fall sharply
Alveolar-to-arterial oxygen difference	3–30 mmHg	>450 mmHg (on high concentrations of O_2)	The A-a DO_2 is the difference between the alveolar O_2 tension (PAO_2) and the arterial oxygen tension (PaO_2), and is a measure of the ease with which the administered oxygen diffuses into the pulmonary capillary blood
Arterial/alveolar PO_2	0.75	<0.15	The PaO_2/PAO_2 ratio is the proportion of oxygen in the alveolus that eventually gains entry into the pulmonary capillary blood. The PaO_2 is easily read out from the ABG, but the PAO_2 cannot be directly measured and needs to be calculated from the alveolar gas equation (see section 7.1)
PaO_2/FIO_2	475	<200	The PaO_2/FIO_2 ratio obviates the need to calculate PAO_2 (which can be something of an effort for those who are mathematically challenged!)

means that the gas exchange mechanisms in the lung are deranged to a degree that cannot be supported by external oxygen devices alone, and that intubation and ventilation is required for effective support.

It is important to emphasize that the criteria for intubation and ventilation are meant to serve as a guide to the physician who must view them in the context of the clinical situation. Conversely, the patient does not necessarily have to satisfy every criterion for intubation and ventilation in order to be a candidate for invasive ventilatory management. Importantly, improvement or worsening in the trends within these numbers provide the key to judgment in a borderline situation. It must also be pointed out that with the advent of noninvasive positive pressure ventilation as a potential tool for the treatment of early respiratory failure, some of the criteria for the institution of mechanical ventilatory support may need to be revisited. These issues have been discussed in Chap. 13.

References

1. Brochard L. Profuse diaphoresis as an important sign for the differential diagnosis of acute respiratory distress. *Intensive Care Med*. 1992;18:445
2. Comroe JH, Botelho S. The unreliability of cyanosis in the recognition of arterial anoxemia. *Am J Med Sci*. 1947;214:1–6
3. Gibson GJ, Pride NB, Davis JN, et al Pulmonary mechanics in patients with respiratory muscle weakness. *Am Rev Respir Dis*. 1977;115:389–395
4. Gilston A. Facial signs of respiratory distress after cardiac surgery: a plea for the clinical approach to mechanical ventilation. *Anaesthesia*. 1976;31:385–397
5. Hess DR, Branson RD. In: Hess DR, MacIntyre NR, Mishoe SC, et al, eds. *Respiratory care: principles and practices.* Philadelphia: WB Saunders; 2003
6. Kacmarek RM, Cheever P, Foley K, et al Deterination of vital capacity in mechanically ventilated patients: a comparison of techniques. *Respir Care*. 1990;35(11):129

7. Lundsgaard C, Van Slyke DD. Cyanosis. *Medicine*. 1923;2:1–76
8. Manthous CA, Hall JB, Kushner R, et al The effect of mechanical ventilation on oxygen consumption in critically ill patients. *Am J Respir Crit Care Med*. 1995;151:210–214
9. Medd WE, French EB, McA Wyllie V. Cyanosis as a guide to arterial oxygen desaturation. *Thorax*. 1959;14:247–250
10. Mithoefer JC, Bossman OG, Thibeault DW, Mead GD. The clinical estimation of alveolar ventilation. *Am Rev Respir Dis*. 1968;98:868–871
11. Perrigault PF, Pouzeratte YH, Jaber S, et al Changes in occlusion pressure (P0.1) and breathing pattern during pressure support ventilation. *Thorax*. 1999;54:119–123
12. Semmes BJ, Tobin MJ, Snyder JV, Grenvik A. Subjective and objective measurement of tidal volume in critically ill patients. *Chest*. 1985;87:577–579
13. Slutsky AS. Mechanical ventilation. American College of Chest Physicians' Consensus Conference. *Chest*. 1993;104:1833
14. Strohl KP, O'Cain CF, Slutsky AS. Alae nasi activation and nasal resistance in healthy subjects. *J Appl Physiol*. 1982;52:1432–1437
15. Tobin MJ, Guenther SM, Perez W, et al Konno-Mead analysis of ridcage- abdominal motion during successful and unsuccessful trials of weaning from mechanical ventilation. *Am Rev Respir Dis*. 1987;135:1320–1328
16. Tobin MJ, Jenouri GA, Watson H, Sackner MA. Noninvasive measurement of pleural pressure by surface inductive plethysmography. *J Appl Physiol*. 1983;55:267–275
17. Tobin MJ, Mador MJ, Guenther SM, et al Variability of resting respiratory drive and timing in healthy subjects. *J Appl Physiol*. 1988;65:309–317
18. Tobin MJ. Respiratory muscles in disease. *Clin Chest Med*. 1988;9:263–286
19. Tobin MJ. Noninvasive monitoring of ventilation. In: Tobin MJ, ed. *Principles and Practice of Intensive Care Monitoring*. New York: NcGraw-Hill; 1998:465–495
20. Tobin MJ, Perez W, Guenther SM, et al Does rib cage-abdominal paradox signify respiratory muscle fatigue? *J Appl Physiol*. 1987;63:851–860

Chapter 3
Physiological Considerations in the Mechanically Ventilated Patient

3.1 The Physiological Impact of the Endotracheal Tube

The volume of the upper airway is approximately 72 mL in the adult subject.[64] An endotracheal tube of 8 mm internal diameter cuts down this volume by 55–60 mL or by approximately 1 mL/kg body weight.[26] By thus reducing the upper airway volume – and the dead-space – this can increase the alveolar ventilation. In health, it appears that the volume of the upper airway can change by as much as 50% by mere changes in head position. Therefore, the diminution in airway volume that occurs when an endotracheal tube is placed may not be greatly beyond the physiological changes that occur in the innate airway.[64] In fact, the interposition of a Y-connector *adds* approximately 75 mL of dead-space to the circuit, and so the impact of the endotracheal tube in reducing the dead-space is largely negated.

One of the important functions of the glottis is to regulate the flow of air in and out of the lungs. By varying its aperture, the glottis retards the rate at which the deflating lung returns to functional residual capacity (FRC).[20] Since the glottis, by narrowing during expiration, reduces the *rate* of return to FRC but does not influence the *dimensions* of the FRC itself, it is unlikely that bypassing the glottis by the endotracheal tube will result in any reduction in the FRC.[3,4]

A. Hasan, *Understanding Mechanical Ventilation*,
DOI: 10.1007/978-1-84882-869-8_3,

Poiseuille's law states that the resistance (R_{aw}) to the flow of fluids through a long and narrow tube is proportional to the length of the tube (l) and the viscosity of the fluid (η).

Significantly, resistance is inversely proportional to the fourth power of the radius (r). This means that small changes in the radius can have inordinate effects on airway resistance.[6,13]

Poiseuille's law applies to the continuous flow of fluids at low flow rates (laminar flow) in long straight tubes.

The endotracheal tube, however, is neither long nor straight. The length of an endotracheal tube is typically 24–26 cm. This length may not suffice for the conditions for laminar flow to develop, as demanded by Poiseuille's classic equation. Bends in the endotracheal tube interfere with laminar flow and produce turbulence, as do the almost ubiquitous secretions that are adherent to its luminal surface.[84] Moreover, the flow within the endotracheal tube is not constant: a high flow rate engenders further turbulence.

Turbulent rather than laminar flow is therefore the rule in the endotracheal tube, and this adds to the airflow resistance.[46] Increased resistance to the airflow translates into increased work of breathing. Contributing to the work of breathing, as an independent factor, is the bend in the tube itself.[73] The endotracheal tube is especially liable to become sharply angulated when the nasotracheal route is preferred. Any kinking of the tube or biting upon it by the patient is liable to compromise the tubal diameter and has a major impact on airflow resistance.

Despite the fact that Poiseuille's equation may not be relevant in its totality in clinical situations, the effect of variation in endotracheal tube radius can have a tremendous effect on airway resistance.[50]

Interestingly, the replacement of the relatively straight endotracheal tube with the shorter but more angulated tracheostomy tube (of an identical internal diameter) appears to confer no additional advantage with respect to airflow resistance: in experimental animals, the work of breathing in either situation remains the same.[72] Owing to its shorter length, the tracheostomy tube can be expected to offer less resistance to airflow, compared to the endotracheal tube. In fact, the additional turbulence in airflow produced by the crook in the tracheostomy tube negates the advantage of its shorter length.

Box 3.1 Poiseuille's Law

According to Poiseuille's law, the resistance to air flow varies as a function of tube diameter. Poiseuille's law is summarized by the equation

$$R_{aw} = 8\,\eta l/\pi r^4$$

where R_{aw} is the resistance to flow of fluids (in this case, air) within long and narrow tubes (airways), η is the viscosity of the fluid (air) flowing within the tubes (airways), r is the radius of the tubes (airways).

In the clinical context, the length of the airways and the viscosity of the air cannot vary. The only variable is the radius of the tubes, which, of course, is proportional to the airway diameter. If, hypothetically speaking, airway radius were to be halved, the airflow resistance calculated as per Poiseuille's formula would go up 16-fold because airway radius is raised to the power of 4. What this means is that even a slight narrowing in the diameter of either the patient's intrinsic airways or in the endotracheal tube is likely to amplify airway resistance greatly.

3.2 Positive Pressure Breathing

In the spontaneously breathing individual, inspiration is active. The descent of the diaphragm during inspiration increases the vertical size of the thorax; contraction of the scalenii increases the anteroposterior thoracic diameter (by elevating the ribs by a pump-handle movement), and contraction of the parasternal group of muscles increases the transverse thoracic diameter (by a bucket-handle movement). The overall result is an increased intrathoracic volume, and a fall in intrathoracic pressure (ITP) secondary to it. From its usual end-expiratory level of –5 cm H_2O, the intrapleural pressure falls to –10 cm H_2O at the height of inspiration. As a result, the alveolar pressure becomes negative relative to atmospheric pressure, and air flows into the bronchial tree, and through it, to the alveoli. Exhalation is passive and returns the intrathoracic volume to FRC at the end of tidal expiration.

During positive pressure breathing (PPB), inspiration occurs when the central airway pressure is raised above atmospheric pressure, impelling the air into the respiratory tract. As in the spontaneously breathing subject, expiration is passive.

The commonly encountered intrathoracic pressures during breathing have been defined in Fig. 3.1.

Four types of pressure gradients are encountered within the lung[70] (see Fig. 3.2). The transpulmonary pressure (P_{TA}), also known as the lung distending pressure, is the pressure difference between the alveolar pressure (P_{ALV}) and intrapleural pressure (see also Chap 8). Lung inflation occurs when the P_{TA} increases. During spontaneous breathing and negative pressure ventilation, it is the drop in intrathoracic pressure that causes the P_{TA} to increase; on the other hand, the increase in P_{TA} during PPB occurs as a result of an increase in P_{ALV} (see Fig. 3.2). P_{TA} is unchanged when forced inspiratory or expiratory efforts are made against the closed glottis, and so there is no bulk airflow, respectively, in or out of the lungs.

The pressure required for overcoming resistance and elastance during lung inflation can now be worked out (Figs. 3.3 and 3.4).

The major difference between physiological breathing and positive pressure ventilation lies in the intrathoracic pressures during inspiration. In the spontaneously breathing subject, the intrathoracic pressure during inspiration is negative to the atmospheric pressure. In the mechanically ventilated patient on positive pressure ventilation, intrathoracic pressure is positive – this has far reaching implications on the respiratory and circulatory systems (Fig. 3.5).

In the normal lung, in an erect individual, there exists a vertical gradient in the pleural pressure. Intrapleural pressure is more negative at the lung apices than at the bases, primarily because of the effect of the weight of the lung. Intrapleural pressure falls by approximately 0.25 cm of H_2O for each centimeter of lung height. This gradient is also influenced by the hilar attachments of the lung, the shape of the thorax (which

Airway Opening Pressure (P_{awo}) *Syn:* Airway pressure (P_{aw}), Mouth pressure (P_M), Upper airway pressure, proximal airway pressure, mask pressure	• This is the pressure applied at the airway opening (mouth or the patient tube) • In the absence of positive pressure breathing (through endotracheal tube, tracheostomy tube or noninvasively by mask), the P_{aw} is equal to atmospheric pressure
Body surface pressure (P_{bs})	• The pressure at the body surface • Again this pressure is equal to atmospheric pressure unless the patient's body is subjected to negative pressure (as within a negative pressure ventilator **see chapter 14)** or a positive pressure (hyperbaric chamber)
Intrapleural pressure (P_{pl})	• The pressure within the pleural space • During spontaneous breathing this is normally, minus 5cm H_2O at end-exhalation, and minus 10 cm H_2O at end-inspiration. • The surrogate measurement for P_{pl} is esophageal pressure (P_{es}) which can be measured using an esophageal balloon
Alveolar pressure (P_A or P_{ALV}) *Syn:* Intrapulmonary pressure, Lung pressure	• During spontaneous breathing, alveolar pressure is negative to the atmospheric pressure during inspiration (minus 1 cm H_2O), and positive to atmospheric pressure during exhalation (1 cm H_2O)

FIGURE 3.1. Intrathoracic pressures.

is more tapered toward the top) and the abdominal contents (which push upward upon the lung bases).

As the negativity of intrapleural pressure is greater in the upper regions of the lung, the alveoli in the upper lung zones will be larger and more patent than those in the lower zones. During a normal inspiration, the alveoli in the lower lung

Trans-airway pressure (P_{TA}) The difference between the airway opening pressure (P_{awo}) and the alveolar pressure (P_{ALV}): $P_{TA} = P_{awo} - P_{ALV}$	• It is the pressure responsible for driving the bulk flow through the airways. • Produced by the resistance to airflow within the conducting airways.
Transpulmonary pressure (P_{TP}) *Syn* Transalveolar pressure (P_A), Alveolar distending pressure: The difference between the alveolar pressure (P_{ALV}) and the intrapleural pressure (P_{PL}): $P_{TP} = P_{ALV} - P_{PL}$	• The pressure required to distened the lung • When P_{TP} increases, the lung distends • P_{TP} can be made to increase by either increasing the P_{alv} (by positive pressure ventilation) or by decreasing the P_{PL} (by negative pressure ventilation). See also **fig. 3.4**
Trans-Thoracic Pressure (P w or p_{TT}) The difference between the alveolar pressure (P_{ALV}) and the body surface pressure (P_{bs}): $P_{TT} = P_{ALV} - P_{bs}$	• It is the pressure required to distend the lungs along with the thoracic cage.
Transrespiratory-system pressure The difference between the airway opening pressure (pressure at the mouth or patient tube) and the pressure at the body surface): $P_{TR} = P_{awo} - P_{bs}$	• It is the pressure required to expand the lungs (pressure required to overcome elastance), and also to produce airflow (pressure required to overcome resistance). • P_{TR} therefore has two components: Transairway pressure (P_{TA}) which performs the resistive work, and transthoracic pressure (P_{TT}) which performs the elastic work.

FIGURE 3.2. Pressure gradients within the thorax.

zones (which are of relatively smaller end-expiratory volume) are capable of greater expansion, and so comparatively more inspired air goes to the dependent zones. The lower lung

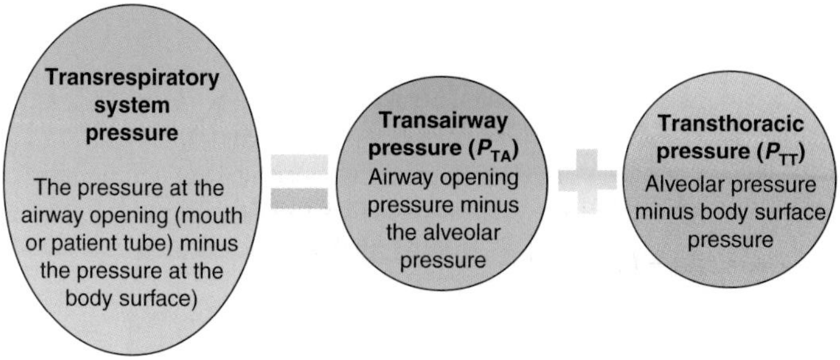
Transrespiratory system pressure
The pressure at the airway opening (mouth or patient tube) minus the pressure at the body surface)
=
Transairway pressure (P_{TA})
Airway opening pressure minus the alveolar pressure
+
Transthoracic pressure (P_{TT})
Alveolar pressure minus body surface pressure

FIGURE 3.3. Distending pressures of the respiratory system.

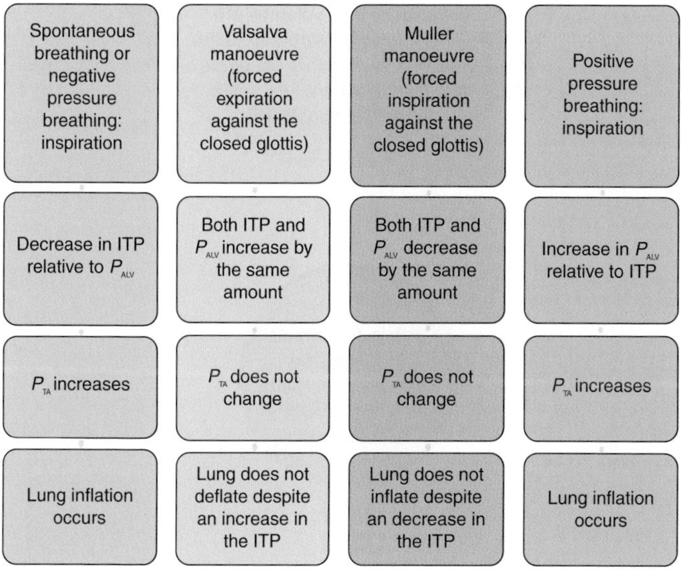
Spontaneous breathing or negative pressure breathing: inspiration
Valsalva manoeuvre (forced expiration against the closed glottis)
Muller manoeuvre (forced inspiration against the closed glottis)
Positive pressure breathing: inspiration
Decrease in ITP relative to P_{ALV}
Both ITP and P_{ALV} increase by the same amount
Both ITP and P_{ALV} decrease by the same amount
Increase in P_{ALV} relative to ITP
P_{TA} increases
P_{TA} does not change
P_{TA} does not change
P_{TA} increases
Lung inflation occurs
Lung does not deflate despite an increase in the ITP
Lung does not inflate despite an decrease in the ITP
Lung inflation occurs

FIGURE 3.4. Intrathoracic pressures during spontaneous and positive pressure breaths.

regions due to gravitational effects are also better perfused, and since they are better ventilated as well, there is more complete matching of ventilation and perfusion in these areas.

When the patient is ventilated with positive pressure breaths, the normal intrapleural pressure gradient is reduced. Also, as the alveolar units in the nondependent regions of the lung are more compliant than those in the dependent areas, they are

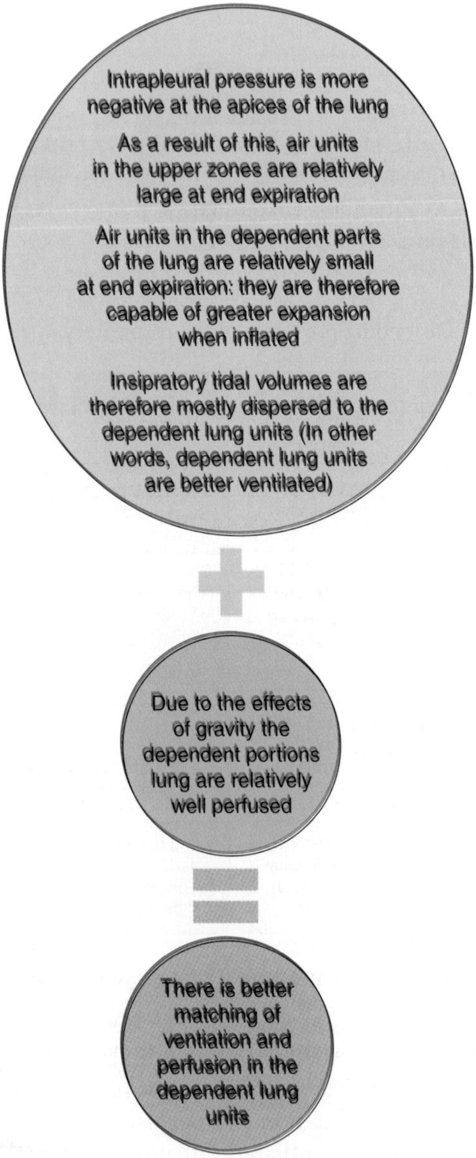
Intrapleural pressure is more negative at the apices of the lung
As a result of this, air units in the upper zones are relatively large at end expiration
Air units in the dependent parts of the lung are relatively small at end expiration: they are therefore capable of greater expansion when inflated
Insipratory tidal volumes are therefore mostly dispersed to the dependent lung units (In other words, dependent lung units are better ventilated)
Due to the effects of gravity the dependent portions lung are relatively well perfused
There is better matching of ventiation and perfusion in the dependent lung units

FIGURE 3.5. Matching of ventilation and perfusion during spontaneous breathing.

preferentially ventilated with positive pressure breaths. The increased ventilation to these relatively poorly perfused areas results in wasted ventilation. In other words, alveolar dead-space increases.

With those modes of ventilation, that do not require active participation from the patient's inspiratory muscles, lack of diaphragmatic contractility encourages regional closure of alveoli at the lung bases; though ventilation in these areas is compromised, perfusion is still intact, and shunting of blood occurs causing a further derangement in blood gases (Fig. 3.6).

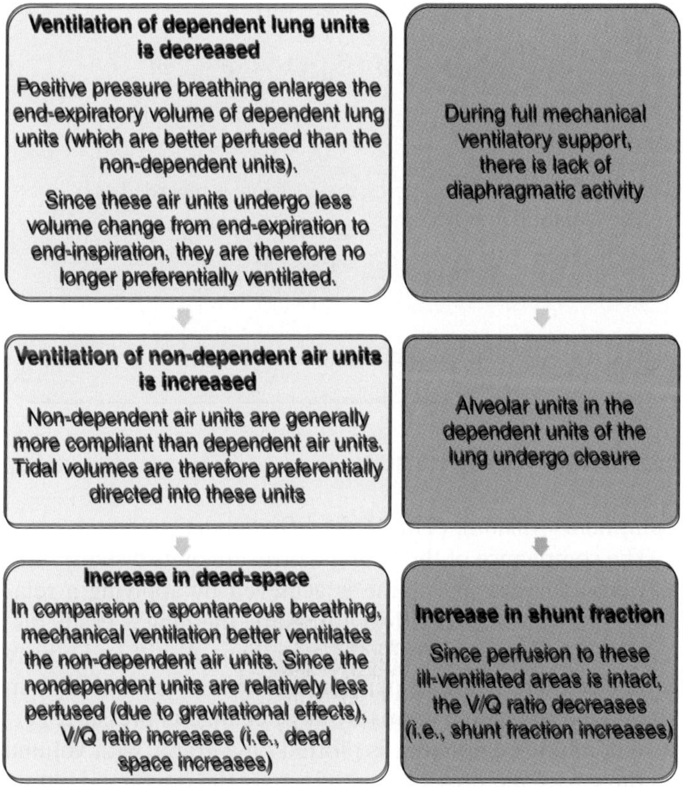
Ventilation of dependent lung units is decreased
Positive pressure breathing enlarges the end-expiratory volume of dependent lung units (which are better perfused than the non-dependent units).
Since these air units undergo less volume change from end-expiration to end-inspiration, they are therefore no longer preferentially ventilated.
During full mechanical ventilatory support, there is lack of diaphragmatic activity
Ventilation of non-dependent air units is increased
Non-dependent air units are generally more compliant than dependent air units. Tidal volumes are therefore preferentially directed into these units
Alveolar units in the dependent units of the lung undergo closure
Increase in dead-space
In comparsion to spontaneous breathing, mechanical ventilation better ventilates the non-dependent air units. Since the nondependent units are relatively less perfused (due to gravitational effects), V/Q ratio increases (i.e., dead space increases)
Increase in shunt fraction
Since perfusion to these ill-ventilated areas is intact, the V/Q ratio decreases (i.e., shunt fraction increases)

FIGURE 3.6. Matching of ventilation and perfusion during positive pressure breathing.

Nevertheless, despite the potential regional derangements in pulmonary physiology that occur as a consequence of PPB, the overall benefits of mechanical ventilation brought about by the restoration and maintenance of alveolar patency and by the elevation of mean alveolar pressures usually override its potential drawbacks.

Box 3.2 Pressure Required for Overcoming Resistance and Elastance

$$P_{TR} = P_{TA} + P_{TT},$$

Since

$$P_{TA} = P_{awo} - P_{ALV}, \text{ and } P_{TT} = P_{ALV} - P_{bs}$$

Substituting,

$$P_{TR} = P_{awo} - P_{ALV} + \mathrm{P}_{ALV} - P_{bs}$$

Since P_{bs} is atmospheric pressure, its value is regarded as 0. The equation now becomes:

$$P_{TR} = P_{awo} - P_{ALV} + \mathrm{P}_{ALV} - 0$$

$$P_{TA} = P_{awo}$$

P_{awo} is read off the ventilator panel

3.3 Lung Compliance

Compliant = yielding (The Oxford Dictionary).

The compliance of the lung is a measure of its distensibility. If a large change in volume is achieved by applying a relatively small amount of airway pressure, the lung is easily distensible and is said to be highly compliant. A stiff and poorly compliant lung resists expansion and only a small change in volume occurs with a relatively large change in pressure.

When lung compliance is plotted on a graph, with volume on the *y*-axis and pressure on the *x*-axis, the pressure–volume curve that is obtained is relatively flat and horizontal in its upper and lower portions, and steep and vertical in between.

In health, the lung operates on the middle steep part of the pressure–volume curve. At very low and very high lung volumes, the lung operates on the lower and upper flat portions of the curve, respectively, where the pressure required to bring about a given change in volume is considerable. Here, consequently, respiratory mechanics are inefficient and the work of breathing is high.

The total compliance of the respiratory system is the result of summation of the effects of lung compliance and thoracic wall compliance.

Compliance has two components, static and dynamic.

3.3.1 Static Compliance

The term compliance when used alone and in an unqualified manner (i.e., without a prefix) usually refers to static compliance. Static compliance is the true measure of distensibility of the respiratory system (lung + chest wall).

The *change* in volume between the beginning and end of a tidal breath (ΔV) is the tidal volume itself (V_t). The change in the pressure required (ΔP) to accomplish this change in volume is the plateau pressure when the lung is at rest. If there is any applied PEEP or auto-PEEP, this value must be subtracted from the plateau pressure to give the true ΔP (otherwise, there will be a spurious decrease in measured compliance).

With rare exception, the chest wall compliance remains stable within fairly narrow limits, and this is true in most clinical situations. It is rather the compliance of the lung parenchyma which varies, and underlines any change in the compliance of the respiratory system as a whole.

Another factor that influences the measured compliance of the respiratory system in the ventilated patient is the elastic pressure exerted by the ventilator tubing on the air in the ventilator circuit. This too, like thoracic wall compliance, remains fairly constant in a given patient.

In a mechanically ventilated patient with an essentially normal chest wall and lungs, the static compliance of the respiratory system is usually in the range of 70–100 mL/cm

H_2O. When the static compliance decreases to approximately 25 mL/cm H_2O, the work of breathing will appreciably increase. Patients in acute respiratory failure on mechanical ventilation can have a four to sixfold increase in work of breathing.[43] Most pulmonary disorders (with the notable exception of emphysema) can reduce lung compliance. In emphysema, although static compliance is high because of the overall effect of loss of elastic recoil, dynamic compliance is often low on account of the airways obstruction and because of loss of traction of elastic tissue on the airways (Fig. 3.7).

Lung compliance is reduced in infiltrative lung diseases. In particular, interstitial fibrosis produces a fall in lung compliance because of the excessive collagen deposition within the lung. Collagen has different length–tension relationships as compared to elastin and markedly increases lung stiffness. Pulmonary fibrosis of a lesser degree can also occur as a consequence of the chronic lung congestion produced by a stenotic mitral valve.

In pulmonary edema, the fall in lung compliance is often out of proportion to the decrease in FRC that it produces. The disproportionate fall in lung compliance in pulmonary edema probably results from the alteration in the properties of surfactant or from an alteration in alveolar geometry.

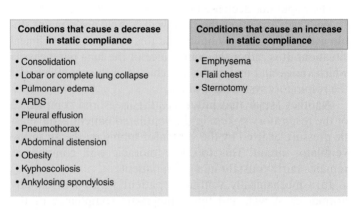

Conditions that cause a decrease in static compliance	Conditions that cause an increase in static compliance
• Consolidation	• Emphysema
• Lobar or complete lung collapse	• Flail chest
• Pulmonary edema	• Sternotomy
• ARDS	
• Pleural effusion	
• Pneumothorax	
• Abdominal distension	
• Obesity	
• Kyphoscoliosis	
• Ankylosing spondylosis	

FIGURE 3.7. Conditions that affect static compliance.

Extrapulmonary conditions may interfere with lung expansion: pleural disorders (pleural effusions, pneumothoraces) oppose lung expansion as do abdominal conditions that impair diaphragmatic movement (ascites and obesity), as well as disorders of the chest wall. In obese individuals, the low respiratory system compliance is probably attributable to a stiff chest wall along with a degree of basal atelectasis.

Mathematically, compliance is the change in volume divided by the change in the pressure that has brought about this volume change and is denoted by the formula:

$$\Delta V/\Delta P$$

Box 3.3 Calculation of Static Compliance in the Ventilated Patient

Static compliance can be measured on the ventilator as follows:

$$C_{\text{stat}} = V_t/(P_{\text{pl}} - \text{PEEP}),$$

where

V_t = tidal volume

P_{pl} = plateau pressure

PEEP = positive end-expiratory pressure

Box 3.4 Respiratory System Compliance

The compliance of the respiratory system is the result of the combined effects of lung compliance and thoracic wall compliance, and this is shown in the equation:

$$1/C_{\text{resp}} = 1/C_{\text{lung}} = 1/C_{\text{chest wall}}'$$

where

C_{resp} = compliance of the respiratory system,

C_{lung} = lung compliance,

$C_{\text{chest wall}}$ = chest wall compliance.

3.3.2 Dynamic Compliance

In contrast to static compliance, which is a measure of lung distensibility during static conditions, dynamic compliance (dynamic effective compliance, DEC) is the compliance measured while air is still flowing through the bronchial tree. Since dynamic compliance is measured during airflow, it reflects not only the lung and chest wall stiffness, but also the airway resistance, against which distending forces have to act. Because dynamic compliance is a measure of both static compliance and airflow resistance, it can be regarded as a measure of impedance. Thus, factored into the measurement of dynamic compliance is the resistance collectively imposed by the endotracheal tube, ventilator circuitry, exhalation valves, heat-moisture exchangers, and the patient's own airways – in addition to the stiffness of the lung and chest wall due to the etiologies already mentioned above. In other words, dynamic compliance falls when *either* lung stiffness *or* airway resistance increases.

Restating the above, static compliance reflects the distensibility of the respiratory system, and dynamic compliance reflects impedance (which is a measure of both compliance and resistance). When the lungs or chest wall are stiff, both static compliance and dynamic compliance decrease, whereas in states of high airway resistance (without significant dynamic hyperinflation) only dynamic compliance decreases. This logic is often made use of to diagnose and differentiate the various pulmonary derangements that can occur in the ventilated patient (Figs. 3.8 and 3.9).

When the lung becomes overdistended as by the delivery of inappropriately high tidal volumes static compliance falls. In the presence of obstructive airway disease, issues may be confounded when severe airway obstruction leads to air-trapping within the lung, and the lung as a result becomes overdistended. When dynamic hyperinflation occurs, the hyperinflated lung operates at the top of the pressure–volume curve, where it is relatively noncompliant; thus airway obstruction by itself results in a fall in *dynamic*

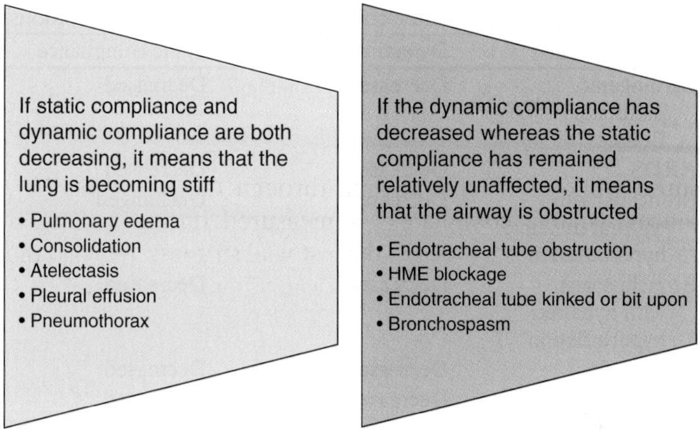
If static compliance and dynamic compliance are both decreasing, it means that the lung is becoming stiff
• Pulmonary edema
• Consolidation
• Atelectasis
• Pleural effusion
• Pneumothorax
If the dynamic compliance has decreased whereas the static compliance has remained relatively unaffected, it means that the airway is obstructed
• Endotracheal tube obstruction
• HME blockage
• Endotracheal tube kinked or bit upon
• Bronchospasm

FIGURE 3.8. Relationship between static and dynamic compliance.

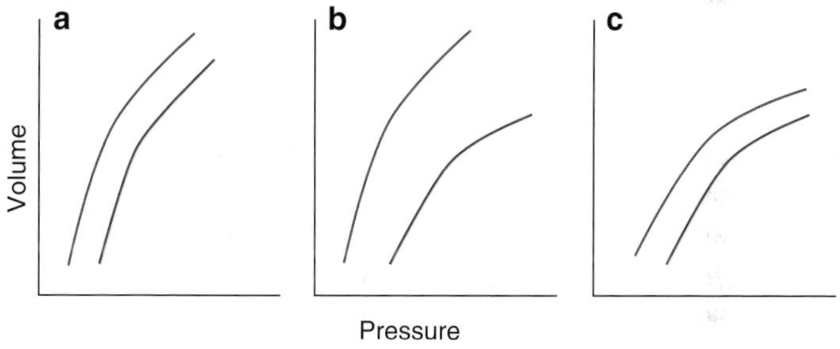
a
b
c
Volume
Pressure

FIGURE 3.9. Lung compliance in health and disease. *Panel a*: the normal pressure–volume curve. Dynamic compliance is represented by the *blue line* and static compliance by the red. *Panel b*: airway obstruction. A fall in dynamic compliance is seen – the static compliance remains more or less unaltered. *Panel c*: stiff lungs. Both static and dynamic compliance have fallen.

compliance, but when it results in dynamic hyperinflation, the *static* compliance too falls. These differences can be easily appreciated where ventilator graphics are displayed (Chap 8) (Table 3.1).

TABLE 3.1. Static and dynamic compliance in various lung conditions.

Lung condition	Dynamic compliance	Static compliance
Cardiogenic pulmonary Edema	Decreased	Decreased
ARDS	Decreased	Decreased
Bronchospasm without dynamic hyperinflation	Decreased	Unchanged
Bronchospasm with dynamic hyperinflation	Decreased	Decreased
Atelectasis	Decreased	Decreased
Pneumonia	Decreased	Decreased
Pneumothorax	Decreased	Decreased
Tube obstruction	Decreased	Unchanged
Pulmonary embolism	Unchanged	Unchanged

Box 3.5 Calculation of Dynamic Compliance in the Ventilated Patient

Dynamic compliance can be measured using a similar equation to that used for the measurement of static compliance. In the equation for dynamic compliance, however, peak inflation pressures (P_{pk}) are used instead of plateau pressures (P_{pl}):

$$C_{dyn} = V_t/(P_{pk} - PEEP),$$

where

V_t = tidal volume,
P_{pk} = peak airway pressure,
PEEP = positive end-expiratory pressure.

3.4 Airway Resistance

Airway resistance occurs as a result of the friction between the air molecules and the walls of the tracheobronchial tree, and to some extent, as a result of the friction between the air molecules themselves. For airway resistance to exist, there must be airflow; airflow occurs on account of a pressure differential between the alveolar and atmospheric pressure.

The possibilities and the limitations of Poiseuille's law, when applied to the respiratory system, have been discussed in an earlier section. It was stated that airflow resistance is directly proportional to the length of the tube (airway) and the viscosity of the fluid flowing through it (air); airflow resistance varies inversely as the fourth power of the radius of the airway. If Poiseuille's law could indeed be applied to the respiratory tract, it could be argued that in a given patient, the length of the system cannot be changed since neither the bronchial tubes nor the ventilator tubings are capable of significantly varying their length.

As to air viscosity, whatever be the relative percentages of oxygen and nitrogen inspired (in other words, whatever be the FIO_2 inhaled), the viscosity of the resultant mixture will remain more or less unaltered. Mixtures of helium and oxygen (Heliox: usually 80% He and 20% O_2) are on rare occasions used to ventilate patients with severe obstructive airway disease, and since this mixture has less viscosity compared to air, laminar airflow replaces turbulent airflow and airway resistance falls.

The remaining variable is the radius. Radius is a powerful determinant of airway resistance, since the latter is inversely proportional to the *fourth* power of the radius. In effect, if the radius is halved, airway resistance increases 16-fold (and not twofold as would be anticipated). In other words, relatively minor decrements in airway radius vastly increase the airway resistance, to the detriment of lung mechanics.

The distending pressures that are required to deliver a given tidal volume within a given inflation time are proportional to the total elastance (the elastic load) and the total resistance (resistive load) and can be summarized by the equation:

$$P_{tot} = P_{el} + P_{res}$$

P_{el} (elastance) is the pressure required to counter the elastic recoil of the chest wall and lungs. Elastance increases progressively as the lungs are inflated above their resting position (FRC); pulmonary elastance is inversely proportional to the compliance of the respiratory system. P_{res} (airway resistance) is the cumulative resistance offered by the patient's airways, endotracheal tube (or tracheostomy tube) and ventilation circuits; it is also proportional to the flow rate, which adds yet another dimension: the higher the flow rate, the higher will be the resistance.

More than 90% of the normal airway resistance originates in airways which are more than 2.0 mm in diameter. Although the large airways are (obviously!) wider than small airways – and would therefore be expected to have a lower resistance compared to the latter – the cumulative cross-sectional area of the small airways (diameter $<$ 2.0 mm) far exceeds the cumulative cross-sectional area of the large airways.

Therefore, if a pathological process were to involve the larger central airways, the smaller overall cross-sectional area of these airways would lead to an earlier rise in airways resistance, than would the involvement of smaller airways. Conversely, any lung pathology confined to the small airways would need to be quite extensive for a significant compromise to occur.

As stated, the resistance to airflow (R_{aw}) through the tracheobronchial tree occurs as a result of friction between the air molecules and the walls of the tracheobronchial tree, and also as a result of friction between the air molecules themselves. It is obvious then, that for airflow resistance to exist, flow must be present. The driving pressure across a tube is a function of the difference between the pressures at its ends. The driving pressure during inspiration in a patient who is not being given positive pressure breaths is dependent upon the difference between the atmospheric pressure (P_{atm}) and the alveolar pressure (P_{ALV}). In a patient breathing spontaneously, inhalation is initiated by the contraction of the inspiratory muscles, which expand the thoracic cage and cause the intrathoracic pressure to become negative. When the intraalveolar pressure becomes negative relative to atmospheric pressure, a gradient is established across the tracheobronchial tree and a driving force for inspiration is created.

Box 3.6 Calculation of Airflow Resistance

The resistance to airflow can be expressed by dividing the driving force by the flow across the airways:

$$P_{atm} - P_{ALV}/V,$$

where

P_{atm} = atmospheric pressure
P_{ALV} = alveolar pressure
V = flow

The tracheobronchial tree has an intrathoracic part and an extrathoracic part. The diameter of the airway does not remain constant at all phases of respiration. During spontaneous inspiration, the negative intrapleural pressure dilates the intrathoracic airways. The airways return to their resting diameter at the end of expiration. Airway resistance being largely dependent upon, the caliber of the airways, R_{aw} in these airways tends to be higher during expiration than during inspiration.

Nor is the airway diameter constant during all phases of inspiration; the higher the lung volume, the greater tends to be the traction on the airway, pulling it open. Thus, airway diameter tends to be greater and airway resistance lower, at high lung volumes. In a given patient, measurement of R_{aw} at different lung volumes would therefore result in discrepancies and lead to erroneous conclusions.

To eliminate this potential source of error and to allow for uniformity, R_{aw} is often reported as specific airway resistance. Specific airway resistance is arrived at by dividing R_{aw} by the lung volume at which R_{aw} was measured. The advantage here is that comparisons can now be made. Resistance can be compared at different lung volumes in a given person; also R_{aw}

can be compared between different persons at different lung volumes.

Box 3.7 Calculation of Airway Resistance (R_{aw}) in a Ventilated Patient

$$R_{AW} = P_{PK} - P_{PL}/V,$$

where

P_{pk} = peak inflation (peak airway) pressure,
P_{pl} = pause pressure or plateau pressure,
V = flow.

Example: If in a given situation,
P_{pk} = 40 cm H_2O,
P_{st} = 38 cm H_2O,
V = 60 L/min (i.e., 1 L/s),
R_{aw} will be:
= 40 − 38/1
= 2 cm H_2O/L/s.

Normal R_{aw} ranges from 0.6 to 2.4 cm H_2O/L/s. With an endotracheal tube in situ, this can increase to 6 cm H_2O/L/s or more. In cases of widespread airway narrowing (as in obstructive lung disease), airway resistance may be as high as 3–18 cm H_2O/L/s.

The causes of increased R_{aw} have been dealt with earlier, and treatment strategies directed at decreasing the impact of airways obstruction will be covered in a subsequent section.

3.5 Time Constants of the Lung

In most diseases, the involvement of the lung is not uniform. Regional differences in compliance and resistance occur. Owing to this, alveoli in different parts of the lung behave differently; diseased alveoli take longer to fill and to empty. The rate of filling of an individual lung unit is referred to as its time constant. A time constant is the product of the resistance and compliance of a particular lung unit. It has been estimated that it takes the equivalent of five time constants for the lung to completely fill (or to empty).

In the time afforded by one time constant, 63% of the lung will fill (or empty); two time constants allow 86% of the inspiratory or expiratory phase to be completed; three time constants allow for 95%, and four time constants for 98%.

Thus, mathematically speaking, five times the product of compliance and resistance would approximate the time required for complete filling or emptying of the respective lung units.[16]

Box 3.8 Time Constants of the Lung Example:

A lung unit with a normal airway resistance of 1 cm $H_2O/L/s$ and a normal compliance of 0.1 L/cm H_2O would have a time constant of:

$$= 1 \times 0.1$$
$$= 0.1 \text{ s}$$

Five times this is 0.5 s, which would be the time required for this unit to fill or empty satisfactorily (see text). This information comes useful while setting a ventilator's inspiratory and expiratory time.

Since diseased air units take longer to fill, deliberately prolonging the inspiratory time may enable such units to participate more meaningfully in gas exchange. These issues have been discussed in Chaps. 5 & 9.

3.6 Alveolar Ventilation and Dead-Space

The total surface area of the alveolar epithelium is about 72–80 m^2. Approximately 85–95% (about 70 m^2) of this is in contact with pulmonary capillaries: this constitutes the alveolocapillary interface.

The part of the inspired gas that does not come into contact with the pulmonary capillary bed is termed the dead-space. Dead-space may exist on account of several reasons.

3.6.1 Anatomical Dead-Space

The space within the conducting airways (from the mouth and the nose down to the terminal bronchi) constitutes the anatomical dead-space. Conducting airways merely conduct air down to the respiratory zone of the lung, and by themselves, play no role in gas exchange. The volume of the conducting airways is approximately 150 mL in an adult. Thus, of a tidal breath of 450 mL, only 300 mL will participate in gas exchange, 150 mL being contained within the dead-space. This 150 mL of anatomical dead-space can be cut down to about 60% by tracheotomy.

3.6.2 Alveolar Dead-Space

Alveolar dead-space is created when nonperfused alveoli are ventilated.

3.6.3 Physiological Dead-Space

Physiological dead-space is the sum of the alveolar and the anatomical dead-spaces. It is that part of an inspired breath that takes no part in gas exchange (Fig. 3.10).

The body defends itself against the formation of alveolar dead-space in the following manner. The CO_2 tension in the atmospheric air is negligible. In contrast, the level of CO_2 in alveolar air is substantial, exerting a partial pressure of approximately 40 mmHg. This CO_2 in the alveolar air originates in the capillary blood and diffuses across the alveolocapillary membrane into the alveoli. The alveolocapillary membrane is highly permeable to CO_2, and as a result of this, the partial pressure of the CO_2 in alveolar air is almost identical to the partial pressure of CO_2 in alveolar capillary blood.

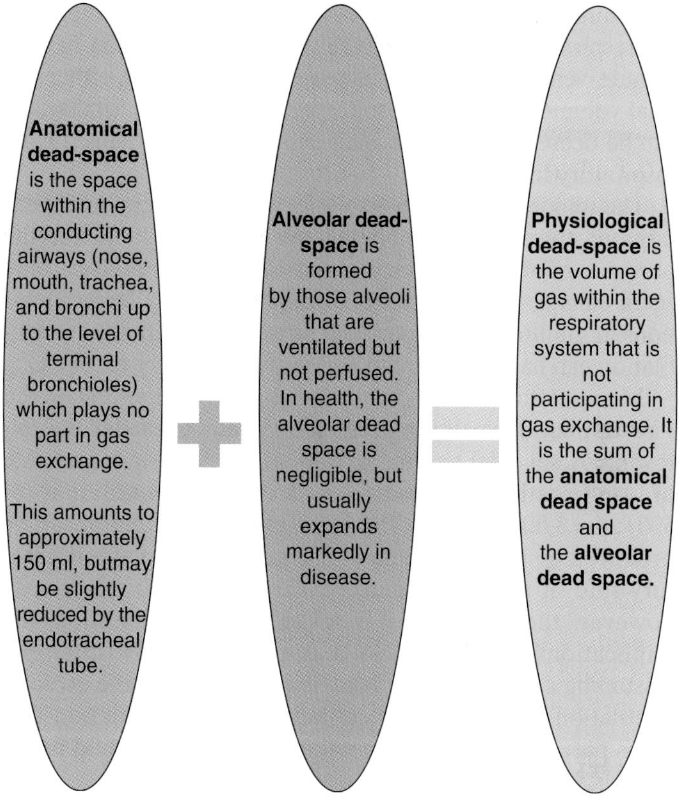
Anatomical dead-space is the space within the conducting airways (nose, mouth, trachea, and bronchi up to the level of terminal bronchioles) which plays no part in gas exchange.
This amounts to approximately 150 ml, butmay be slightly reduced by the endotracheal tube.
Alveolar dead-space is formed by those alveoli that are ventilated but not perfused. In health, the alveolar dead space is negligible, but usually expands markedly in disease.
Physiological dead-space is the volume of gas within the respiratory system that is not participating in gas exchange. It is the sum of the anatomical dead space and the alveolar dead space.

FIGURE 3.10. The components of physiological dead-space.

If an alveolus for some reason loses its blood supply and yet preserves its ventilation, alveolar dead-space is created. In an alveolus that is bereft of its blood supply, CO_2 cannot readily diffuse into the alveolus since its source (the capillary bed) has been obliterated. This results in a drop in the partial pressure of CO_2 within the underperfused alveolus and this causes reflex bronchoconstriction to occur locally, closing off the affected alveolus. By this mechanism, the hypoxemia and hypercapnia that can potentially result from dead-space ventilation are prevented from occurring.

Minute ventilation is the product of the tidal volume times the respiratory rate: it is inversely proportional to the $PaCO_2$. Minute ventilation can be increased by increasing either the tidal volume (V_t) or the respiratory frequency (f). Similarly, it can be decreased by decreasing either the tidal volume or the respiratory frequency.

The minute ventilation also affects the PaO_2 in a nonlinear fashion; however, manipulating the minute volume for the purposes of achieving a change in PaO_2 is undesirable, as only small changes in PaO_2 can be brought about by large alterations in minute ventilation. Such large changes in minute ventilation can have a profound and unwanted effect on $PaCO_2$.

Manipulation of tidal volumes has a different effect on the $PaCO_2$ than does altering respiratory rate. Consider the following: A set tidal volume of 500 mL and a respiratory rate of 10 breaths/min results in a minute ventilation of $500 \times 10 = 5{,}000$ mL/min. The same minute ventilation can be produced by a tidal volume of 250 mL delivered at a respiratory rate of 20 breaths/min, i.e., $250 \times 20 = 5{,}000$ mL/min. If, however, the dead-space is taken into consideration, the implications of these two settings are vastly different. Assuming a physiological dead-space of 150 mL, the alveolar ventilation (the effective ventilation or the ventilation that takes part in gas exchange) in the first example would be:

$$(500 - 150) \times 10 = 3{,}500,$$

and in the second example would be:

$$(250 - 150) \times 20 = 2{,}000.$$

The alveolar ventilation in the first instance would vastly exceed the alveolar ventilation in the second. Since it is the alveolar ventilation that determines the $PaCO_2$, it is crucial to decide how the minute volume should be made up, especially when there is a need to control the $PaCO_2$ tightly, or when $PaCO_2$ control is difficult. It should be appreciated that the $PaCO_2$ is inversely proportional not to all of the minute ventilation, but to that part of the ventilation that is independent of dead-space (i.e., the alveolar ventilation) (Figs. 3.11 and 3.12).

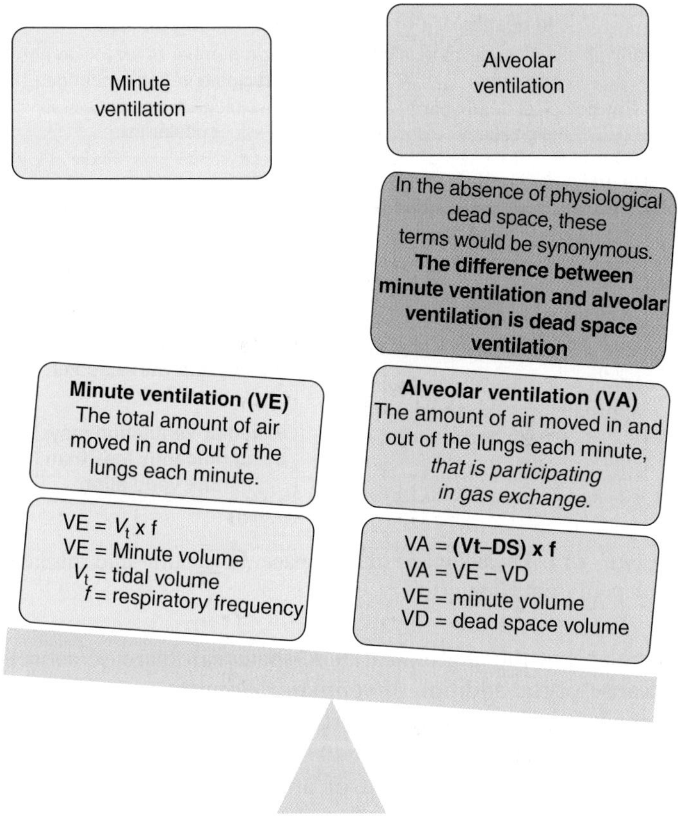
Minute ventilation
Alveolar ventilation
In the absence of physiological dead space, these terms would be synonymous. The difference between minute ventilation and alveolar ventilation is dead space ventilation
Minute ventilation (VE) The total amount of air moved in and out of the lungs each minute.
Alveolar ventilation (VA) The amount of air moved in and out of the lungs each minute, that is participating in gas exchange.
VE = Vt x f
VE = Minute volume
Vt = tidal volume
f = respiratory frequency
VA = (Vt–DS) x f
VA = VE – VD
VE = minute volume
VD = dead space volume

FIGURE 3.11. Alveolar ventilation. (Adapted from Hasan[35])

In normal individuals dead-space is mostly anatomical dead-space, and dead-space ventilation (V_d/V_t) is inversely proportional to the tidal volume. For example, in normal individuals, V_d remaining constant, an increase in V_t will cause a fall in the ratio of V_d to V_t. The normal V_d/V_t ratio is approximately 0.3.

In ventilated individuals the situation can be very different; the amount of dead-space can be very high, to the order of 0.7–0.8, and this can be on account of an increase in the anatomical dead-space or in the alveolar dead-space or both. In ventilated patients, the increase in dead-space is principally

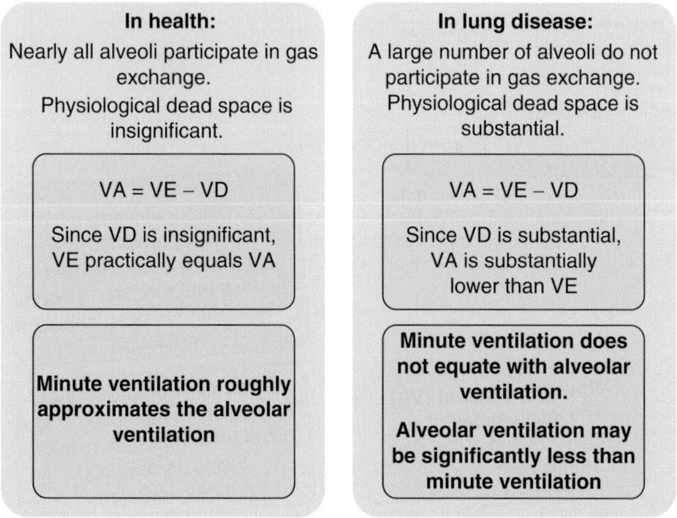
In health:
Nearly all alveoli participate in gas exchange.
Physiological dead space is insignificant.
VA = VE – VD
Since VD is insignificant, VE practically equals VA
Minute ventilation roughly approximates the alveolar ventilation
In lung disease:
A large number of alveoli do not participate in gas exchange.
Physiological dead space is substantial.
VA = VE – VD
Since VD is substantial, VA is substantially lower than VE
Minute ventilation does not equate with alveolar ventilation.
Alveolar ventilation may be significantly less than minute ventilation

FIGURE 3.12. Physiological dead space in health and disease. (Adapted from Hasan[35])

alveolar, but the anatomical dead-space can increase as well because of the addition of ventilator circuitry, heat-moisture exchangers, etc. Tracheostomy can cut down the anatomical dead-space by approximately 40%.

Because of some amount of unavoidable distensibility in the ventilator circuits, a part of the inspired tidal volume is used up in stretching the circuits, and so never reaches the patient's lungs. The volume of the inspiratory breath that is "lost" as a result of tubing compliance (circuit compressibility) is proportional to the difference in airway pressures during the respiratory cycle (i.e., the difference between the peak inspiratory pressure and the PEEP). For every 1 cm H_2O of pressure difference, 3–5 mL of inspiratory tidal volume is lost.[44]

Since the magnitude of V_d/V_t in ventilated patients is high, it cannot be easily overcome by merely increasing the tidal volumes. Moreover, if tidal volumes are increased indiscriminately in an effort to bring down dead-space ventilation, it could increase the risk of barotrauma. Such manipulations

All the exhaled CO_2 comes from the alveolar gas.
None of the exhaled CO_2 comes from the dead-space air.
Therefore,
$V_T = V_A + V_D$
Or tidal volume (V_T) = Alveolar gas volume (V_A) + dead-space gas (V_D)
Rearranging, $V_A = V_T - V_D$ ...(Eq. 1)

$V_T \times FE_{CO_2} = V_A \times FA_{CO_2}$...(Eq. 2)

Where,
V_T = tidal volume
FE_{CO_2} = Fractional concentration of CO_2 in exhaled gas
V_A = Alveolar gas volume
FA_{CO_2} = Fractional concentration of CO_2 in alveolar gas

Substituting the value of VA (Eq. 1) within Eq. 2,

$$V_T \times FE_{CO_2} = (V_T - V_D) \times FA_{CO_2}$$

Therefore,

$$V_D / V_T = (FA_{CO_2} - FE_{CO_2}) / FA_{CO_2}$$

Since the partial pressure of a gas is proportional to its concentration, the equation can be rewritten as "Bohr's equation":

$$V_D / V_T = (PA_{CO_2} - PE_{CO_2}) / PA_{CO_2}$$

And since the PCO_2 of alveolar gas ($PACO_2$) very nearly equals the PCO_2 of arterial gas ($PaCO_2$),

$$V_D / V_T = (PaCO_2 - PE_{CO_2}) / PaCO_2$$

FIGURE 3.13. The simplified Bohr equation. (Adapted from Hasan[35])

could also lead to an expansion in the zone 1 of the lung (the zone in the nondependent part of the lung where no perfusion exists), leading to high *V*/*Q* mismatch, and consequently to hypercarbia. It may be more prudent sometimes to accept some degree of CO_2 retention and allow "permissive" hypercapnia to occur in certain clinical circumstances (see Chapter 9). Conversely, a high V_d/V_t must be anticipated when a high

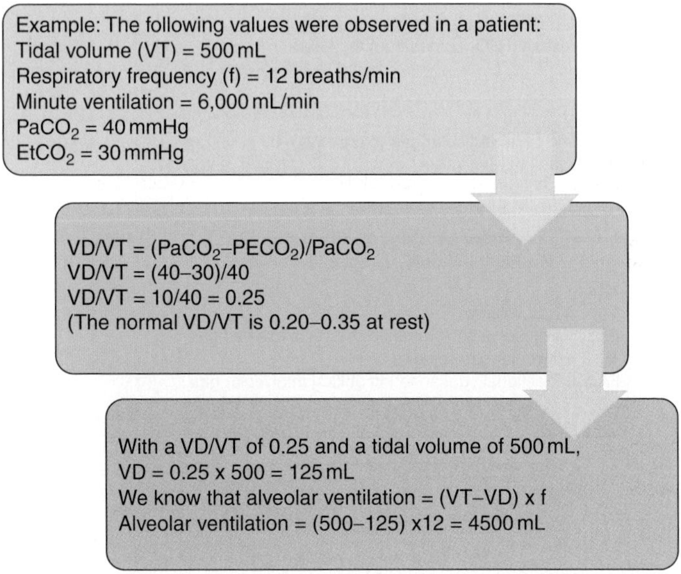
Example: The following values were observed in a patient:
Tidal volume (VT) = 500 mL
Respiratory frequency (f) = 12 breaths/min
Minute ventilation = 6,000 mL/min
$PaCO_2$ = 40 mmHg
$EtCO_2$ = 30 mmHg
VD/VT = ($PaCO_2$–$PECO_2$)/$PaCO_2$
VD/VT = (40–30)/40
VD/VT = 10/40 = 0.25
(The normal VD/VT is 0.20–0.35 at rest)
With a VD/VT of 0.25 and a tidal volume of 500 mL,
VD = 0.25 x 500 = 125 mL
We know that alveolar ventilation = (VT–VD) x f
Alveolar ventilation = (500–125) x12 = 4500 mL

FIGURE 3.14. Calculation of alveolar ventilation. (Adapted from Hasan[35])

minute volume is needed to wash out a rising $PaCO_2$, and appropriate causes sought.

Physiological dead-space can be calculated from Bohr's equation[23] (see Fig. 3.14). $PaCO_2$ (the partial pressure of CO_2 in arterial blood) can be read off the arterial blood gas report, and $PECO_2$ (the partial pressure of CO_2 in the expired air) can be measured by capnometry.

3.7 Mechanisms of Hypoxemia

Five principal mechanisms of hypoxemia exist (see Fig. 3.15).

3.7.1 Hypoventilation

Hypoventilation means a reduction in the bulk flow of air into the lungs. This reduction may be on account of a variety

V/Q mismatch

- There is decreased ventilation relative to perfusion or vice versa. V/Q mismatch is the most commonly encountered mechanism for hypoxemia (see text)

Shunt

- An extreme form of V/Q mismatch. Due to lack of regional ventilation, the blood passing through the pulmonary capillaries fails to get oxygenated (see text)

Hypoventilation

- A decrease in the bulk flow in and out of the lungs leads to a buildup of CO_2 in the blood. The defining feature of hypoventilation is hypercapnia (see text)

Diffusion defect

- A thickening of the alveolo-capillary membrane delays the diffusion of oxygen which conequently has insufficient time to equilibriate with the O_2 in alveolar capillary blood (see text)

Low barometric pressure

- A decreased inspired fraction of O_2 has the same effect as a low barometric pressure

FIGURE 3.15. Mechanisms of hypoxemia. (Adapted from Hasan[35])

of etiologies having their origin at various anatomical sites, both intra and extrapulmonary (see Fig. 3.16).

The level of $PaCO_2$ depends on the balance between CO_2 production and CO_2 elimination. The amount of CO_2 that is produced depends upon the metabolic rate. CO_2 production almost never results in a rise in $PaCO_2$ when ventilatory

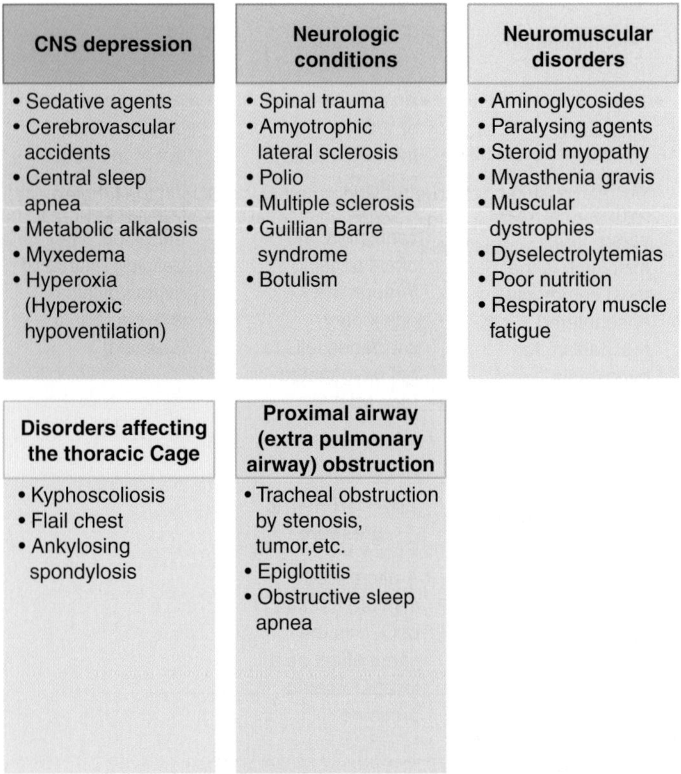
CNS depression
• Sedative agents
• Cerebrovascular accidents
• Central sleep apnea
• Metabolic alkalosis
• Myxedema
• Hyperoxia (Hyperoxic hypoventilation)
Neurologic conditions
• Spinal trauma
• Amyotrophic lateral sclerosis
• Polio
• Multiple sclerosis
• Guillian Barre syndrome
• Botulism
Neuromuscular disorders
• Aminoglycosides
• Paralysing agents
• Steroid myopathy
• Myasthenia gravis
• Muscular dystrophies
• Dyselectrolytemias
• Poor nutrition
• Respiratory muscle fatigue
Disorders affecting the thoracic Cage
• Kyphoscoliosis
• Flail chest
• Ankylosing spondylosis
Proximal airway (extra pulmonary airway) obstruction
• Tracheal obstruction by stenosis, tumor,etc.
• Epiglottitis
• Obstructive sleep apnea

FIGURE 3.16. Mechanisms of hypoventilation. (Adapted from Hasan[35])

mechanisms are intact. Therefore, any rise in $PaCO_2$ almost always means that there is inadequate removal of CO_2 from the circulation by the lungs, i.e., hypoventilation (see Fig. 3.17).

When hypoventilation occurs, there is an elevation of $PaCO_2$ as well as a fall in PaO_2 – the situation of a type II respiratory failure.

The relation of the hypercapnia to the hypoxemia in pure alveolar hypoventilation can be predicted from the alveolar gas equation. Assuming a respiratory quotient of 0.8, the PaO_2 will fall 1.25 mmHg for each 1 mmHg increase in

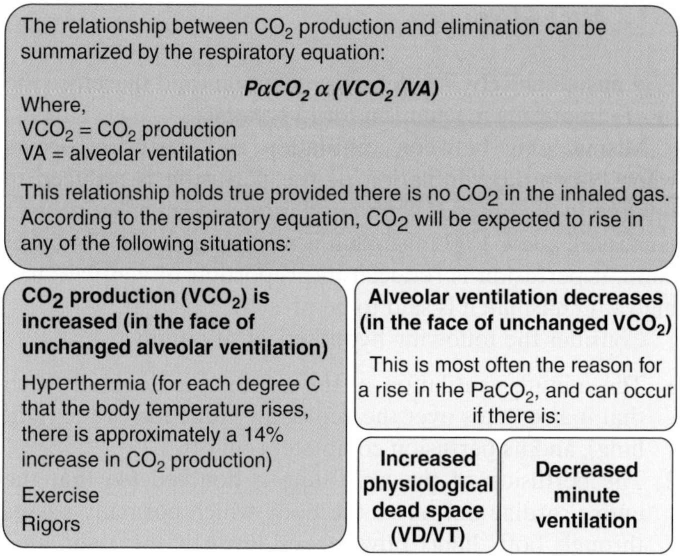
The relationship between CO_2 production and elimination can be summarized by the respiratory equation:
$PaCO_2 \alpha (VCO_2 /VA)$
Where,
VCO_2 = CO_2 production
VA = alveolar ventilation
This relationship holds true provided there is no CO_2 in the inhaled gas. According to the respiratory equation, CO_2 will be expected to rise in any of the following situations:
CO_2 production (VCO_2) is increased (in the face of unchanged alveolar ventilation)
Hyperthermia (for each degree C that the body temperature rises, there is approximately a 14% increase in CO_2 production)
Exercise
Rigors
Alveolar ventilation decreases (in the face of unchanged VCO_2)
This is most often the reason for a rise in the $PaCO_2$, and can occur if there is:
Increased physiological dead space (VD/VT)
Decreased minute ventilation

FIGURE 3.17. CO_2 Production and elimination. (Adapted from Hasan[35])

$PaCO_2$. Since in pure alveolar hypoventilation gas exchange mechanisms are intact (it is the bulk airflow which is inadequate), the A-a DO_2 gradient will remain normal. A rise in $PaCO_2$ that is proportionate to the fall in PaO_2 is the hallmark of hypoventilation, and serves to differentiate it from the other mechanisms of hypoxemia.

If the fall in PaO_2 is out of proportion to the rise in $PaCO_2$, or if the A-a DO_2 gradient is widened, an additional mechanism of hypoxemia is likely to exist in addition to the hypoventilation, and its etiology must be sought.

Again, since the gas exchange mechanisms in states of pure hypoventilation are basically intact, the hypoxemia resulting from hypoventilation should be correctable by increasing the FIO_2. It is far more important, however, to correct the hypoventilation itself by treating the underlying problem, and to support ventilation until the active pathology has been corrected.

3.7.2 V/Q Mismatch

V/Q mismatch is by far the most common (and therefore the most important) mechanism for hypoxemia.

Mismatching between ventilation and perfusion occurs when either the ventilation or the perfusion is reduced in relation to the other. If ventilation is reduced in proportion to perfusion, a low-*V/Q* mismatch is said to exist. On the other hand, if perfusion is reduced in proportion to ventilation, a high *V/Q* mismatch is said to be present.

Consider the following hypothetical situation:

1. The minute ventilation of the *left* lung is doubled (such that it also takes over the ventilatory function of the right lung), and its perfusion completely cut off.
2. The perfusion of the *right* lung is doubled (so that the entire cardiac output of the body which normally passes through both lungs now passes through the right lung alone), and its ventilation completely cut off.

We now have a situation where the *total* minute volume is normal (since the entire minute volume that was being delivered to both lungs is now being supplied to the left lung). The net perfusion of the system is also unchanged (since the amount of blood being delivered to both the lungs put together is now being delivered to the right lung alone). Yet, despite there being no overall change in the amount of ventilation or perfusion, there is a complete mismatch of ventilation and perfusion. Though, overall, such a system does receive normal minute ventilation and perfusion, no part of the blood perfusing the lungs is in contact with the air ventilating the system, and life cannot be possible on account of the asphyxia.[23]

In the example above, the system within the right lung (intact perfusion but no ventilation) is an example of a shunt. The *V/Q* ratio here is $0/q$ (where q represents the quantity of blood perfusing the system), and so the *V/Q* ratio is 0. The left lung (intact ventilation but no perfusion) has a *V/Q* ratio of $v/0$ (where v is the quantity of air ventilating the system). Mathematically, any fraction with a denominator of zero is infinity. This is an example of dead-space ventilation.

Although the situation described above is a clinical impossibility, *regional* areas in the lungs do manifest instances of *V*/*Q* mismatching as outlined above. Intermediate degrees of *V*/*Q* mismatching ranging between 0 and infinity do occur in some regions of the lung; some of these areas have relatively little ventilation and others have relatively little perfusion.

Much of the more common type of *V*/*Q* mismatch is a low-*V*/*Q* mismatch in which ventilation is unevenly distributed to the alveoli, though there is relatively uniform perfusion (poorly ventilated alveoli have low-*V*/*Q* ratios). The blood leaving these alveoli is deficient in oxygen since compromised ventilation has insufficiently oxygenated the blood. Hyperventilation of adjacent alveoli (alveoli with normal *V*/*Q* ratios) will *not* completely compensate for the deficiency in oxygenation produced by the diseased alveoli. The blood that leaves normal alveoli is already well saturated with oxygen, and the oxyhemoglobin dissociation curve is operating at its top flat part where any further addition of oxygen to the blood will add very little to the saturation of hemoglobin.

Hyperventilation will, however, have a different effect. Unlike the oxygen dissociation curve, the carbon dioxide dissociation curve is not sigmoid, but more or less linear, and carbon dioxide is highly diffusible across biological membranes. Hyperventilation will result in washout of carbon dioxide from the alveoli. Hyperventilation of alveoli with normal *V*/*Q* ratios will succeed in lowering the arterial CO_2 tension, though as just discussed, it will not be able to compensate for the hypoxemia that alveoli with low-*V*/*Q* ratios can cause.

It is important to realize that despite the existence of a large *V*/*Q* mismatch, the total alveolar ventilation can be normal, as can the total perfusion: this can be deduced from the hypothetical situation described earlier. What is important, therefore, is the *uniformity* of ventilation and perfusion.

As mentioned earlier, the *V*/*Q* mismatching is the commonest mechanism of hypoxemia, and is ubiquitous in pulmonary pathologies. Virtually, any pulmonary parenchymal disorder is capable of causing a *V*/*Q* mismatch.

3.7.3 Right to Left Shunt

As is apparent from the discussion above, a right to left shunt can be viewed as an extreme example of mismatch, where in respect of a given alveolus, perfusion (*Q*) is preserved, but ventilation (*V*) entirely absent.

The hypoxemia that occurs due to *V*/*Q* mismatch can usually be corrected with moderate concentrations of supplemental oxygen. Hypoventilated alveoli have a lower oxygen tension (PaO_2). If a patient having areas of low-*V*/*Q* mismatch should be made to breathe high concentrations of FIO_2 (100% oxygen, or as close to 100% oxygen as possible) for long enough (e.g., for 10–20 min), the inhaled oxygen will eventually displace the nitrogen even from relatively poorly ventilated alveoli. Enough quantity of this oxygen will be transferred to the blood that is leaving the alveolus, increasing the oxygen saturation of its hemoglobin. This of course is not possible when the conditions of a shunt exist (in alveoli that have *no* ventilation but a preserved perfusion). In these alveoli, the *V*/*Q* ratio is 0 and increasing the concentration of supplemental oxygen will not raise the arterial oxygen tension because the oxygen-enriched air has no access to the blood perfusing the unventilated alveoli. A failure of PaO_2 to rise significantly with 100% O_2 indicates the existence of a shunt fraction of at least 30% of the cardiac output (Fig. 3.18).

Of the mechanisms of hypoxia enumerated above (*V*/*Q* mismatch, shunt, alveolar hypoventilation, and diffusion defect), the right to left shunt is the only cause of arterial hypoxemia that is refractory to correction by oxygen supplementation. Disorders that produce a right to left shunt involve either filling up of alveoli with exudate (ARDS, lobar pnemonia) or with thin fluid (cardiogenic pulmonary edema), or closure of alveoli (atelectasis). Pulmonary emboli can also produce right to left shunting by reflex closure of alveoli (though by compromising perfusion rather than ventilation, they would intuitively be expected to produce an increase in dead-space ventilation). The hypoxemia in pulmonary embolism occurs as a result of a combination of several mechanisms. Intracardiac right to left shunts and intrapulmonary

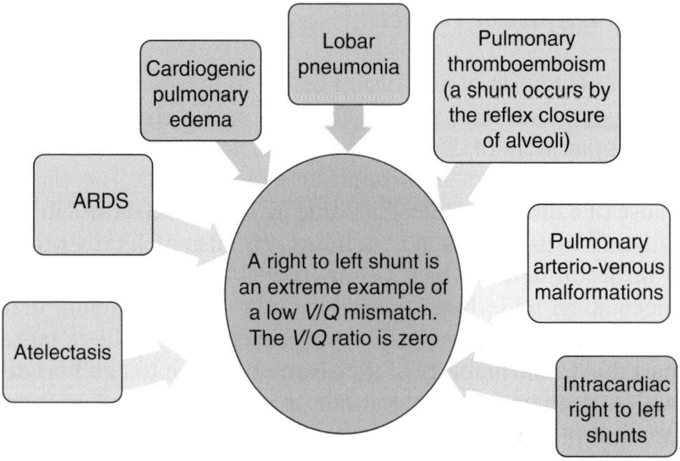
Cardiogenic pulmonary edema
Lobar pneumonia
Pulmonary thromboemboism (a shunt occurs by the reflex closure of alveoli)
ARDS
A right to left shunt is an extreme example of a low *V/Q* mismatch. The *V/Q* ratio is zero
Pulmonary arterio-venous malformations
Atelectasis
Intracardiac right to left shunts

FIGURE 3.18. Disorders associated with intrapulmonary shunting of blood.

arteriovenous malformations are also capable of producing large shunts.

Box 3.9 The Shunt Equation

$$QS/QT = CcO_2 - CaO_2) - (CcO_2\} - CvO_2)$$

where

QS/QT = shunt fraction,

CcO_2 = end capillary O_2 content,

CaO_2 = arterial oxygen content,

CvO_2 = mixed venous oxygen content

Helps quantify the degree of the right to left shunt.

CaO_2 is easily obtained by measurement of PaO_2 from an ABG sample.

CcO_2 may be arrived at by using the alveolar gas equation to calculate alveolar O_2 tension (PaO_2). PaO_2 is assumed to reflect the O_2 tension in the capillary blood.

CvO_2 is determined by sampling mixed venous blood; this requires the placement of a Swan–Ganz (PA) catheter.

3.7.4 Diffusion Defect

The contribution of a diffusion defect to hypoxemia in disorders commonly met with in the ICU is poorly understood, and impairment of diffusion is thought not to be the predominant mechanism of hypoxemia in ICU patients. The classic cause of a diffusion defect is fibrosing alveolitis (diffuse interstitial fibrosis), but even here it is a *V*/*Q* mismatch rather than a diffusion defect which is now thought to be the principal mechanism underlying the hypoxemia. The hypoxemia that occurs during exercise in fibrosing alveolitis may be in large part due to the inability of the alveolar oxygen to equilibriate with oxygen in the red blood cells in pulmonary capillaries on account of the rapidity of pulmonary blood flow (Fig. 3.19).

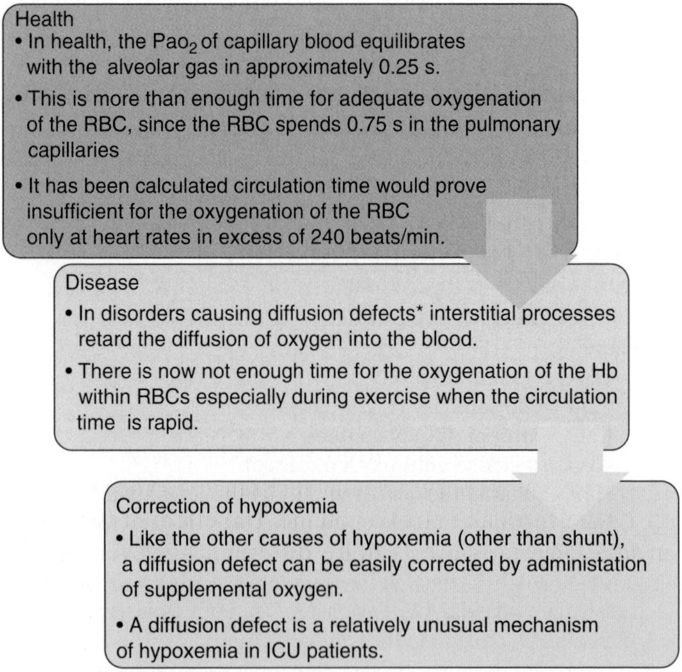
Health
• In health, the Pao_2 of capillary blood equilibrates with the alveolar gas in approximately 0.25 s.
• This is more than enough time for adequate oxygenation of the RBC, since the RBC spends 0.75 s in the pulmonary capillaries
• It has been calculated circulation time would prove insufficient for the oxygenation of the RBC only at heart rates in excess of 240 beats/min.
Disease
• In disorders causing diffusion defects* interstitial processes retard the diffusion of oxygen into the blood.
• There is now not enough time for the oxygenation of the Hb within RBCs especially during exercise when the circulation time is rapid.
Correction of hypoxemia
• Like the other causes of hypoxemia (other than shunt), a diffusion defect can be easily corrected by administation of supplemental oxygen.
• A diffusion defect is a relatively unusual mechanism of hypoxemia in ICU patients.

FIGURE 3.19. Diffusion defect. (Adapted from Hasan[35])

Identification of the mechanism producing hypoxemia helps narrow down the etiologic possibilities in a given clinical situation. It also helps predict the effect of an applied therapeutic measure. For example, supplemental oxygen is generally ineffective in the situation of a right to left shunt, and specific treatment directed to the causative pathology may prove superior to supportive therapy.

The systemic and pulmonary blood vessels respond differently to hypoxia. Hypoxia induces systemic blood vessels to dilate, but it constricts the pulmonary blood vessels[53] (see Fig. 3.20).

Mechanical ventilation has a major role to play in reversing the underlying pathology in this setting: by improving oxygenation it reverses the hypoxic pulmonary vasoconstriction: PEEP recruits and stabilizes collapsed alveoli.

3.8 Hemodynamic Effects

Hypotension in a patient who has been started on positive pressure ventilation is a common occurrence. PPB is associated with a rise in intrathoracic pressure, which decreases the venous return from the extrathoracic veins to the right side of the heart. The resultant fall in right ventricular output impairs the filling of the left ventricle, and the cardiac output consequently decreases. These events are augmented by the application of external PEEP, or in the presence of spontaneous PEEP ($PEEP_i$); the effects are also amplified in the presence of hypovolemia.

The increase in alveolar pressure due to PPB distends alveoli, compressing the alveolar blood vessels. This leads to a rise in pulmonary vascular resistance, further decreasing right ventricular stroke volume. The effect of the raised intrathoracic pressure is quite different, however, on the extrapulmonary intrathoracic vessels – quite the opposite of that on the alveolar vessels – and the left ventricular output is liable to increase by this mechanism (see Fig. 3.21). It is difficult to predict which of these effects will dominate in a given patient, and cardiac output may actually improve

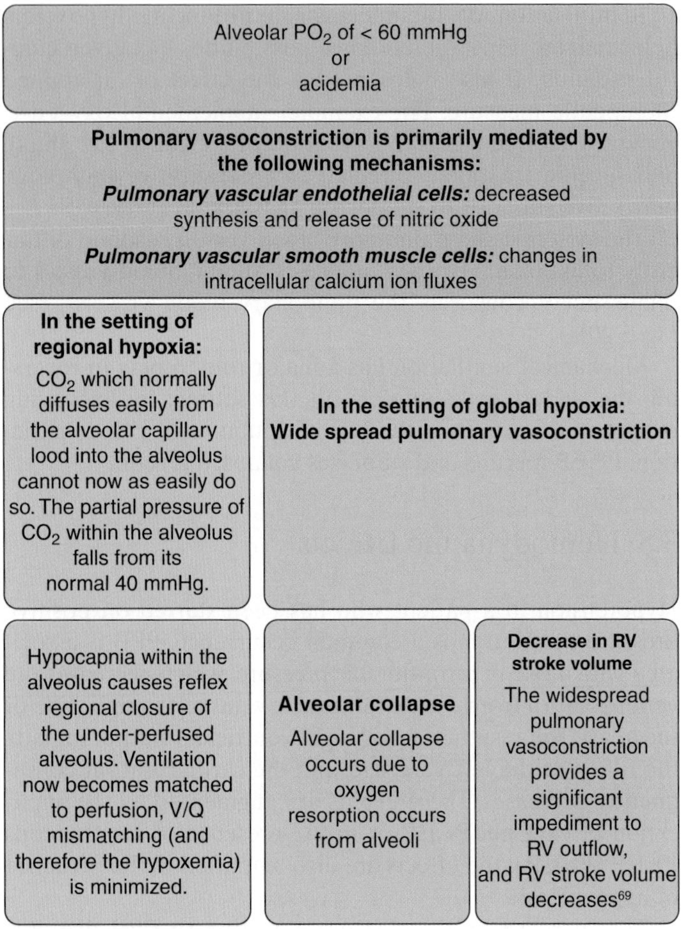
Alveolar PO2 of < 60 mmHg
or
acidemia
Pulmonary vasoconstriction is primarily mediated by the following mechanisms:
Pulmonary vascular endothelial cells: decreased synthesis and release of nitric oxide
Pulmonary vascular smooth muscle cells: changes in intracellular calcium ion fluxes
In the setting of regional hypoxia:
CO2 which normally diffuses easily from the alveolar capillary lood into the alveolus cannot now as easily do so. The partial pressure of CO2 within the alveolus falls from its normal 40 mmHg.
In the setting of global hypoxia: Wide spread pulmonary vasoconstriction
Hypocapnia within the alveolus causes reflex regional closure of the under-perfused alveolus. Ventilation now becomes matched to perfusion, V/Q mismatching (and therefore the hypoxemia) is minimized.
Alveolar collapse
Alveolar collapse occurs due to oxygen resorption occurs from alveoli
Decrease in RV stroke volume
The widespread pulmonary vasoconstriction provides a significant impediment to RV outflow, and RV stroke volume decreases69

FIGURE 3.20. Pulmonary vasoconstriction with hypoxia. (Adapted from Hasan[35])

with the commencement of mechanical ventilation (see Chap. 8).

There is yet another mechanism that influences the effect of mechanical ventilation upon the circulation: the phenomenon of ventricular interdependence. A substantial increase in pulmonary vascular resistance by the mechanism stated

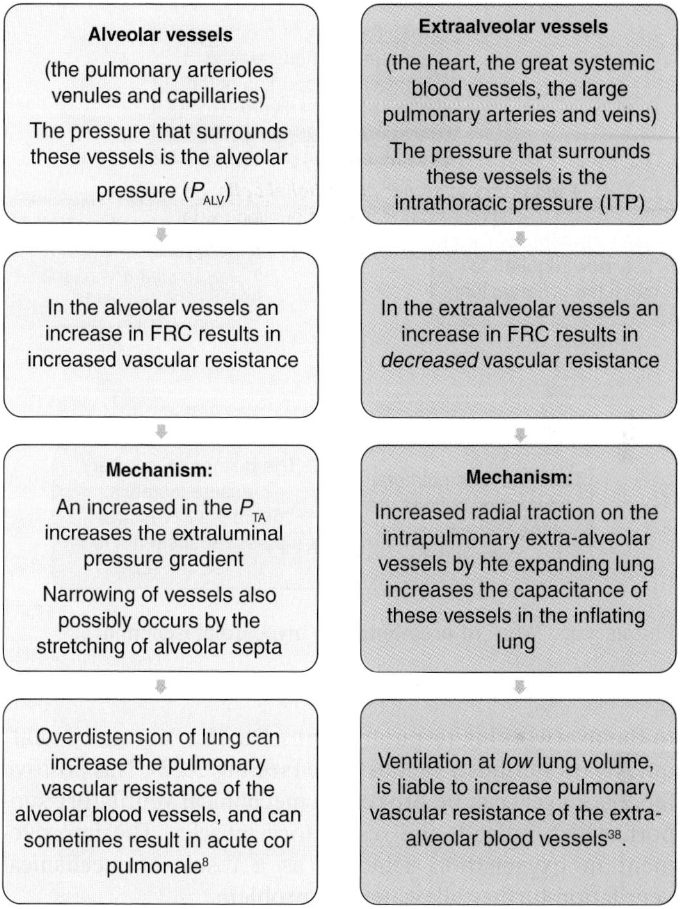
Alveolar vessels
(the pulmonary arterioles venules and capillaries)
The pressure that surrounds these vessels is the alveolar pressure (P_{ALV})
In the alveolar vessels an increase in FRC results in increased vascular resistance
Mechanism:
An increased in the P_{TA} increases the extraluminal pressure gradient
Narrowing of vessels also possibly occurs by the stretching of alveolar septa
Overdistension of lung can increase the pulmonary vascular resistance of the alveolar blood vessels, and can sometimes result in acute cor pulmonale[8]
Extraalveolar vessels
(the heart, the great systemic blood vessels, the large pulmonary arteries and veins)
The pressure that surrounds these vessels is the intrathoracic pressure (ITP)
In the extraalveolar vessels an increase in FRC results in *decreased* vascular resistance
Mechanism:
Increased radial traction on the intrapulmonary extra-alveolar vessels by hte expanding lung increases the capacitance of these vessels in the inflating lung
Ventilation at *low* lung volume, is liable to increase pulmonary vascular resistance of the extra-alveolar blood vessels[38].

FIGURE 3.21. Effect of increase in FRC on alveolar and extraalveolar vessels.

above may shift the interventricular septum to the left, narrowing the lumen of the left ventricle and preventing the left ventricle from filling properly during diastole. This can also contribute to the fall in cardiac output.

When the work of breathing is increased for any reason, a significant proportion of the cardiac output can be diverted

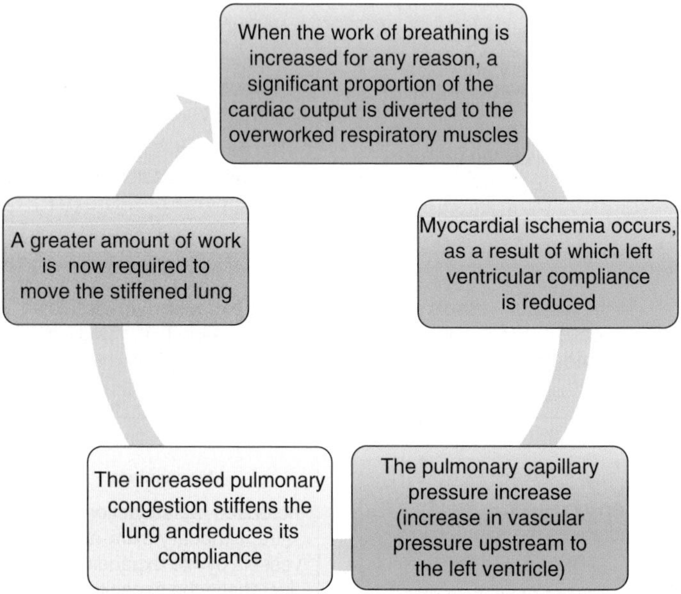
When the work of breathing is increased for any reason, a significant proportion of the cardiac output is diverted to the overworked respiratory muscles
Myocardial ischemia occurs, as a result of which left ventricular compliance is reduced
The pulmonary capillary pressure increase (increase in vascular pressure upstream to the left ventricle)
The increased pulmonary congestion stiffens the lung andreduces its compliance
A greater amount of work is now required to move the stiffened lung

FIGURE 3.22. Work of breathing and myocardial ischemia.

to the overworking respiratory muscles. The "coronary steal" quickly establishes a vicious cycle (see Fig. 3.22). This positive feedback cycle can be broken by mechanical ventilatory support, which unloads the respiratory muscles. The improvement in oxygenation achieved as a result of mechanical ventilation further alleviates the problem.

It is when the lung is yielding and highly compliant that the effects of the raised airway pressures due to positive pressure ventilation are most apparent on the vasculature, and on the other neighboring structures. A pliable and compliant lung easily transmits pressures to nearby structures resulting in more hemodynamic compromise. When the lungs are stiff and poorly compliant, they provide a buffer of sorts against the transmission of this pressure to the intrathoracic structures, and so afford a measure of protection against hemodynamic compromise.

A poorly compliant *chest wall* (as in the setting of a fibrothorax), by encompassing the system within its rigid confines, enables a buildup of pressure within its unyielding walls, and easily enables transmission of airway pressures to the surrounding structures. This predisposes to circulatory compromise. On the other hand, a highly compliant chest wall (as in patients who have had a sternotomy) enables "decompression" of the chest, transmitting relatively little pressure to the intrathoracic vasculature.

Not only may the circulatory dynamics be adversely affected by mechanical ventilation, but the accuracy of their monitoring also influenced. For example, the measurement of pulmonary capillary wedge pressure may be falsely high in mechanically ventilated patients. An approximation of the true pulmonary capillary wedge pressure may be made by halving the measured PEEP level and subtracting the resultant from the measured pulmonary capillary wedge pressure. This holds good for lungs with normal compliance. For lungs that are poorly compliant, the PEEP level should probably be divided by four and the resulting figure subtracted from the measured pulmonary capillary wedge pressure.[56]

Box 3.10 Transmission of Alveolar Pressure to the Pleural Space

How much of the alveolar pressure is eventually transmitted to the pleural space is summarized by the equation:

$$\Delta P_{pl} = \Delta P_{ALV}[C_l/C_l + C_w)],$$

where

ΔP_{pl} = change in pleural pressure
ΔP_{ALV} = change in alveolar pressure
C_l = compliance of the lungs
C_w = compliance of the chest wall

3.9 Renal Effects

The renal dysfunction that the PPB produces seems ascribable in large part to the decrease in cardiac output.[74] Positive pressure ventilation has been shown to redistribute renal blood flow to the juxtamedullary nephrons and this has been causally linked by some investigators to the renal dysfunction.[27,33]

Mechanical ventilation by increasing intrathoracic pressure decreases venous return; the consequent rise in inferior vena-caval pressure can raise the renal venous pressure. Although this could theoretically result in renal dysfunction, it is again unlikely that by itself, the moderate rise in renal venous pressure that commonly occurs with mechanical ventilation could significantly impact renal function. Experimentally, it has been shown that stimulation of the renal sympathetic nerves can result in diminished renal blood flow and a reduced sodium excretion.[51,67] It has been proposed that the reduced firing of carotid baroreceptors that PPB produces could result in increased renal sympathetic stimulation, thereby producing a fall in renal blood flow (Fig. 3.23).

Changes in the renin–angiotensin–aldosterone axis that are produced by PPB have also been cited by some investigators as being casually linked to the renal dysfunction, though concrete evidence in this respect has been hard to come by.[7]

Hypercapnia can promote the secretion of hydrogen ions into the glomerular filterate in lieu of bicarbonate and sodium: the conservation of the latter can result in salt and water retention. Both hypercapnia and hypoxia can independently decrease renal perfusion, and stimulate the renin–angiotensin–aldosterone axis.[65]

Antidiuretic hormone (ADH) is believed to mediate at least some of the effects of PPB on renal dysfunction. The physiological function of ADH is the conservation of body water. ADH promotes the resorption of the glomerular filtrate from the collecting ducts of the nephron into the renal interstitium and thence back into the systemic circulation. The resorption of salt-poor fluid results in the excretion of a concentrated urine.

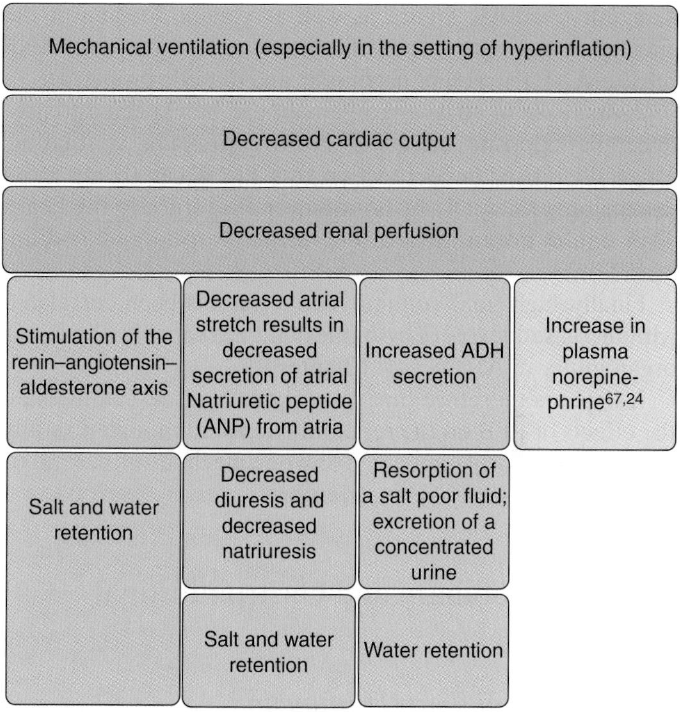
Mechanical ventilation (especially in the setting of hyperinflation)
Decreased cardiac output
Decreased renal perfusion
Stimulation of the renin–angiotensin–aldesterone axis
Decreased atrial stretch results in decreased secretion of atrial Natriuretic peptide (ANP) from atria
Increased ADH secretion
Increase in plasma norepine-phrine67,24
Salt and water retention
Decreased diuresis and decreased natriuresis
Resorption of a salt poor fluid; excretion of a concentrated urine
Salt and water retention
Water retention

FIGURE 3.23. Mechanisms of fluid retention during mechanical ventilation.

The use of positive pressure ventilation has also been shown to increase serum ADH levels,[5,36] but such results have not been consistently reproducible.[67] It is also possible that the rise in ADH levels associated with PPB is a compensatory response that is directed toward the restoration of the cardiac output in mechanically ventilated patients. This is certainly plausible, and the fact that ADH also has a vasoconstrictor effect lends credence to this theory.

Atrial natriuretic peptide (ANP), which is a hormone that has its origin in the atrial chambers of the heart, also seems to participate in the complex interplay of factors that predispose to renal dysfunction in the setting of PPB. ANP is released from its storage sites within atria in response to atrial distension.

Congestive cardiac failure as well as volume loading of the circulation can cause atrial distension and so promote ANP release. ANP has potent natriuretic and diuretic properties.

A decrease in atrial engorgement can be expected to produce the opposite effects.[2,51] Positive pressure ventilation, especially if used in conjunction with PEEP, can *reduce* atrial distension, principally by limiting venous return to the heart. This could potentially affect urine output and sodium excretion.

Finally, high tidal volume ventilation has been correlated with increased levels of cytokines that are capable of causing organ injury in ARDS (see Chapter 9)

It appears therefore that several mechanisms can mediate the effects of PPB on the renal function, and though no study till date has clearly implicated any one mechanism, several or all these factors may be contributory.

3.10 Hepatobiliary and Gastrointestinal Effects

3.10.1 Hepatobiliary Dysfunction

Liver function is often compromised in critically ill patients. As in respect of the kidney, the reduction in hepatic perfusion appears to be secondary to the decrease in cardiac output that PPB produces.

The liver has a dual blood supply, and although the hepatic artery provides but a third of the blood supply of the liver, it accounts for as much as half of the oxygen supply. Reduction in both hepatic arterial and portal blood flow has been documented in mechanically ventilated patients.[10,55] The decline in hepatic arterial flow appears to strongly correlate with use of PEEP.[9] Hepatic vascular resistance is also elevated in mechanically ventilated patients. A decrease in venous return to the heart (on account of PPB) by increasing the inferior venacaval pressure can elevate the hepatic venous pressure, and this could play a part in hepatic dysfunction as well.[55]

The diaphragm itself is pushed lower into the abdomen in mechanically ventilated patients, but this is unlikely to cause hepatic dysfunction by compressive effects upon the hepatic parenchyma.[42] Resistance to bile flow through the common bile duct has also been shown to increase with the application of PEEP, but the significance of this is presently unclear.[41,42]

3.10.2 Gastrointestinal Dysfunction

Clinicians are familiar with increased incidence of GI bleeding in patients on mechanical ventilation. Gastrointestinal stress ulceration most often accounts for this bleeding and probably results from a reduction in mucosal blood flow that PPB produces.[42] Along with a reduction in arterial perfusion of the gut, PPB can decrease venous return to the heart, and this can promote ischemia of the gut mucosa as well.

References

1. Abraham E, Yoshihara G. Cardiorespiratory effects of pressure controlled ventilation in severe respiratory failure. *Chest.* 1990;98:1445–1449
2. Andrivet P, Adnot S, Brun–Buisson C, et al Involvement of ANF in the acute antidiuresis during PEEP ventilation. *J Appl Physiol.* 1988;65:1967–1974
3. Annest SJ, Gottlieb M, Paloski WH, et al Detrimental effects of removing end-expiratory pressure prior to endotracheal extubation. *Ann Surg.* 1980;191:539
4. Baier H, Wanner A, Zarzecki S, et al Relationships among glottis opening respiratory flow, and upper airway resistance in humans. *J Appl Physiol.* 1977;43:603
5. Baratz R, Ingraham R. Renal hemodynamics and antidiuretic hormone release associated with volume regulation. *Am J Physiol.* 1960;198:565–570
6. Bedford RF. Circulatory responses to tracheal intubation. *Probl Anesth.* 1988;2:201

7. Berry A. Respiratory support and renal function. *Anesthesiology*. 1981;55:655–667
8. Block AJ, Boyson PG, Wynne JW. The origins of cor pulmonale, a hypothesis. *Chest*. 1979;75:109–114
9. Bonnet F, Richard C, Glaser P, et al Changes in hepatic flow induced by continuous positive pressure ventilation in critically ill patients. *Crit Care Med*. 1982;10:703–705
10. Brendenberg C, Paskanik A. Relation of portal hemodynamics to cardiac output during mechanical ventilation with PEEP. *Am Surg*. 1983;198:218–222
11. Broseghini C, Brandolese R, Poggi R, et al Respiratory mechanics during the first of mechanical ventilation in patients with pulmonary edema and chronic airway obstruction. *Am Rev Respir Dis*. 1988;138:355–361
12. Bynum LJ, Wilson JE, Pierce AK. Comparison of spontaneous and positive pressure breathing in supine normal subjects. *J Appl Physiol*. 1976;41:341–347
13. Chen CT, Toung TJK, Donham RT, et al Fentanyl dosage for suppression of circulatory response to laryngoscopy and endotracheal intubation. *Anesthesiol Rev*. 1986;13:37
14. Clements JA, Tierney DF. Alveolar instability associated with altered surface tension. In: Fenn WO, Rahn H, eds. *Handbook of Physiology, Respiration*, vol. 1. 1964: American Physiology Society; 1964:1565–1583
15. Clements JA, Husted RF, Johnson RP, et al Pulmonary surface tension and alveolar stability. *J Appl Physiol*. 1961;16:444–450
16. Criner JC, D'Alonzo GE. *Pulmonary Pathophysiology*. Madison: Fence Creek Publishing; 1999
17. Crotti S, Pelosi P, Mascheroni D, et al The effect of extrinsic PEEP on lung inflation and regional compliance in mechanically ventilated patients: a CT scan study. *Inten Care Med*. 1995;21:135
18. Dawson CA, Grimm DJ, Linehan JH. Lung inflation and longitudinal distribution of pulmonary vascular resistance during hypoxia. *J Appl Physiol*. 1979;47:532–536
19. Dubois AB. Resistance to breathing. In: Fenn WO, ed. *Handbook of Physiology, Respiration*, vol. 1. Washington, DC: American Physiology Society; 1964:451–462
20. England SJ, Bartlett D. Influence of human vocal cord movements on airflow resistance during apnea. *J Appl Physiol*. 1982;52:773
21. Fewell J, Bond G. Role of sinoaortic baroreceptors in initiating the renal response to continuous positive pressure ventilation in the dog. *Anesthesiology*. 1980;52:408–413

22. Fleury B, Murciano D, Talamo C, et al Work of breathing in patients with obstructive pulmonary disease in acute respiratory failure. *Am Rev Respir Dis*. 1985;131:822–827
23. Forster RE II, DuBois AB, Briscoe WA, Fisher AB, eds. *The Lung: Physiological Basis of Pulmonary Function Tests*. Chicago: Yearbook Medical Publishers; 1986
24. Frage D, de la Coussaye JE, Beloucif S, Fratacci MD, Payen DM. Interactions between hormonal modifications during peep-induced antidiuresis and antinatriuresis. *Chest*. 1995;107:1095–1100
25. Freeman C, Cicerchia E, Demers RR, Sakklad M. Static compliance, effective compliance and dynamic effective compliance as indicators of elastic recoil in the presence of lung disease. *Crit Care Med*. 1976;21(4):323
26. Gal TS. How does tracheal intubation alter respiratory mechanics? *Probl Anesth*. 1988;2:191
27. Gammanpila S, Bevan D, Bhudu R. Effect of positive and negative expiratory pressure on renal function. *Br J Anesth*. 1977;49:199–205
28. Gattinoni L, Pesenti A, Avalli L, et al Pressure-volume curve of total respiratory system in acute respiratory failure: computed topographic scan study. *Am Rev Respir Dis*. 1987;136:730–736
29. Gay CG, Rodarte JR, Hubmayer RD. The effects of positive expiratory pressures on isovolume flow and dynamic hyperinflation in patients receiving mechanical ventilation. *Am Rev Respir Dis*. 1989;139:621–626
30. Gottfried SB, Reissman H, Ranieri VM. A simple method for the measurement of intrinsic positive end-expiratory pressure during controlled and assisted modes of mechanical ventilation. *Crit Care Med*. 1992;5:621–629
31. Gottfried SB. The role of PEEP in the mechanically ventilated COPD patient. In: Marini JJ, Roussos C, eds. *Ventilatory Failure*. Springer: New York; 1991:392–394
32. Grant BJB, Lieber BB. Compliance of the main pulmonary artery during the ventilatory cycle. *J Appl Physiol*. 1992;72: 535–542
33. Hall S, Johnson E, Hedley-Whyte J. Renal hemodynamics and function with continuous positive pressure ventilation in dogs. *Anesthesiology*. 1984;41:452–461
34. Harrison RA. In respiratory procedures and monitoring. *Crit Care Clin*. 1995;11(1):151
35. Hasan A, ed. *Handbook of Blood Gas/Acid-Base Interpretation*. London: Springer; 2009

36. Hemmer M, Viquerat C, Suter P, et al Urinary antidiuretic hormone excretion during mechanical ventilation and weaning in man. *Anesthesiology*. 1980;52:395–400
37. Hoffman RA, Ershowsky P, Krieger BP. Determination of auto-PEEP during spontaneous and controlled ventilation by monitoring changes in end-expiratory thoracic gas volume. *Chest*. 1989;96:613–616
38. Howell JBL, Permutt S, Proctor DF, et al Effect of inflation of the lung on different parts of the pulmonary vascular bed. *J Appl Physiol*. 1961;16:71–76
39. Hurst JM, Branson RD, Davis K Jr, et al Cardiopulmonary effects of pressure support ventilation. *Arch Surg*. 1989;124:1067–1070
40. Johnson E, Hedley-Whyte J. Continuous positive pressure ventilation and portal flow in dogs with pulmonary edema. *J Appl Physiol*. 1982;33:385–389
41. Johnson E, Hedley-Whyte J. Continuous positive-pressure ventilation and choledo-choduodenal flow resistance. *J Appl Physiol*. 1985;39:937–942
42. Johnson E. Splanchnic hemodynamic response to passive hyperventilation. *J Appl Physiol*. 1975;38:156–162
43. Jubran A, Tobin JM. Pathophysiologic basis of acute respiratory distress in patients who fail a trial of weaning from mechanical ventilation. *Am J Respir Care Med*. 1997;155:906–915
44. Kacmerek RM, Venegas J. Mechanical ventilatory rates and tidal volumes. *Respir Care*. 1987;32:466–475
45. Kaneko K, Milic-Emili J, Dolovich MB, et al Regional distribution of ventilation and perfusion as a function of body position. *J Appl Physiol*. 1966;21:767–777
46. Kaplan JD, Schuster DP. Physiological consequences of tracheal intubation. *Clin Chest Med*. 1991;12:3
47. Katz M, Shear L. Effect of renal nerves on renal nerves on renal hemodynamics. *Nephron*. 1976;14:246–256
48. Kawagoe Y, Permutt S, Fessler HE. Hyperinflation with intrinsic PEEP and respiratory muscle blood flow. *J Appl Physiol*. 1994;77:2440–2448
49. Kimball WR, Leith DE, Robins AG. Dynamic hyperinflation and ventilatory dependence in chronic obstructive pulmonary disease. *Am Rev Respir Dis*. 1982;126:991–995
50. Kriet JW, Eschenbacker LW. The physiology of spontaneous and mechanical ventilation. *Clin Chest Med*. 1988;9:11
51. Leithner C, Frass M, Pacher R, et al Mechanical ventilation with PEEP decreases release of alpha-atrial natriuretic peptide. *Crit Care Med*. 1987;15:484–488

52. Lessard MR, Lofaso F, Brochard L. Expiratory muscle activity increases intrinsic positive end-expiratory pressure independently of dynamic hyperinflation in mechanically ventilated patients. *Am J Respir Crit Care Med*. 1995;151:562–569
53. Madden JA, Dawson CA, Harder DR. Hypoxia-induced activation in small isolated pulmonary arteries from the cat. *J Appl Physiol*. 1985;59:113–118
54. Maltais F, Reissmann H, Navalesi P, et al Comparison of static and dynamic measurements of intrinsic PEEP in mechanically ventilated patients. *Am J Respir Crit Care Med*. 1994;150:1318–1324
55. Manny J, Justice R, Hechtman H. Abnormalities in organ blood flow and its distribution during PEEP. *Surgery*. 1979;85:425–432
56. Marini JJ, O'Quin R, Culver BH, et al Estimation of transmural cardiac pressures during ventilation with PEEP. *J Appl Physiol*. 1982;53:384
57. Marini JJ, Ravenscraft SA. Mean airway pressure: physiologic determinants and clinical importance: 2. Clinical implications. *Crit Care Med*. 1992;20:1604–1616
58. Matamis D, Lemaire F, Harf A, et al Total respiratory pressure-volume curves in the adult respiratory distress syndrome. *Chest*. 1984;86:58–66
59. Mathru M, Rao TL, El-Etr AA, et al Hemodynamic response to changes in ventilatory patterns in patients with normal and poor left ventricular reserve. *Crit Care Med*. 1982;10:423–426
60. Matuschak G, Pinsky M, Rogers R. Effects of PEEP on hepatic blood flow and performance. *J Appl Physiol*. 1987;62:1377–1383
61. Mead J. Respiration: pulmonary mechanics. *Am Rev Physiol.*. 1973;35:169–192
62. Michard F, ChemLa D, Richard C, et al Clinical use of respiratory changes in arterial pulse pressure to monitor the hemodynamic effects of PEEP. *Am J Respir Crit Care Med*. 1999;159:935
63. Ninane V, Yernault JC, De Troyer A. Intrinsic PEEP in patients with chronic obstructive pulmonary disease: role of expiratory muscles. *Am Rev Respir Dis*. 1999;148:1037–1042
64. Nunn JF, Campbell EJM, Peckett BW. Anatomical subdivision of the volume of respiratory dead space and effects of position of the jaw. *J Appl Physiol*. 1959;14:174
65. Pannu N, Mehta RL. Effect of mechanical ventilation on the kidney. *Best Pract Res Clin Anesthesiol*. 2004;18:189–203
66. Payen D, Farge D, Beloucif S, et al No involvement of ADH in acute antidiuresis during PEEP ventilation in humans. *Anesthesiology*. 1987;66:17–23

67. Payen DM, Brun-Buisson CJL, Carli PA, et al Hemodynamic, gas exchange, and hormonal consequences of LBPP during PEEP ventilation. *J Appl Physiol.* 1987;62:61–70
68. Pepe PE, Marini JJ. Occult positive end-expiratory pressure in mechanically ventilated patients with airflow obstruction. *Am Rev Respir Dis.* 1982;126:166–170
69. Piene H, Sund T. Does pulmonary impedance constitute the optimal load for the right ventricle? *Am J Physiol.* 1982;242: H154-H160
70. Pilbeam SP. Basic terms and concepts of mechanical ventilation. In: Pilbeam SP, Cairo JM, eds. *Mechanical Ventilation – Physiological and Clinical Applications.* Missouri: Mosby; 2006:15–30
71. Pinsky MR. The effects of mechanical ventilation on the cardiovascular system. *Crit Care Clinics.* 1990;6:663–678
72. Plost J, Campbell SC. The non-elastic work of breathing through endotracheal tubes of various sizes [abstract]. *Am Rev Respir Dis.* 1984;129:A106
73. Predley TJ, Drazen JM. Aerodynamic theory. In: Fisherman AP, Mackem PT, Mead J, eds. *Handbook of Physiology, Vol 3, Pt 1.* Bethesda: American Physiologic Society; 1986:41
74. Priebe H, Heimann J, Hedley-Whyte J. Mechanisms of renal dysfunction during PEEP ventilation. *J Appl Physiol.* 1981;50: 643–649
75. Quist J, Pontoppidan H, Wilson RS, et al Hemodynamic responses to mechanical ventilation with PEEP. *Anesthesiology.* 1971;42:45
76. Rahn H, et al The pressure volume diagram of the lung and thorax. *Am J Physiol.* 1946;146:161–178
77. Ranieri VM, Suter PM, Trotorella C, et al Effect of mechanical ventilation on inflammatory mediators in patients with acute respiratory distress syndrome: a randomized controlled trial. *JAMA.* 1999;282:54–61
78. Rossi A, Gottfried SB, Zocchi L, et al Measurement of static lung compliance of the total respiratory failure during mechanical ventilation: the effect of intrinsic positive end-expiratory pressure. *Am Rev Respir Dis.* 1985;131:672–677
79. Slutsky AS. Mechanical ventilation. American College of Chest Physicians' Consensus Conference. *Chest.* 1993;104: 1833
80. Straus C, Louis B, Isabey D, et al Contribution of the endotracheal tube and the upper airway to breathing workload. *Am J Respir Crit Care Med.* 1998;157:23–30

81. Teboul JL, Besbes M, Andrivet P, et al A bedside index assessing the reliability of pulmonary artery occlusion pressure measurements during mechanical ventilation with positive end-expiratory pressure. *J Crit Care*. 1992;7:22
82. Tobin MJ, Jenouri G, Birch S, et al Effect of positive end-expiratory pressure on breathing patterns of normal subjects and intubated patients with respiratory failure. *Crit Care Med*. 1983;11:859–867
83. Wood LDH, Engel LA, Griffin P, et al Effect of gas physical properties and flow on lower pulmonary resistance. *J Appl Physiol*. 1975;41:234–244
84. Yung MV, Snowden SL. Respiratory resistance of tracheostomy tubes. *Arch Otolaryngol*. 1984;110:591

Chapter 4
The Conventional Modes of Mechanical Ventilation

4.1 Mechanical Ventilators

The care of the patient in the ICU is, to say the least, extremely demanding. Mechanically ventilated patients are at high risk of mortality, not only from the primary condition for which they have been ventilated, but also from complications arising directly or indirectly from mechanical ventilation itself. Techniques for mechanically ventilating patients are even now evolving, and modes of ventilation are frequently chosen based not only on the lung pathology, hemodynamics, oxygenation, and lung mechanics, but also on clinician familiarity. It is generally accepted that current modes of mechanical ventilation are inadequate in many respects, and there is much room for improvement.

Before further discussion on the topic, it is necessary to define a few important concepts. In essence, mechanical ventilators are devices that enable gas to flow into the patient's airways in a regulated manner. For air to flow into the patient's lungs during inspiration, there must exist a gradient between the pressure within the ventilator's inspiratory circuit and the patient's alveoli. Ventilators are classified as positive pressure or negative pressure devices depending upon how they bring about the flow of air into the patient's lungs.

Positive pressure devices work by generating positive pressure at the airway opening and so drive air into the patient's lungs. Negative pressure ventilators, on the other hand, act by

A. Hasan, *Understanding Mechanical Ventilation*,
DOI: 10.1007/978-1-84882-869-8_4,

enclosing the patient's torso within a sealed box within which negative pressure is generated by means of a vacuum device. The thorax expands passively, secondary to the pressure drop outside the chest, and the negativity of alveolar pressure so produced pulls air into the patient's lungs. Negative pressure ventilators have been discussed in Chap. 14 Positive pressure ventilation can be applied in an invasive manner (where positive pressure is transmitted to the patient's airway through the endotracheal tube) or noninvasively by means of a securely fitting nasal or orofacial mask. A low pressure cuff around the endotracheal tube affords a seal between the endotracheal tube and the tracheal wall.

The physiologic impact of the endotracheal tube and positive-pressure breathing has been discussed in Chap. 3 Noninvasive ventilation has been discussed in Chap. 13.

4.1.1 Open-Loop and Closed-Loop Systems

Closed-loop ventilators are sophisticated microprocessor-controlled devices, which constantly monitor the ventilator-aided respirations; sophisticated feedback systems modify the operator-determined characteristics of delivered breaths. In-built alarms alert the operator should the breaths not be delivered in accordance with the ventilator settings. Open-loop systems also continuously provide feedback data, but otherwise lack artificial intelligence, and are not capable of spontaneously restoring breath characteristics should these deviate from the intended.

4.1.2 Control Panel

Ventilator parameters are set or modified through the control panel. In essence, four basic variables are operator-controlled: volume, flow, pressure, and time, and the interactions between these govern the characteristics of ventilator-driven breaths.

4.1.3 Pneumatic Circuit

Oxygen and compressed air from wall outlets are mixed to give the prescribed FIO_2 in a blender; the air then enters a system of tubes comprising the ventilator's internal and external circuits. The air is conducted to the patient's airways through the inspiratory circuit. The exhaled air is received back into the ventilator through the expiratory circuit and is subsequently discharged through the expiratory port to the exterior.

4.1.3.1 The Internal Circuit

The system of tubes and valves within the ventilator itself constitutes the internal circuit of the ventilator. Ventilators may be categorized into single or double-circuit systems depending upon whether the internal circuit allows the gas to go directly from the power source to the patient or is used to operate a bellows, respectively. In the latter case, the gas from the power source is used to compress a bag or bellows which routes the air to the patient via a separate circuit.

4.1.3.2 The External Circuit

The corrugated polyvinyl tubes along with their connections that connect the ventilator to the patient tube (endotracheal or tracheostomy tube) constitute the external circuit.

4.1.4 The Expiratory Valve

During a ventilator-driven inspiration, it is essential to ensure that airflow is directed to the patient's airways in a controlled manner. Closure of an internally situated exhalation valve directs air to the patient during inspiration. The valve opens periodically after each inspiration, thereby permitting exhalation.

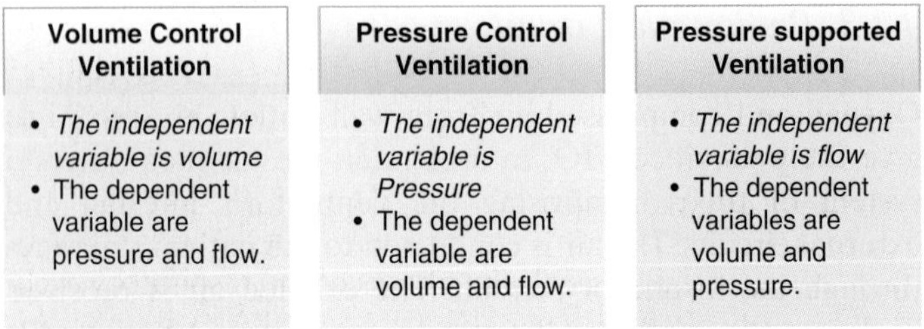
Volume Control Ventilation
The independent variable is volume
The dependent variable are pressure and flow.
Pressure Control Ventilation
The independent variable is Pressure
The dependent variable are volume and flow.
Pressure supported Ventilation
The independent variable is flow
The dependent variables are volume and pressure.

FIGURE 4.1. Control variables in different modes of ventilation.

4.1.4.1 Phases of the Respiratory Cycle

Each ventilator-controlled respiratory cycle can be divided into four phases[49] (Fig. 4.1).

Box 4.1 The Four Phases of the Respiratory Cycle

1. Changeover from expiration to inspiration
2. Inspiration
3. Changeover from inspiration to expiration
4. Expiration

4.1.5 Variables

Variables are elements of a breath that a ventilator can control during breath delivery.

There are two kinds of variables, *control variables* and *phase variables*.

4.1.5.1 Control Variables

Only one of the three control variables – volume, pressure, or flow – can be used to control the shape of a breath.[1] This controlling variable is called *independent variable*; the other

[1]In the older jet ventilators, *time* used to be the independent variable.

two variables automatically become *dependent variables*. According to the independent variable selected, the ventilator is classified as a volume, pressure, or flow controller.

4.1.5.2 Phase Variables

How the ventilator controls the phases of the respiratory cycle depends upon the phase variables [21]. Four phase variables are recognized: trigger variable, limit variable, cycle variable, and baseline variable.

4.1.6 The Trigger Variable ("Triggering" of the Ventilator)

Triggering is the mechanism that the ventilator uses to cycle from expiration to inspiration. A ventilator-driven breath may be delivered regardless of patient effort; on the other hand, it may be patient initiated (patient-triggered). When triggered, the ventilator detects the onset of a patient-initiated inspiration (by detecting changes in pressure or flow that occur within the ventilator circuit), and delivers a breath in synchrony with the patient's inspiratory effort. Either a pressure, flow or volume target can be used to initiate inspiration (see Fig. 4.2).

The trigger variable The variable involved in the initiation (triggering) of inspiration			
Pressure as a trigger variable:	Flow as a trigger variable:	Volume as a trigger variable:	Time as a trigger variable:
The pressure drop in the circuit as a result of the patient's attempt to inhale is sensed by the ventilator, and the ventilator delivers a breath in response to it	The flow into the circuit as a result of the patient's attempt to inhale is sensed by the ventilator, and the ventilator delivers a breath in response to it	The volume change in the circuit as a result of the patient's attempt to inhale is sensed by the ventilator, and the ventilator delivers a breath in response to it	The breath is triggered according to a preset frequency, and is delivered at regular intervals of time, independent of the patient effort

FIGURE 4.2. The trigger variable.

4.1.7 Limit Variable

The value of the limit variable cannot be exceeded at any time during inspiration (Fig. 4.3). By definition, time cannot be a limit variable. Once the limit variable is reached, inspiration does *not* end: the remainder of the breath is regulated within the set limit of this variable.[12]

4.1.8 Cycle Variable

The changeover from inspiration to expiration and from expiration to inspiration is called cycling. Ventilators use different ways to cycle between inspiration and expiration (Fig. 4.4).

4.1.8.1 Volume-Cycled Breath

The inspiratory breath is terminated after a specified volume has been delivered to the patient. When the inspiratory tidal volume is delivered at a low flow rate, inspiration will necessarily take longer. The addition of an inspiratory pause (which is considered a part of inspiration) extends

The limit variable The value of this variable cannot be exceeded at any time during inspiration		
Pressure as a limit variable	**Volume as a limit variable**	**Flow as a limit variable**
The set upper pressure limit cannot be exceeded during the inspiration	The set volume limit cannot be exceeded during the inspiration	The flow limit cannot be exceeded during the inspiration
e.g., Pressure control ventilation or Pressure Support ventilation	e.g., Volume control ventilation	e.g., Volume control ventilation

FIGURE 4.3. The limit variable.

The cycle variable The variable used to end inspiration, viz, to cycle off from inspiration to expiration.			
Volumed	**Time**	**Flow**	**Pressure**
The ventilator cyclesfrom inspiration to expiration after a preset volume has been delivered (e.g., in the volume control mode) If an inspiratory pause has been set,expiration does not immediately follow the delivery of a breath; the breath by definition now becomes time cycled rather than volume cycle	The ventilator cycles from inspiration to expiration after a preset inspiratory time has elapsed (e.g., pressure control mode)	When the flow during inspiration falls to a certain level (typically 25% of the peak inspiratory flow), the ventilatorcycles from inspiration to expiration (e.g., pressure support ventilation)	During volume-controlled ventilation, if the airway pressure exceeds the set maximum airway pressure limit, the ventilator will cycle to expiration regardless ofthe tidal volume that has been delivered to the patient

FIGURE 4.4. The cycle variable.

the inspiratory time. Because the pause time must be specified, the breath becomes time-cycled, though volume-limited.

4.1.8.2 Flow-Cycled Breath

The ventilator cycles to expiration once the flow has decreased to a certain level, which is either an absolute value (e.g., 5 L/min) or a fraction of the peak flows achieved (usually 25% of the peak inspiratory flows). Such a mechanism is operative during the pressure support ventilation, in which patient effort and lung characteristics determine the tidal volume, airway pressure, and inspiratory time (see section 4.4).

4.1.8.3 Time-Cycled Breath

The inspiratory time is preset, and at the predesignated time, the ventilator cycles from inspiration to expiration. Pressure control ventilation is an example of time-cycled ventilation where the airway pressure is held constant at a desired level throughout inspiration. In the pressure control mode, both airway pressure and inspiratory time are physician-preset, so the tidal volume will vary depending upon the resistance and compliance of the lung (see section 4.8).

4.1.8.4 Pressure-Cycled Breath

When a ventilator is set to pressure cycle, it will do so when a predesignated pressure level is reached. Appropriate setting of this pressure level will prevent the airway pressure from rising to an inordinate level, and so, will protect the lung against pressure-induced lung injury. It is important to note that pressure cycling can occur during volume-targeted ventilation as well. If the airway pressure exceeds the set maximum airway pressure limit, the ventilator will cycle to expiration regardless of the tidal volume that has been delivered to the patient. Under such circumstances, high airway pressures may result in premature termination of inspiratory breaths, causing the delivered minute volume to fall – with consequent hypoventilation.

4.1.9 Baseline Variable

This is the variable that is controlled at end exhalation. Most often, the baseline variable controlled is pressure. The end-expiratory pressure may be set to zero (ZEEP), or a positive pressure may be created at end-expiration (PEEP) by the closure of the expiratory valve before the lung has quite emptied (Fig. 4.5).

The baseline variable (e.g., pressure): The varible (most often pressure) that is controlled at end-exhalation	
ZEEP	**PEEP**
Baseline pressure set to zero relative to atmospheric pressure	Baseline pressure set positive relative to atmospheric pressure

FIGURE 4.5. The baseline variable.

4.1.10 Inspiratory Hold

Once the inspiratory tidal volume has been delivered, the air may briefly be held within the patient's lungs by using the inspiratory hold option. The inspiratory hold is used when the plateau airway pressure needs to be calculated (see section 8.2.1.1).

4.1.11 Expiratory Hold and Expiratory Retard

Expiratory hold (or expiratory pause) is utilized for the purpose of measuring the pressure within airways during a state of no-flow (see p...). Expiratory *retard* was once employed with the intent of slowing down the expiratory flow and to so mimic the physiological effects of pursed-lip breathing (as in emphysematous subjects). Expiratory retard is no longer used; rather, a small amount of PEEP ("physiological PEEP") is used to accomplish the same purpose (see p...Chaps. 5 and 8). In fact, the ventilator circuit and the expiratory valves themselves engender a measure of expiratory flow resistance,

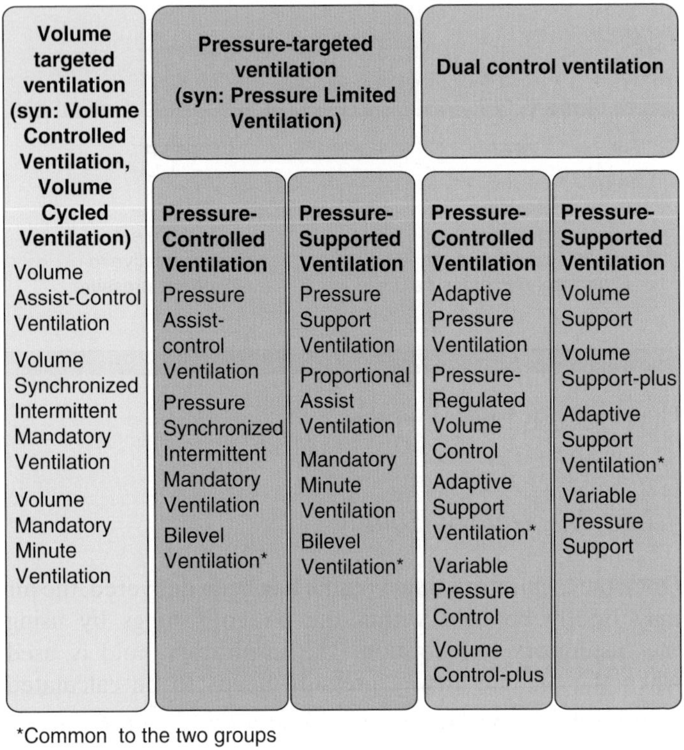
Volume targeted ventilation (syn: Volume Controlled Ventilation, Volume Cycled Ventilation)
Volume Assist-Control Ventilation
Volume Synchronized Intermittent Mandatory Ventilation
Volume Mandatory Minute Ventilation
Pressure-targeted ventilation (syn: Pressure Limited Ventilation)
Pressure-Controlled Ventilation
Pressure Assist-control Ventilation
Pressure Synchronized Intermittent Mandatory Ventilation
Bilevel Ventilation*
Pressure-Supported Ventilation
Pressure Support Ventilation
Proportional Assist Ventilation
Mandatory Minute Ventilation
Bilevel Ventilation*
Dual control ventilation
Pressure-Controlled Ventilation
Adaptive Pressure Ventilation
Pressure-Regulated Volume Control
Adaptive Support Ventilation*
Variable Pressure Control
Volume Control-plus
Pressure-Supported Ventilation
Volume Support
Volume Support-plus
Adaptive Support Ventilation*
Variable Pressure Support
*Common to the two groups

FIGURE 4.6. The baseline variable.

and this produces much the same effects as a small degree of expiratory retard.

4.2 Volume-Targeted Modes

These have been summarized in Fig. 4.6.[36]

4.2.1 Volume Assist-Control Mode (ACMV, CMV)

This is the mode used most often at the initiation of mechanically ventilated support to a patient.

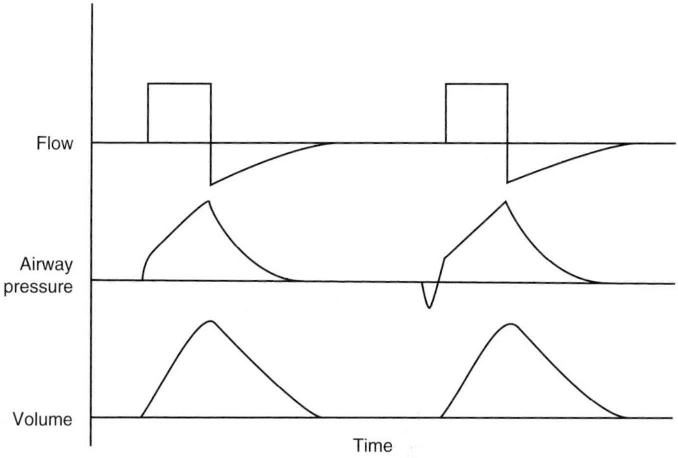
Flow
Airway pressure
Volume
Time

FIGURE 4.7. Volume-targeted ventilation: The assist-control mode.

In the critical care unit, the initiation of mechanical ventilatory support to a patient is usually undertaken when the patient is very sick or unstable. Under such circumstances, it is desirable that the patient be spared any undue excess of work of breathing that could impose a major burden on his cardiorespiratory system (Fig. 4.7).

The ACMV mode ensures this. The physician determines the tidal volume and the respiratory rate according to the needs of the patient. The preset tidal volume – or the guaranteed tidal volume (say, 500 mL) – is delivered at the set rate (say, 12 breaths/min). This guarantees the patient a minimum minute ventilation of 500 mL times 12 breaths/min = 6,000 mL/min.

The advantage of assist-control ventilation is that full ventilatory support is potentially assured, provided that the backup rate has been set high enough. Assist-control ventilation rests the patient and relieves him of most of the work of breathing. While guaranteeing the basic ventilatory requirements, the ACMV does not preclude spontaneous breathing by the patient, who is allowed to breathe above the set rate. Therefore, ACMV responds to the dynamic needs of the patient, in that the respiratory rate is controlled by the patient according to his needs (e.g.,

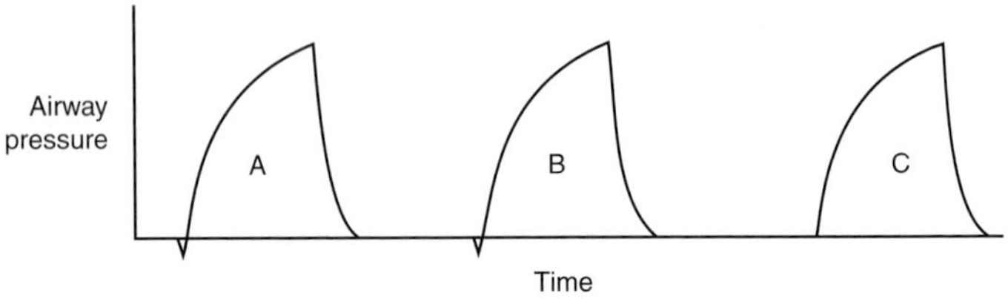
Airway
pressure
A
B
C
Time

FIGURE 4.8. Assist-Control ventilation. Breaths A and B are patient-triggered: note the negative deflection preceding each ventilator-driven positive-pressure breath. Breath C is ventilator-triggered, the patient having failed to initiate inspiration on his own.

the pyrexial patient – whose CO_2 production is high – breathes more frequently to enable washout of CO_2) (Fig. 4.8).

Close matching of the ventilator's settings to the patient's requirements demands careful attention to the physiological variables discussed later in this book. The mode is often uncomfortable to the patient whose respiratory drive demands higher tidal volumes than those that have been preset. The lack of adaptability of the assist-control mode to a changing clinical situation can result in other problems. For example, in obstructive airways disease, with widespread airway narrowing, the available expiratory time frequently proves insufficient for the complete exhalation of the preset tidal volumes. Air trapping results, and can lead not only to an increase in the intrathoracic pressure, but also to a worsening in lung compliance. Moving noncompliant lungs can impose an additional inspiratory load on the patient and increase the work of breathing further (Fig. 4.9).

Although an advantage of the assist mode is that the work of breathing is performed mainly by the ventilator (once it has been triggered), it is the patient who has to expend energy to trigger the ventilator. If the trigger sensitivity is set at too high a level, the energy required to trigger the ventilator can be considerable, leading to substantial work of breathing.

Nor does the patient's inspiratory effort cease once the ventilator is triggered. Neuronal input to the respiratory muscles can continue for a variable period while the

Advantages	Disadvantages
• Minute ventilation is guaranteed • The set tidal volume is guaranteed • The patient can choose to overbreathe the set respiratory rate • Each breath is delivered in synchrony with the patient's spontaneous effort; this makes for more comfortable breathing • The mode affords rest to the patient and unloads the respiratory muscles	• The breathing schedule is relatively rigid. Alkalosis may occur if the set respiratory rate is too high. • Airway pressures may rise if lung mechanics are poor: dynamic hyperinflation can occur. • The work of breathing can be high if the trigger sensitivity or flow settings are not appropriately adjusted • Sedation often required • Due to prolonged unloading of the respiratory muscles, atrophy is possible

FIGURE 4.9. Advantages and disadvantages of the Volume-Targeted Assist-Control Mode.

ventilator is yet in the process of delivering the inspiratory breath. When the set inspiratory time on the ventilator does not match the patient's neuronal inspiratory time, patient-ventilator asynchrony can occur.

A ventilator-delivered inspiratory breath can sometimes coincide with the patient's effort at expiration, resulting in "clashing" of breaths with patient-ventilator incoordination. It is also possible that a patient with a high respiratory drive might make ineffectual attempts at inspiration while awaiting the next breath from the ventilator; this can increase the work of breathing, increase the level of discomfort, and have a negative impact on the hemodynamic status.

Such a patient might require considerable sedation, and at times, pharmacological paralysis. The use of pharmacological paralysis has important implications. Inadvertent disconnection of the paralyzed – and therefore apneic – patient from the ventilator would certainly be catastrophic if unrecognized.

On the other hand, if the set minute volume exceeds that which is required to keep the patient's $PaCO_2$ within a reasonable range, respiratory alkalosis can occur with its attendant consequences. The patient whose respiratory drive is increased because of fever or discomfort is also liable to develop respiratory alkalosis.

If ACMV is used at the predominant mode of ventilation for a prolonged time, the lack of stimulus to the patient's respiratory muscles can result in respiratory muscle atrophy. Hence, although suitable for the ventilation of the newly intubated "unstable" patient, ACMV does not fulfill the needs of an ideal long-term ventilation mode for most others.

For graphical representation of ACMV mode see Fig. 4.7 & 4.8.

Box 4.2 Assist Control

Example:

If a tidal volume of 500 mL at a backup rate of 10 breaths/min were to be set for a patient breathing spontaneously at 20 breaths/min, the ventilator would deliver 500 mL for each breath triggered by the patient.

If the patient's respiratory rate were to fall for some reason, to say, 5 breaths/min, the ventilator backup would then kick in and provide 5 extra breaths/min, each of a tidal volume of 500 mL, to realize the 10 breaths/min requirement.

Should the patient not breathe at all, the set tidal volumes would again be delivered at the backup rate, in this case, 10 breaths/min.

4.3 Intermittent Mandatory Ventilation

Initially, the IMV mode was used principally as a weaning mode.

In this mode, a certain number of breaths are preset by the physician. These mandatory (compulsory) breaths are compulsorily given to the patient, irrespective of the patient's own demands. The physician sets the tidal volume and the respiratory frequency: *mandatory breaths* are delivered to the patient intermittently, at equal intervals of time.

In between the mandatory breaths, the patient may breathe at his desired respiratory rate. The tidal volume of the *spontaneous breaths* will depend on the strength of the patient's inspiratory effort. When the patient cannot generate sufficient inspiratory force to generate satisfactory tidal volumes during his spontaneous breaths, alveolar hypoventilation can occur – unless the backup (mandatory) rate has been set high enough to take care of most of the minute ventilation of itself.

Just as in the *control mode* of ventilation, if any asynchrony occurs between the patient's spontaneous inspiration and the ventilator-delivered breath, there can be "clashing" or "breath-stacking." As a result of an innovation designed to prevent patient-ventilator asynchrony, the ventilator detects the onset of the patient's spontaneous inspiratory effort and delivers the mandatory breath in synchrony with it, in a similar manner to that in the assist-control mode. Such a mode of ventilation is called synchronized intermittent mandatory ventilation (SIMV) mode (Fig. 4.10). The SIMV is much more comfortable for the patient than is the IMV mode.

At this juncture, it is relevant to recall the discussion on dead space ventilation (section 3.6.3). The conducting airways play no part in gas exchange, and the space within them is termed the

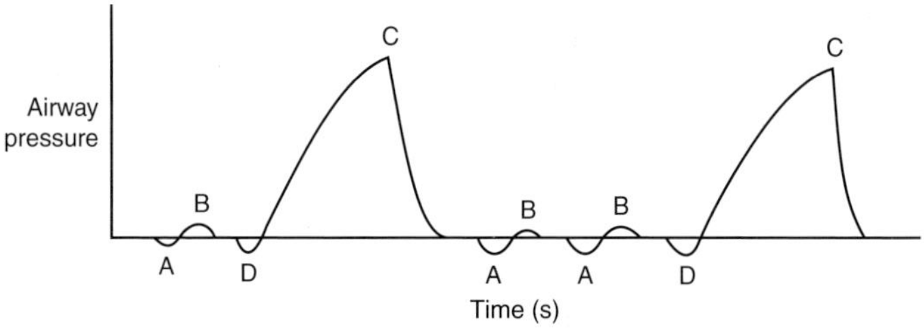

Airway pressure
C
C
B
B
B
A
D
A
A
D
Time (s)

FIGURE 4.10. Synchronized Intermittent Mandatory Ventilation. The gentle undulations about the baseline (A and B) represent the patient's spontaneous breaths. C is the mandatory ventilator-driven breath, which is synchronized with the patient's inspiratory effort (D). Within a timing window activated at periodic intervals of time, the patient's inspiratory ort is sensed by the ventilator and the mandatory breath delivered in synchrony with it.

anatomical dead space. For obvious reasons, anatomical dead space does not change, except – as in mechanically ventilated patients – if an endotracheal tube is in place. The endotracheal tube being of smaller volume than the upper airway, which it bypasses, slightly cuts down the anatomical dead space.

Alveolar dead space is formed by such alveoli that are ventilated but not perfused. The anatomical dead space and the alveolar dead space together comprise the physiological dead space.

In normal individuals, alveolar dead space is negligible. In a diseased lung, however, there is considerable expansion in the alveolar dead space due to the general inhomogeneity of ventilation; as a result, the physiological dead space increases.

Alveolar ventilation is determined by how much the delivered tidal volume exceeds the dead space. If the *spontaneous* breaths on the SIMV mode are around 150–200 mL in volume, they will not exceed the dead space by much, and therefore, will not participate in meaningful alveolar ventilation. To boost the volume of these spontaneous breaths, external pressure support may be applied, resulting in a combination of these two modes – the SIMV + PSV mode.

There are important differences between the SIMV mode and the assist-control mode. In the SIMV mode, the mandatory breaths are set by the physician. During the *mandatory* breaths, the patient is delivered the *preset tidal volumes*, but the tidal volumes of the *spontaneous* breaths depend upon the strength of the inspiratory effort. On the other hand, each breath in the assist-control mode will have a tidal volume equal to the preset tidal volume, be it a patient-triggered breath or a backup breath. In the SIMV mode, the patient is delivered the full complement of the preset mandatory breaths irrespective of how many additional spontaneous breaths he chooses to take; in the assist-control mode, the patient determines his own respiratory rate so long as he is breathing spontaneously at a rate above the backup rate. If the patient's respiratory frequency on the assist-control mode should for some reason fall below the minimum (backup) rate, the machine ensures a secured level of ventilation by delivering the minimum number of (backup) breaths (Fig. 4.11).

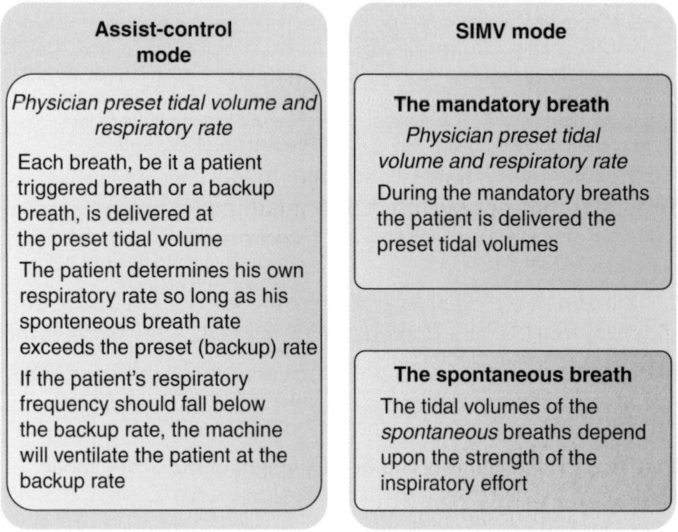
Assist-control mode
Physician preset tidal volume and respiratory rate
Each breath, be it a patient triggered breath or a backup breath, is delivered at the preset tidal volume
The patient determines his own respiratory rate so long as his sponteneous breath rate exceeds the preset (backup) rate
If the patient's respiratory frequency should fall below the backup rate, the machine will ventilate the patient at the backup rate
SIMV mode
The mandatory breath
Physician preset tidal volume and respiratory rate
During the mandatory breaths the patient is delivered the preset tidal volumes
The spontaneous breath
The tidal volumes of the spontaneous breaths depend upon the strength of the inspiratory effort

FIGURE 4.11. Comparison of the Assist Control and the SIMV mode.

An advantage of the SIMV mode is that it allows the patient to use his respiratory muscles (by breathing spontaneously in between the mandatory breaths). This is a distinct advantage during long-term mechanical ventilation where disuse atrophy of the respiratory muscles can occur; and this can certainly be an advantage during the time of weaning, when the ventilatory burden can gradually be transferred from the machine to the patient by gradually decreasing the number of mandatory breaths and encouraging the patient to breathe on his own (see discussion below) (Fig. 4.12).

Notably, the assist-control mode is very different in this respect. In the assist-control mode, at least in theory, apart from expending energy in triggering the ventilator, the patient performs very little of the work of breathing, since additional breathing in between machine delivered breaths is not possible. Once triggered, the ventilator is responsible for the entire inspiratory work of breathing from then on, enabling tired respiratory muscles to rest. Therefore, the assist-control mode is used in situations where a greater degree of respiratory

Advantages	Disadvantages
• The mandatory breath is delivered in synchrony with patient-effort (SIMV). This makes for greater comfort during breathing	• The work of breathing can be high if the trigger sensitivity and the flow are inappropriate to the patient's needs
• In between the mandatory breaths, the patient can breathe at his preferred respiratory rate, tidal volume and flow	• Hypoventilation is possible if the patient is not capable of spontaneous breathing, and the mandatory breath rate has not been set high enough
• The patient's respiratory muscles remain active, and so disuse atrophy is less common	• Excessive work of breathing is possible during spontaneous breaths unless an adequate level of pressure support is applied

FIGURE 4.12. Advantages and disadvantages of the SIMV mode.

support is needed, and should be expected to completely fulfill the ventilatory requirements of the patient.

The intent in the SIMV mode is different. It is the patient who is encouraged to perform more of the work of breathing, with the mandatory backup rate serving as a buffer for his minute ventilation and preventing the patient from entirely taking upon himself the burden of his work of breathing. One advantage of the SIMV mode is that the patient can increase or decrease the volume and frequency of his spontaneous breaths in accordance with his requirements. As a result, alkalosis is usually less of a problem. Although setting a high enough mandatory breath rate can completely satisfy the ventilatory requirements of the patient, this is usually not the intent of this mode. The objective, as mentioned above, is to make the patient perform at least some of the work of breathing, and to enable this to happen, the minute ventilation provided by the mandatory breaths is deliberately set at a level below the minute ventilation requirements of the patient.

The generation of a spontaneous breath in the SIMV mode requires the creation of a negative intrathoracic pressure by contraction of the inspiratory muscles. Thus, the spontaneous breaths are generated in a fashion more akin to physiological breathing. As a consequence of this, there is not as much a rise in the intrathoracic pressure as there would have been should all breaths be positive-pressure breaths (the latter, of course, is the case in the assist-control mode). Logically, therefore, the magnitude of hemodynamic compromise caused by this mode should be relatively less.

The advantage that the SIMV mode has over the assist-control mode in respect of circulatory hemodynamics appears to be operative only as long as less than half of the minute volume is provided in the form of positive-pressure breaths: when more than half of the minute volume is made up by the mandatory breaths, the hemodynamic advantage is lost. These are, however, vexatious issues, and it may well be that the hemodynamic advantage gained by the use of a low backup rate in the SIMV mode is offset by the increased work of breathing necessitated by breathing at a high spontaneous rate (when the mandatory rate is low). In fact, SIMV breathing can lead to an undesirable increase in oxygen consumption, which may even exceed the O_2 consumption that occurs in assist-control mode. When at least 80% of the minute volume is provided by mandatory SIMV breaths, patients can be considered to be fully supported. When this is the case, there may be no special advantage of either mode (SIMV or assist-control) over the other.

4.4 Pressure–Support Ventilation

During pressure–supported ventilation (PSV), the ventilator augments the inspiratory effort of the patient with positive pressure support. Exhalation is passive. Since the level of the pressure support is physician-preset – given a constant strength of inspiratory effort on the part of the patient – the tidal volumes can be made to rise or fall by varying the level of the pressure support. In other words, the level of pressure support determines the tidal volumes (Fig. 4.13).

With the onset of inspiration, the airway pressure rapidly rises, and this level of pressure is maintained at a plateau for most of inspiration. When the airflow begins to slow down

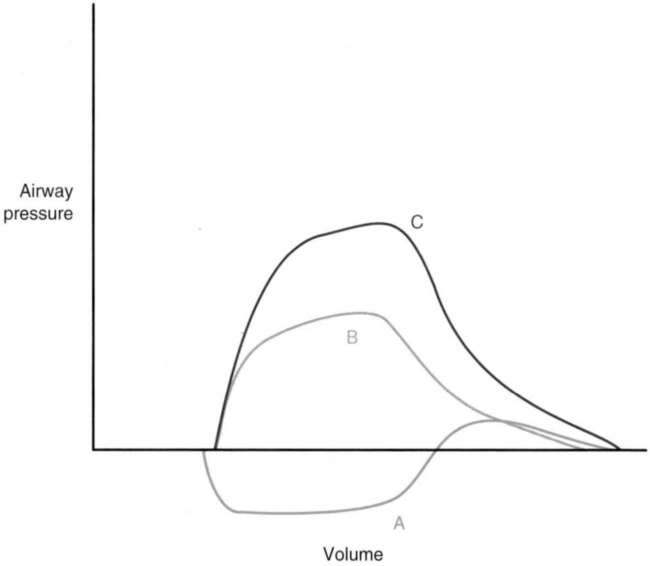
Airway
pressure
C
B
A
Volume

FIGURE 4.13. Pressure Support mode. Airway pressure during an unassisted breath is represented by the *green line* (A). Airway pressure during pressure supported breaths is represented by the *pink* (B) and *red* (C) lines.

toward the end of inspiration, the ventilator cycles to expiration and allows exhalation to occur passively. The flow threshold that determines this cycling to expiration is 25% of the peak flow for most ventilators. In other words, cycling to expiration occurs when the airflow during the deceleration phase of inspiration falls to 25% of its peak level.

Although flow cycling is the norm in PSV, time cycling is used as a *backup* method of cycling. During flow-cycled breaths, in the presence of a leak in the circuit, the ventilator may fail to cycle from inspiration to expiration. A backup cycling mechanism provides protection: the breath is automatically terminated after a certain inspiratory time has elapsed – usually 3–5 s.

In order for the ventilator to deliver an inspiratory breath, it is necessary that the patient first "demand" a breath from

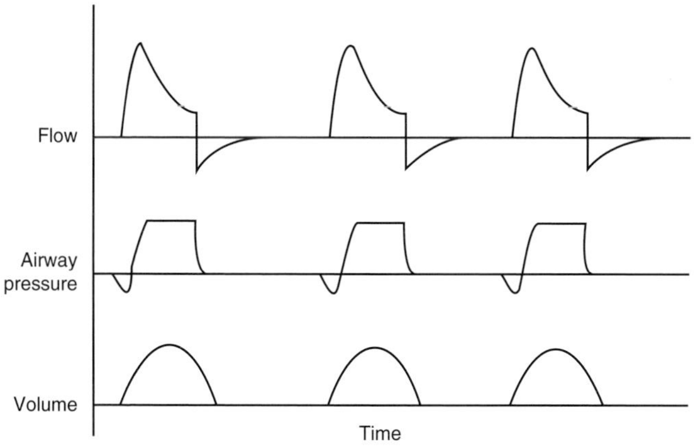
Flow
Airway pressure
Volume
Time

FIGURE 4.14. Pressure Support Ventilation

the ventilator by attempting to initiate inspiration. The ventilator senses the transient dip in airway pressure that the patient's effort at inspiration produces, and instantly delivers the pressure-supported breath. PSV, therefore, will work only if the patient is able to trigger the ventilator on his own (Fig. 4.14).

Within the PSV mode, the patient can breathe at the respiratory rate that he chooses. The patient also controls the inspiratory time and inspiratory flow rate of each breath. This is an important distinction from the Pressure *Control* mode (see later). Since the patient can control the depth, length, and flow profile of each breath, PSV tends to be a relatively comfortable and well-tolerated mode. Because it is the patient who decides when to initiate a breath, there is better synchronization with the ventilator.

By supporting the inspiratory effort of the patient, PSV minimizes the work of breathing. With enhancement of tidal volumes, the respiratory rate falls; this is a sign of more comfortable breathing. A low level of pressure support (e.g., 5–10 cm H_2O) generally suffices to negate the additional resistance imposed by an endotracheal tube (since the lumen of the endotracheal tube is much smaller than that of the innate airway) (Fig. 4.15).

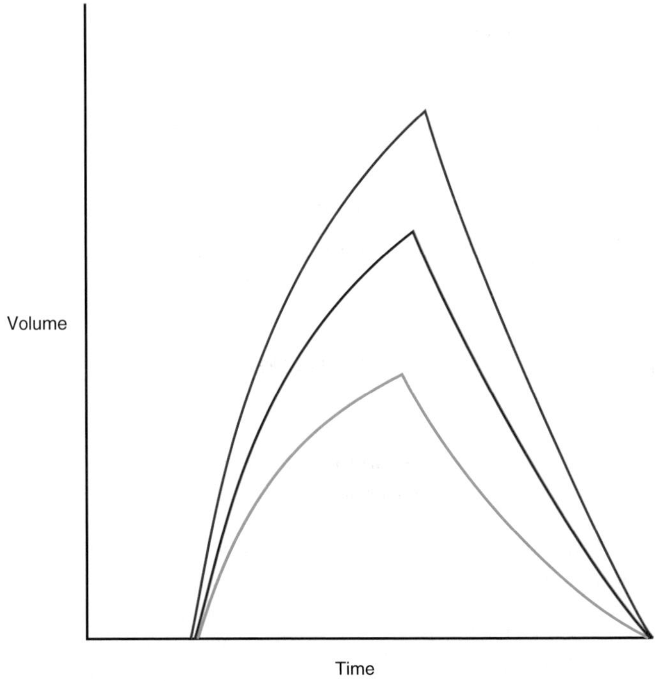
Volume
Time

FIGURE 4.15. Pressure Support Ventilation. With increasing levels of applied pressure support, the tidal volumes can be made to rise.

PSV allows considerable flexibility in ventilatory support: high levels of pressure support are capable of providing virtually full ventilatory support. When the pressure support is set to a level that offsets the additional resistance imposed by the endotracheal tube and the ventilator circuitry, a breathing pattern very similar to physiological breathing can be achieved (Fig. 4.16).

The disadvantages of PSV stem from the fact that the state of respiratory system is usually dynamic and varies constantly. Within the PSV mode, it is only pressure that is assured (to the patient) and not tidal volumes: if the lung becomes stiff (e.g., pulmonary edema) or obstructed (e.g., bronchospasm or secretions obstructing the endotracheal tube) for any reason, tidal volumes will fall.

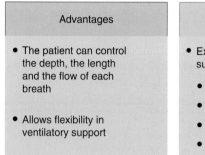

Advantages	Disadvantages
• The patient can control the depth, the length and the flow of each breath • Allows flexibility in ventilatory support	• Excessive levels of support can result in: • Respiratory alkalosis • Hyperinflation • Ineffective triggering • Apneic spells[31]

FIGURE 4.16. Advantages and disadvantages of the Pressure Support mode.

Falling tidal volumes by decreasing the minute ventilation can result in hypoventilation. Provided the respiratory drive is intact, the patient can be expected to defend his minute ventilation by raising his spontaneous respiratory rate to compensate for the falling tidal volumes. A rising spontaneous respiratory frequency in a patient on PSV should therefore draw one's attention to the possibility of worsening respiratory mechanics.

By the same token, PSV is generally poorly tolerated in patients with active bronchospasm for the reason that the set level of PSV may be inadequate to deliver adequate tidal volumes in a patient with high intrinsic airway resistance.

Although the PSV mode probably approximates physiological breathing more than several other modes do, it can still provoke patient-ventilator asynchrony. As mentioned earlier, cycling from inspiration to expiration occurs when the inspiratory flow has fallen to a certain predesignated level, usually 25% of the peak flow rate. In COPD patients, airway narrowing is widespread throughout the tracheobronchial tree, and can be considerable in the small airways. This results in slow emptying of the lungs, and a longer time is required for expiration. Also, it takes longer for the lungs to fill during inspiration. The flow rate may continue to be relatively high even late in the inspiratory phase. Inspiration is, therefore,

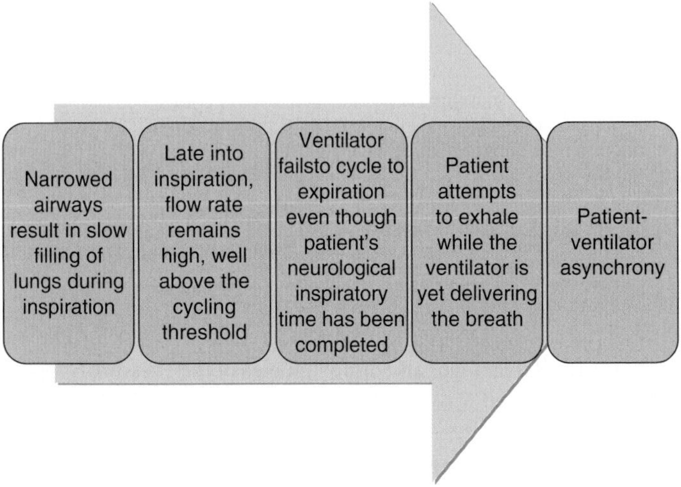
Narrowed airways result in slow filling of lungs during inspiration
Late into inspiration, flow rate remains high, well above the cycling threshold
Ventilator failsto cycle to expiration even though patient's neurological inspiratory time has been completed
Patient attempts to exhale while the ventilator is yet delivering the breath
Patient-ventilator asynchrony

FIGURE 4.17. Patient-ventilator asynchrony in COPD patients with the PSV mode.

considerably prolonged due to the failure of airflow to fall to the predesignated threshold of 25% of the peak expiratory flow rate, even after a substantial time has been spent in inspiration. It is common, then, for COPD patients to try to commence expiration while the ventilator is still delivering a breath (Fig. 4.17).

4.5 Continuous Positive Airway Pressure

In the spontaneously breathing individual, active inspiration is followed by passive expiration, at the end of which the airway pressure falls to the atmospheric level – the pressure at the mouth. Since the pressure at the two ends of a tube must be equal for airflow to cease, at end-expiration, alveolar pressure must necessarily equate with the atmospheric pressure. At end-expiration, alveolar pressure is low, but alveoli are prevented from collapsing completely because of the surfactant within them. When alveoli are diseased, they tend to

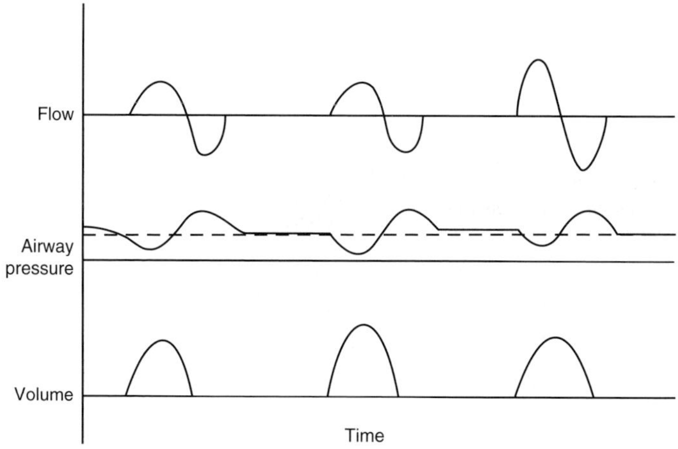
Flow
Airway pressure
Volume
Time

FIGURE 4.18. Continuous Positive Airway Pressure.

collapse prematurely. Hypoxia due to V/Q mismatch and shunting will then occur, as the blood brought to the collapsed alveoli returns – without being oxygenated – to the heart via the pulmonary veins.

Diseased alveoli have a tendency to collapse completely as they are deficient in surfactant, and if they are allowed to completely close, the magnitude of the force required to reopen them is likely to be considerable (see LaPlace's law p. 484). In other words, it takes much more pressure to expand a diseased lung by a given volume, than it does to expand a normal lung by the same volume. The ratio ΔV/ΔP (change in volume for a given change in pressure) for a diseased lung is low. This means that the increase in volume is relatively small for a given increase in pressure, and this reflects a poorly compliant system (Fig. 4.18).

Whenever compliance decreases for any reason the work of breathing increases. The high pressure required to open up the completely closed alveoli repetitively during each respiratory cycle can overdistend the healthier and more compliant alveoli, predisposing to volutrauma and barotrauma (see Chapter 10).

Advantages	Disadvantages
• Stabilization of the upper airway • Alveolar recruitment improves oxygenation • Increase in FRC improves lung compliance • Decrease in microatelectasis, macroatelectasis. • Decreased work of breathing by improving compliance and preventing atelectasis • Decreased work of breathing in the setting of intrinsic PEEP	• Air leaks during noninvasive CPAP • Problems related to interfaces • Dynamic hyperinflation, if level of CPAP has been set inappropriately high

FIGURE 4.19. Advantages and disadvantages of the CPAP mode.

If the diseased alveoli can be prevented from collapsing entirely, this will save the lungs from the high distending pressures. By elevating the end-expiratory pressure to above the atmospheric pressure, continuous positive airway pressure (CPAP) internally splints the lungs, keeping the unstable alveolar units from collapsing. The recruitment of previously collapsed alveolar units increases the functional residual capacity (FRC).

By this, two advantages accrue: firstly, the restoration of ventilation to the perfused areas reverses the hypoxemia. Secondly, the compliance improves, since with the active participation of additional alveoli in ventilation, a greater change in volume is now possible for a given change in pressure. With an improvement in pulmonary compliance, the work of breathing decreases (Fig. 4.19).

CPAP can be used both in intubated and nonintubated patients. Nasal and oronasal CPAP masks enable the administration of positive end-expiratory pressure to the patient's lungs in a noninvasive manner. Since the aim of the CPAP is solely to maintain a positive pressure in the airways at the end of expiration, CPAP does not provide the kind of intermittent positive pressure during *inspiration* in the manner that PSV does. For CPAP to be used successfully, the patient needs to have the capacity to breathe spontaneously. The addition of inspiratory pressure support on top of the CPAP (the Bi-PAP mode) helps the patient with an inadequate respiratory effort.

Disadvantages of CPAP include its propensity to produce hyperinflation. Hyperinflation can not only increase the pressure gradient between the alveolar and the proximal airways making inspiration difficult but also make the lungs stiffer (the lungs operate on the higher, stiffer part of the pressure volume curve). Consequently, the work of breathing during inspiration increases. The work of breathing performed during expiration can increase as well (see section 9.5), and the expiratory muscles of the patient may then come into play.

4.6 Bilevel Positive Airway Pressure

The patient is ventilated at two different levels of CPAP; the switchover from one to the other level of CPAP is synchronized with the patient. Pressure–support can be added at one or both the levels of the CPAP used.

4.7 Airway Pressure Release Ventilation (APRV)

[*Syn:* CPAP with release, Intermittent CPAP, variable positive airway pressure (VPAP)].

APRV is available in Drager's Evita 2 Dura and Evita 4, and BiLevel-Puritan Bennet 840.

APRV involves the periodic release of pressure while breathing in the CPAP mode. The release in pressure may be time-cycled, or may be allowed to occur after a predesignated number of breaths; the latter mode has been termed intermittent mandatory airway pressure release ventilation (IMPRV): like SIMV, the mandatory breaths can be synchronized to the patient's inspiratory effort.

CPAP breaths are given at two levels of pressure – P_{high} and P_{low}. Mandatory breaths begin with the timed closure of a release valve, and the pressure rises from P_{low} to P_{high}. At this elevated level of CPAP (P_{high}), the patient is allowed to breathe spontaneously. The release in pressure is usually time-cycled, and at the end of the mandatory breath, the opening of the release valve drops the pressure back to P_{low} for a brief period of time – usually 1–2 s – during which interval again the patient is allowed to breathe spontaneously. The drop in airway pressure from P_{high} to P_{low} allows greater washout of CO_2 to occur. In paralyzed patients, the mode becomes identical to the PC-IRV mode.

The indications for APRV are similar to those for pressure-controlled ventilation (PCV) – i.e., ALI and ARDS – though the mode can be used with milder disease as well. The mode is capable of providing either partial or full ventilatory support.

The particular advantage of APRV is that it allows IRV – and therefore recruitment – in spontaneously breathing patients. Patients often synchronize well with the machine, reducing the need for heavy sedation or paralysis. Airway pressures are, overall, lower.

Since exhalation is abbreviated, the disadvantage, of course, is that air trapping can occur or worsen in those patients who have airflow limitation. Tidal volumes can be inconsistent when respiratory mechanics are unstable, and in such situations close monitoring is necessary.

4.7.1 Bi-PAP

Bi-PAP is a term used by a specific manufacturer (Respironics) to describe the noninvasive application of positive airway pressure (pressure support or pressure control) on top of a baseline CPAP (noninvasive CPAP and Bi-PAP have been dealt with in Chap. 13).

4.8 Pressure-Controlled Ventilation

In PCV, the physician only indirectly controls the tidal volume. A certain pressure limit is set. During a ventilator-delivered inspiration, as air is driven into the lungs, airway pressure rises, rapidly reaching the preset pressure control level. This pressure is maintained for the duration of inspiration. The pressure limit, the respiratory frequency, and the inspiratory time are physician-preset.

Within a given inspiratory time, a higher set pressure limit will allow greater filling of the lungs: more air can enter the lungs before the airflow begins to slow, and so the tidal volumes are larger. Thus in a given patient with stable lung mechanics, the tidal volume increases if the upper pressure limit has been set high and decreases if it has been set at a low level.

For a given pressure control limit and inspiratory time, the ventilator will be able to push in a more air if the lungs are healthy and distensible than if they are stiff and noncompliant. For this reason, tidal volumes in airways obstruction will be low: airway pressure rises much more quickly when air is pushed into the narrowed airways – the pressure limit is reached relatively early during inspiration.

From the point that the pressure limit is reached, inspiratory flow slows down progressively so that the set pressure level is maintained in spite of the distending lungs. Slower flow within the available inspiratory time will result in smaller tidal volumes.

The advantage in PCV lies in the guarantee that the peak pressure will remain at – and never exceed – the set pressure limit. The risk of barotrauma and of other adverse events related to high intrathoracic pressures is, thus, minimized. The relative importance of peak pressure as compared to pause pressure in the genesis of barotrauma has been discussed in Chapter 10.

The major disadvantage of PCV is that in a patient with unstable or changing lung mechanics, any significant fluctuation in the lung compliance or airway resistance will directly affect the delivered tidal volumes. Tidal volumes can vary substantially with changes in compliance or resistance, producing undesirable changes in minute ventilation (Fig. 4.20).

The use of a decelerating waveform during volume-controlled ventilation can, to an extent, mimic the pressure and flow characteristics of PCV. It should be appreciated that pressure control ventilation is time-cycled, which means that the inspiratory breath is terminated after a preset time has

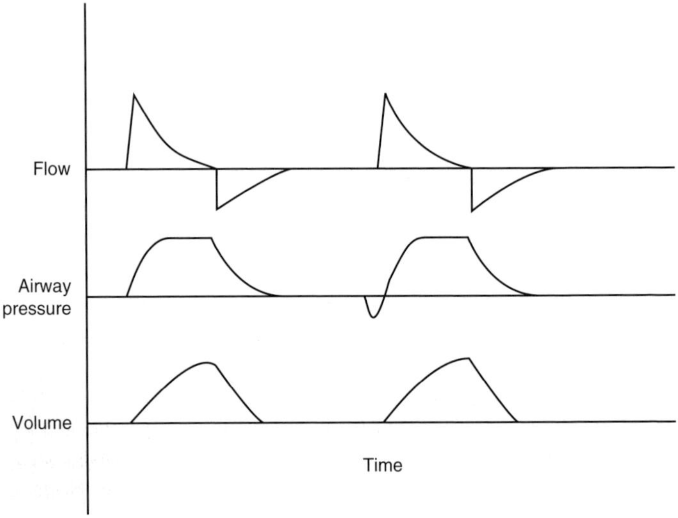
Flow
Airway pressure
Volume
Time

FIGURE 4.20. Pressure control ventilation.

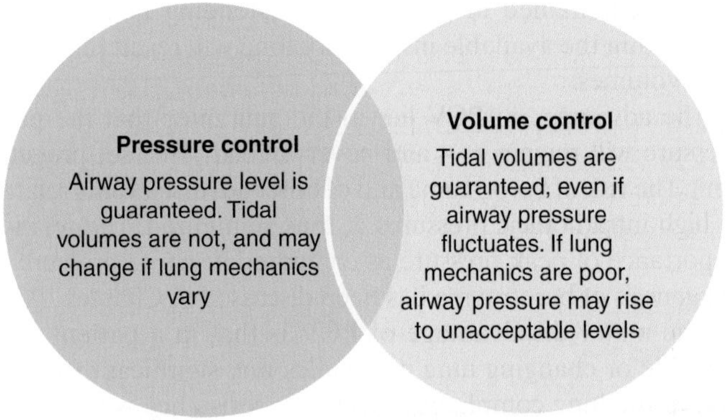
Pressure control
Airway pressure level is guaranteed. Tidal volumes are not, and may change if lung mechanics vary
Volume control
Tidal volumes are guaranteed, even if airway pressure fluctuates. If lung mechanics are poor, airway pressure may rise to unacceptable levels

FIGURE 4.21. Goals of the Volume Control mode and the Pressure Control mode.

elapsed, whereas volume control ventilation is volume-cycled, meaning that inspiration is completed only when the preset tidal volume has been delivered; also, the goals of the two modes are very different (see Fig. 4.21).

4.8.1 Proportional Assist Ventilation (PAV)

In essence, this mode (available within the Evita 4 ventilator) is very similar to the proportional pressure support mode. With this innovative approach, the pressure flow and volume delivery are dictated by the patient's efforts. In addition, the clinician determines how much the ventilator must amplify these variables in response to the patient's inspiratory effort and the prevailing lung mechanics.

The ventilator augments flow (which overcomes the resistive work) and volume (which overcomes the elastic work). The augmentation of flow and volume is in direct proportion to the patient's effort; an intact respiratory drive is, therefore, essential to the successful deployment of this mode. The ventilator monitors patient's lung mechanics on a real-time basis, and shapes the contours of the waveform on a breath to breath basis (Fig. 4.22).

Ventilator settings are targeted at overcoming a specific fraction of the elastic and resistive work of breathing. A typical initial setting of 80% will ensure that the ventilator performs 80% of the work. If respiratory mechanics – and therefore the work of breathing – then change, the patient will still perform no more than 20% of the overall work. The PAV mode is, therefore, most frequently used with the intent of counterbalancing the patient's work of breathing. Since it is the patient who controls the variables (tidal volume,

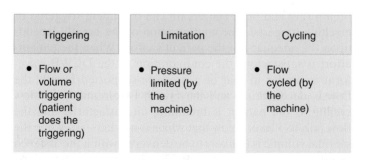

Triggering	Limitation	Cycling
• Flow or volume triggering (patient does the triggering)	• Pressure limited (by the machine)	• Flow cycled (by the machine)

FIGURE 4.22. Ventilator variables with the proportional assist mode.[36]

inspiratory flow, inspiratory time, and expiratory time), the mode promotes better patient-ventilator synchrony.

The obvious downside of the mode is that it cannot be applied in patients with a deficient respiratory drive. On the other hand, excessive assist ("runaway") may occur if lung mechanics suddenly improve. Excessive assist can also occur when air leaks are present, and autocycling can occur.

4.9 Dual Breath Control

Modern ventilators now incorporate complex computer-based algorithms, and are capable of simultaneously controlling two variables.[32]

Intrabreath control (dual control within a single breath, DCWB): During a part of an essentially pressure-targeted breath, flow is controlled.

Interbreath control (dual control from breath to breath, DCBB): The configuration of a pressure-targeted breath is manipulated to deliver a targeted tidal volume.

4.9.1 Intrabreath Control

4.9.1.1 Syn: Dual Control Within a Breath (DCWB)

The clinician sets the minimum tidal volume and backup breath rate and flow. The breath can be patient-triggered or machine-triggered. The configuration of the breath depends upon the adequacy of the patient's effort. When the patient-effort is satisfactory, the configuration of the DCWB waveform is similar to that of a pressure-supported breath: the flow is decelerating, and the breath is terminated by flow cycling. If the patient is breathing unsatisfactorily and the flow falls to a level below that which is needed – i.e., when the set tidal volume is unlikely to be delivered within the assigned inspiratory time – the machine delivers a controlled breath that is flow-targeted and volume-cycled, akin to a CMV breath (Fig. 4.23).

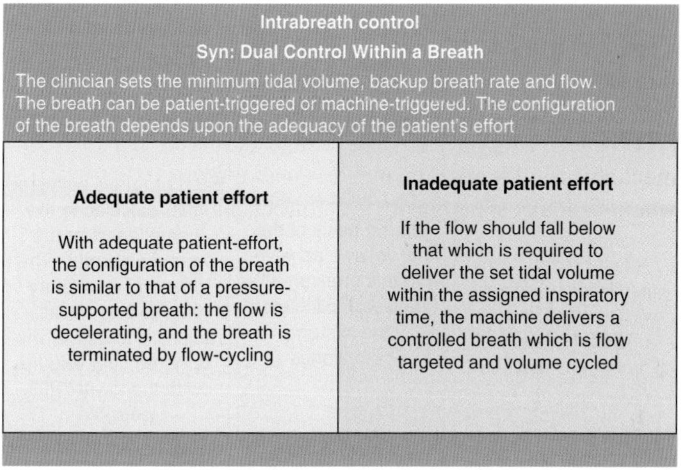
Intrabreath control
Syn: Dual Control Within a Breath
The clinician sets the minimum tidal volume, backup breath rate and flow. The breath can be patient-triggered or machine-triggered. The configuration of the breath depends upon the adequacy of the patient's effort
Adequate patient effort
With adequate patient-effort, the configuration of the breath is similar to that of a pressure-supported breath: the flow is decelerating, and the breath is terminated by flow-cycling
Inadequate patient effort
If the flow should fall below that which is required to deliver the set tidal volume within the assigned inspiratory time, the machine delivers a controlled breath which is flow targeted and volume cycled

FIGURE 4.23. Intrabreath control.

Examples of modes incorporating the intrabreath (DCWB) control are: volume assured pressure support (VAPS – available in Bird, Viasys), pressure augmentation (PA – available in Bird, Viasys), and machine volume (available in Viasys).

4.9.2 Interbreath (DCBB) Control

During intrabreath (DCBB) control, the flow and inspiratory time are automatically adjusted to deliver the targeted tidal volume with the lowest peak inspiratory pressure possible (Figs. 4.24 and Table 4.1).

4.9.3 Pressure Regulated Volume Control (PRVC)

The PRVC mode is available within the Macquet Servo-300. Allied modes are available in other ventilators: autoflow (Evita Drager 4, Savina), adaptive pressure ventilation (Hamilton Galileo), and variable pressure control (Venturi). In the Macquet Servo-300, the mode can only be used with CMV. In the other ventilators it can be used with SIMV as well.

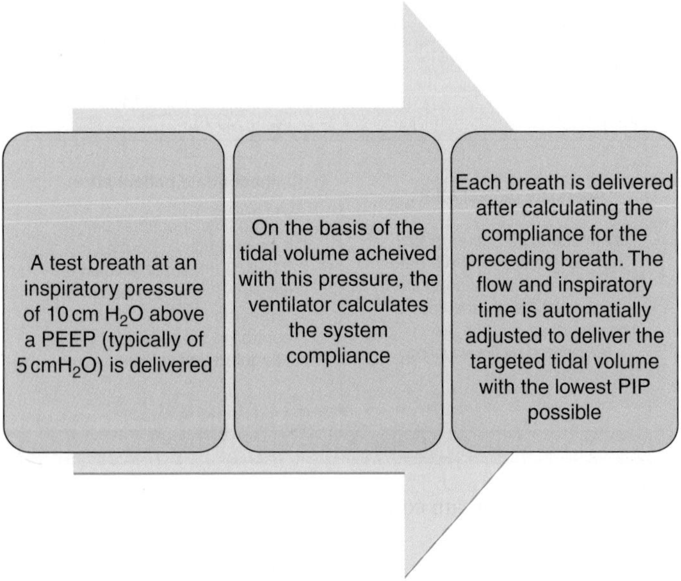
A test breath at an inspiratory pressure of 10 cm H_2O above a PEEP (typically of 5 cmH_2O) is delivered
On the basis of the tidal volume acheived with this pressure, the ventilator calculates the system compliance
Each breath is delivered after calculating the compliance for the preceding breath. The flow and inspiratory time is automatially adjusted to deliver the targeted tidal volume with the lowest PIP possible

FIGURE 4.24. Typical algorithm of interbreath (DCBB) control.

A test breath at an inspiratory pressure of 10 cm H_2O above a PEEP (typically of 5 cm H_2O) is delivered. On the basis of the tidal volume generated with this pressure, the ventilator calculates the system compliance. Each breath is delivered after calculating the compliance for the preceding breath. Three further tidal test breaths are delivered sequentially at about 75% of the pressure it would take to achieve the set tidal volume. The flow and inspiratory time are automatically adjusted to deliver the targeted tidal volume with the lowest PIP possible.

The algorithm for a PRVC breath is given in Fig. 4.24 above.

The flow is decelerating and the pressure waveform is square (if it is not, a higher tidal volume should be considered). The mode therefore should properly be considered a variant of the Pressure Control mode. Inspiratory flow is

TABLE 4.1 Modes with interbreath control[32].

Interbreath control mode	Manufacturer	Trigger variable	Cycle variable
Volume support	Macquet, Puritan-Bennet	Patient triggered	Flow cycled
Minimum mandatory ventilation	Hamilton	Patient triggered	Flow cycled
Flow-cycled, pressure-regul ated volume control	Viasys	Patient triggered	Flow cycled
Pressure-regulated volume control	Macquet, Viasys	Patient or machine-triggered	Time cycled
Adaptive Pressure Ventilation	Hamilton	Patient or machine-triggered	Time cycled
Volume control-plus	Puritan Bennet	Patient or machine-triggered	Time cycled
Autoflow	Drager	Patient or machine-triggered	Time cycled
Automode	Macquet	A combination of: patient or machine triggered and patient-triggered	Time cycled, flow cycled

matched to the patient's demands and the patient is allowed to overbreathe the set frequency (Fig. 4.25).

The advantage of the PRVC mode is that it minimizes PIPs, while at the same time assuring a constant tidal volume (and therefore a guaranteed minute volume). It therefore has a potential role in those patients whose management is constrained by high airway pressures; those with fluctuating lung

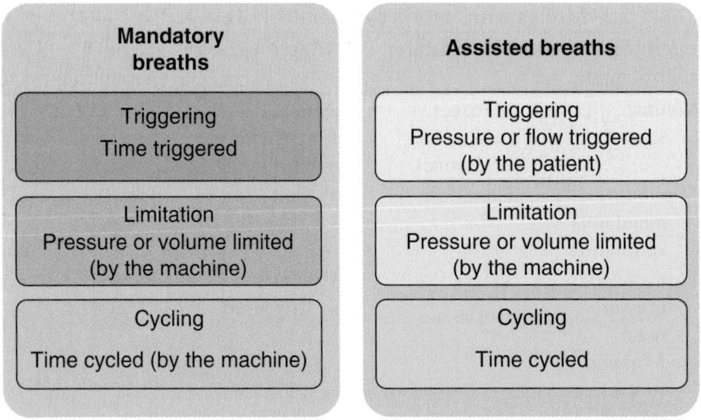
Mandatory breaths
Triggering
Time triggered
Limitation
Pressure or volume limited (by the machine)
Cycling
Time cycled (by the machine)
Assisted breaths
Triggering
Pressure or flow triggered (by the patient)
Limitation
Pressure or volume limited (by the machine)
Cycling
Time cycled

FIGURE 4.25. Variables with the pressure-regulated volume control mode.

mechanics; and those patients requiring high inspiratory flows, variable inspiratory flows, or both.

Disadvantages include variable airway pressures, decrease in the support offered by the ventilator when respiratory rates are high, and air trapping.

4.9.4 Automode

The Macquet Servo 300A incorporates the automode, which allows the patient to switch between a support mode and a control mode. In the absence of triggering – defined in adults by a 12-s apnea – the machine functions in a control mode. When the patient begins to make satisfactory inspiratory efforts – as evinced by two consecutive triggered breaths – the ventilator switches to the support mode. Both control and support settings must individually be programed. A switching of modes is indicated by a blinking light (Fig. 4.26).

Sometimes, auto-triggering is perceived by the ventilator as patient-triggering: the ventilator may respond by switching to the corresponding support mode.

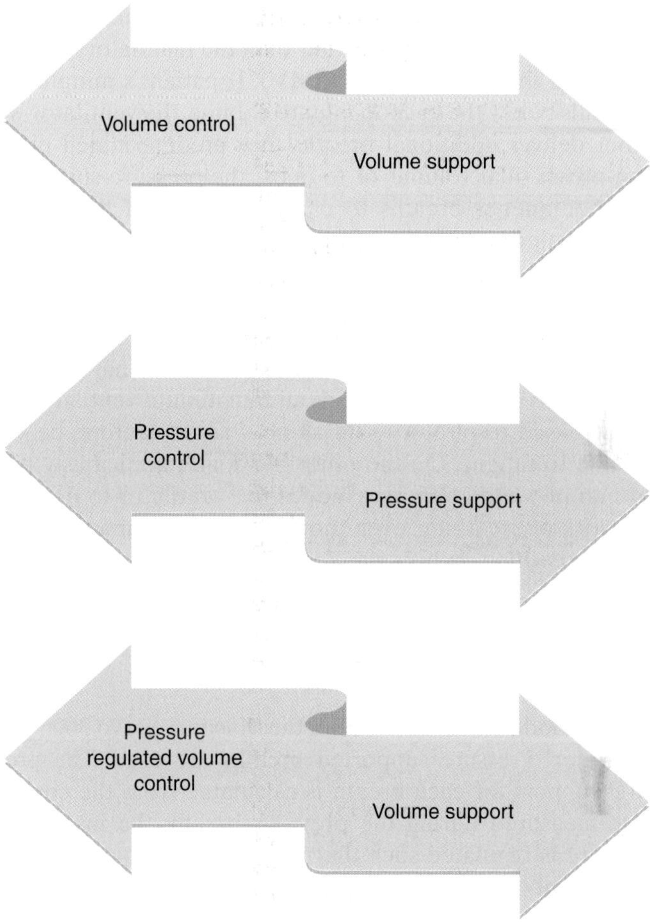
Volume control
Volume support
Pressure
control
Pressure support
Pressure
regulated volume
control
Volume support

FIGURE 4.26. Automode control modes and their corresponding support modes.

4.9.5 *Mandatory Minute Ventilation (MMV)*

Officially, it is the first mode with servo feedback. In a spontaneously breathing patient, backup minute ventilation is set in the SIMV or PSV mode. As long as the patient's minute ventilation exceeds this level, the ventilator makes no extra contribution to the airflow, other than the mandatory breaths (provided the mode used is SIMV). If patient's minute volume falls below the backup minute volume, the ventilator will either deliver additional breaths at a predetermined physician-preset tidal volume, or to boost the pressure-support of the spontaneous breaths to enable delivery of the backup minute volume, depending upon physician preference.

Although much less frequently used today, the MMV mode can be useful in weaning, or in the ventilation of patients with unpredictable respiratory drives.

The most palpable drawback of this mode is that a tachypneic patient can make up the minimum minute ventilation by an increased respiratory rate alone – and therefore, be vulnerable to fatigue. On the other hand, an injudiciously high set minute ventilation may induce the ventilator to do all of the work of breathing, even though the patient may be capable of breathing on his own.

4.9.6 Volume Support (VS)

The VS mode is available within the Macquet Servo 300/300A ventilator. Pressure supported breaths are used. The pressure–support for each breath is calculated from the compliance measured during the previous breath; the inspiratory pressure is regulated such that the set tidal volume is delivered. Tidal volumes are guaranteed. This is, therefore, an example of volume-targeted ventilation within the pressure support mode.

The classic indication for VS is the postoperative patient who is recovering from anesthesia. As the recovering patient makes increasing respiratory efforts, the ventilator gradually backs off on its pressure support: the set tidal volume will be preserved even though the participation of the ventilator is progressively decreasing. The opposite happens if the patient's inpiratory demand decreases; if required, the ventilator can boost up the tidal volume to up to 150% of that which has been set.[36]

The volume support plus (VSP) mode is available in the Puritan Bennet 840 ventilator.

4.9.7 *Adaptive Support Ventilation*[10] *(ASV)*

(*Syn* Adaptive Lung Ventilation)

Considered one of the most sophisticated modes of ventilation in use today, the ASV mode is based on the rationale that optimal breathing patterns depend upon prevailing respiratory system mechanics. With low respiratory system compliance, work of breathing can be minimized by a rapid shallow pattern of breathing, and this is indeed the pattern adopted by patients with stiff lungs. On the other hand, when airflow limitation is present, it is a slower, relatively deep pattern of breathing that results in the least work of breathing [37]: patients with COPD breathe this way. The machine plots respiratory frequency against tidal volume – the curve that is generated represents the minute ventilation. Against the measured respiratory system mechanics, optimal tidal volumes in relation to the respiratory rate are delivered to make up the clinician-preset minute volume.

The clinician keys in the ideal body weight, on the basis of which the ventilator calculates the approximate dead space. Two predetermined settings – pediatric and adult – are configured into the ASV mode. Within the adult setting, a clinician-set minute ventilation of 100% delivers 100 mL/min – this can be adjusted upward or downward (a clinician-preset minute volume of, for instance, 150% will deliver 150 mL/min). At a 100% setting, the pediatric mode correspondingly delivers a minute volume of 20 mL/min, which again can be altered by keying in the desired percent change in minute ventilation.

Initial test breaths measure system compliance and resistance, and check for any prevailing auto-PEEP that might be present. The ventilator then selects appropriate parameters (frequency, upper airway pressure limit, I:E ratio, inspiratory time) for both the mandatory and spontaneous breaths (Fig. 4.27).

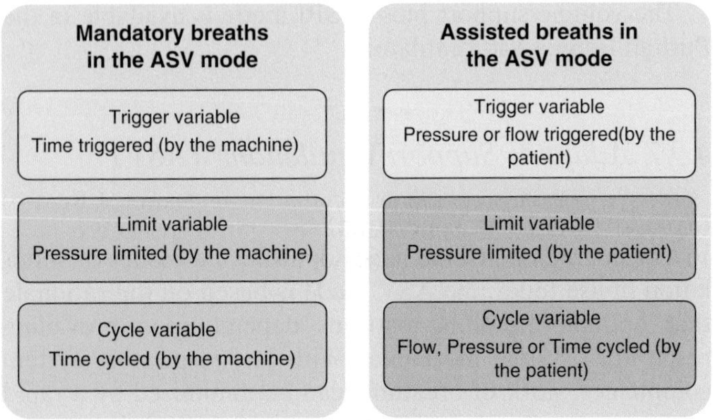
Mandatory breaths in the ASV mode
Trigger variable
Time triggered (by the machine)
Limit variable
Pressure limited (by the machine)
Cycle variable
Time cycled (by the machine)
Assisted breaths in the ASV mode
Trigger variable
Pressure or flow triggered(by the patient)
Limit variable
Pressure limited (by the patient)
Cycle variable
Flow, Pressure or Time cycled (by the patient)

FIGURE 4.27. Adaptive support ventilation.

In the absence of spontaneous triggering, the ventilator delivers machine-triggered time-cycled mandatory breaths. When inspiratory effort is present, patient-triggered flow-cycled breaths are delivered: as just pointed out, the machine boosts spontaneous tidal volumes – by an algorithm which takes into account alveolar volume and dead space – and the number of mandatory breaths is then proportionately decreased.

References

1. Amato MB, Barbas CS, Bonassa J, et al Volume-assured pressure support ventilation (VAPSV): a new approach for reducing muscle workload during acute respiratory failure. *Chest*. 1992;102:1225–1234
2. Ambrosino N, Rossi A. Proportional assist ventilation (PAV): a significant advance or a futile struggle between logic and practice? *Thorax*. 2002;57:272–276
3. Branson R, MacIntyre NR. Dual-control modes of mechanical ventilation. *Respir Care*. 1996;41:294–305
4. Branson RD, Johannigman JA, Campbell RS, et al Closed-loop mechanical ventilation. *Respir Care*. 2002;47:427–453
5. Branson RD, Johannigman JA. What is the evidence base for the newer ventilation modes? *Respir Care*. 2004;49:742–760
6. Brochard L, Harf A, Lorino H, et al Inspiratory pressure support prevents diaphragmatic fatigue during weaning from mechanical ventilation. *Am Rev Respir Dis*. 1989;139:513

7. Brochard L, Rua F, Lorino H, et al Inspiratory pressure support compensates for the additional work of breathing caused by the endotracheal tube. *Anesthesiology*. 1991;75:739
8. Brochard L. Intrinsic (or auto-) positive end-expiratory pressure during spontaneous or assisted ventilation. *Intensive Care Med.* 2002;28:1552–1554
9. Brochard L. Pressure support ventilation. In: Marini JJ, Roussos C, eds. *Ventilatory Failure*. Berlin: Springer; 1991:381–391
10. Brunner JX, Iotti GA. Adaptive support ventilation (ASV). *Minerva Anesthesiol*. 2002;68:365–368
11. Chang DW.Clinical applications of mechanical ventilation3rd Edition, Delmar learning. 2006
12. Chatburn RL. Classification of Mechanical Ventilators. *Respir Care*. 1992;37(9):1009–1025
13. Christopher KL, Neff TA, Bowman JL, et al Intermittent mandatory ventilation systems. *Chest*. 1985;87:625
14. Culpepper JA, Rinaldo JE, Rogers RM. Effects of mechanical ventilator mode on tendency towards respiratory alkalosis. *Am Rev Respir Dis*. 1985;132:1075
15. Davis KJ, Barnson RD, Campbell RS, Porembka DT. Comparison of volume control and pressure control and pressure control ventilation: is flow waveform the difference? *J Trauma*. 1996;41:808–814
16. Desautels DA. Ventilator performance. In: Kirby RR, Smith RA, Desautels DA, editors. Mechanical ventilation. New York: Churchill Livingstone, 1985: 120
17. Dojat M, Brochard L, Lemaire F, et al A knowledge-based system for assisted ventilation of patients in intensive care units. *Int J Clin Monit Comput*. 1992;9:239–250
18. Downs JB, Perkins HM, Model JH. Intermittent mandatory ventilation: an evaluation. *Arch Surg*. 1974;109:519–523
19. Esteban A, Anzueto A, Alia I, et al How is mechanical ventilation employed in the intensive care unit? An international utilization review. *Am J Respir Crit Care Med*. 2000;161: 1450–1458
20. Fabry B, Guttman J, Eberhard L, et al An analysis of desynchronization between the spontaneously breathing patient and ventilator during inspiratory pressure support. *Chest*. 1995;107:1387
21. Fairley HB. Critique of intermittent mandatory ventilation. *Int Anesthesiol Clin*. 1980;18:179–189
22. Fiastro JF, Habib MP, Quan SF. Pressure support compensation for inspiratory work due to endotracheal tubes and demand continuous positive airway pressure. *Chest*. 1988;93:499–505
23. Giuliani R, Mascia L, Recchia F, et al Patient-ventilator interaction during synchronized intermittent mandatory ventilation. *Am J Respir Crit Care Med*. 1995;151:1

24. Groeger JS, Levinson MR, Carlon GC. Assist control versus synchronized intermittent mandatory ventilation during acute respiratory failure. *Crit Care Med*. 1989;17:607–612
25. Hickling KG, Henderson SJ, Jackson R. Low mortality associated with low volume pressure limited ventilation with permissive hypercapnia in severe adult respiratory distress syndrome. *Intensive Care Med*. 1990;16:372
26. Hubmayr RD, Abel MD, Rehder K. Physiologic approach to mechanical ventilation. *Crit Care Med*. 1990;18:103–113
27. Hudson LD, Hurlow RS, Craig KC, et al Does intermittent mandatory ventilation correct respiratory alkalosis in patients receiving assisted mechanical ventilation? *Am Rev Respir Dis*. 1985;132:1071
28. Jaber S, Delay J-M, Matecki S, et al *Volume-guaranteed pressure-support*. 2005;31:1181–1188
29. Jubran A, Van de Graaf WB, Tobin MJ. Variability of patient-ventilator interaction with pressure support ventilation in patients with chronic obstructive pulmonary disease. *Am J Respir Crit Care Med*. 1995;152:129
30. Kondili E, Prinianakis G, Anastasaki M, Georgopoulos D. Acute effects of ventilator settings on respiratory motor output in patients with acute lung injury. *Intensive Care Med*. 2001;27:1147–1157
31. Lofaso F, Isabey D, Lorino H, et al Respiratory response to positive and negative inspiratory pressure in humans. *Respir Physiol*. 1992;89:75–88
32. MacIntyre, N, Branson RD. Feedback enhancement of ventilator breaths. In Principles and Pratice of mechanical ventilation (Ed: Tobin, MJ) McGraw-Hill, 2006
33. Marini JJ, Rodriguez RM, Lamb V. The inspiratory workload of patient-initiated mechanical ventilation. *Am Rev Respir Dis*. 1986;134:902–909
34. Marini JJ, Smith TC, Lamb VT. External work output and force generation during synchronized intermittent mechanical ventilation: Effect of machine assistance on breathing effort. *Am Rev Respir Dis*. 1988;138:1169–1179
35. Mushin WW, Rendell-Baker L, Thompson PW, Mapelson WW. *Automatic Ventilation of the Lungs*. 3rd ed. Oxford: Blackwell Scientific; 1980:62–131
36. Oakes DF, Shortall SP, eds. *Ventilator Management: A Bedside Reference Guide*. 2nd ed. Orono: Health Educator Publications; 2005
37. Otis AB, Fenn WO, Rahn H. Mechanics of breathing in man. *J Appl Physiol*. 1950;2:592–607

38. Petrof BJ, Legare M, Goldberg P, et al Continuous positive airway pressure reduces work of breathing and dyspnea during weaning from mechanical ventilation in severe chronic obstructive pulmonary disease. *Am Rev Respir Dis*. 1990;141:281–289
39. Petty TL. In defense of IMV. *Respir Care*. 1976;21:121–122
40. Petty TL. Intermittent mandatory ventilation-Reconsidered. *Crit Care Med*. 1981;9:620–621
41. Pinsky MR.The effect of mechanical ventilation on the cardiovascular system. Crit Care Clin 1990;6:663–78
42. Prinianakis G, Kondili E, Georgopoulos D. Effects of the flow waveform method of triggering and cycling on patient ventilator interaction during pressure support. *Intensive Care Med*. 2003;29:1950–1959
43. Richard JC, Carlucci A, Breton L, et al Bench testing of pressure support ventilation with three different generations of ventilators. *Intensive Care Med*. 2002;28:1049–1057
44. Rossi A, Polese G, Brandi G. Dynamic hyperinflation. In: Marini JJ, Roussos C, eds. *Ventilatory Failure*. Berlin: Springer; 199:218–1991
45. Sanborn WG. Microprocessor-based mechanical ventilation. *Respir Care*. 1993;38:72–109
46. Sassoon CS, Zhu E, Caiozzo VJ. Assist-control mechanical ventilation attenuates ventilator-induced diaphragmatic dysfunction. *Am J Respir Crit Care Med*. 2004;170:626–632
47. Sassoon CSH, Del Rosario N, Fei R, et al Influence of pressure- and flow-triggered synchronous intermittent mandatory ventilation on inspiratory muscle work. *Crit Care Med*. 1994;22:1933
48. Shapiro M, Wilson RK, Casar G, et al Work of breathing through different sized endotracheal tubes. *Crit Care Med*. 1986;14:1028–1031
49. Sinderby C, Navalesi P, Beck J, et al Neural control of mechanical ventilation in respiratory failure. *Nat Med*. 1999;5:1433–1436
50. Slutsky AS. Mechanical ventilation. American College of Chest Physicians' Consensus Conference. *Chest*. 1993;104:1833
51. Straus C, Louis B, Isabey D, et al Contribution of the endotracheal tube and the upper airway to breathing workload. *Am J Respir Crit Care Med*. 1998;157:23–30
52. Varpula T, Valta P, Niemi R, et al Airway pressure release ventilation as a primary ventilatory mode in acute respiratory distress syndrome. *Acta Anaesthesiol Scand*. 2004;48:722–731
53. Vitacca M. New things are not always better: proportional assist ventilation vs. pressure support ventilation. *Intensive Care Med*. 2003;29:1038–1040

Chapter 5
Ventilator Settings

5.1 Setting the Tidal Volume

Tidal volume is the volume of air moved in and out of the lungs with each breath. Tidal volumes are calculated from the height of the patient. Since in the ICU scenario height can be difficult to measure, ideal body weight is taken as its surrogate (see Fig. 5.1).

5.1.1 Volume-Targeted Ventilation

In volume-targeted ventilation, tidal volumes are physician-preset. Ventilated individuals with normal lungs prefer 2 or 3 times the normal tidal volumes. Therefore, during mechanical ventilation, the tidal volumes traditionally considered appropriate for adults were in the range of 10–15 mL/kg body

Predicted body weight (PBW) in males	Predicted body weight (PBW) in females
• PBW (kg) = 50 + 2.3 (Ht in inches -60)	• PBW (kg) = 45.5 + 2.3 (Ht in inches -60)
• PBW (kg) = 50 + 2.3 [(Ht in cm - 152) /2.54]	• PBW (kg) = 45.5 + 2.3 [(Ht in cm - 152) / 2.54]

FIGURE 5.1. Predicted body weight.

A. Hasan, *Understanding Mechanical Ventilation*,
DOI: 10.1007/978-1-84882-869-8_5,

weight, until it was realized that patients with lung injury do poorly with of even as little as 10 mL/kg per breath. Although there is still debate about what constitute safe tidal volumes in persons with *normal* lungs, it is generally considered unnecessary to exceed 10 mL/kg ideal body weight in these individuals.

It is important that tidal volumes be tailored to the prevailing lung mechanics. For instance, the delivery of high tidal volumes into stiff lungs can increase airway pressures and lead to overdistension. Tidal volumes also require to be curtailed in states of high airway resistance, but for different reasons. When the airways are narrowed, longer inflation and deflation times are required. When tidal volumes are relatively large, there may be insufficient time for the lung to empty and air trapping can result. Intrathoracic pressures will then rise, sometimes to unacceptable levels (see Chap. …).

The tidal volume and respiratory frequency together constitute minute ventilation. $PaCO_2$ can be lowered–by decreasing the minute ventilation–either by decreasing the tidal volume or the respiratory rate. As just mentioned, the size of the tidal volumes is decided upon by factoring in the patient's height (ideal body weight) and lung mechanics, so it is the respiratory rate that is generally manipulated to achieve the desired change in minute ventilation – unless other issues (such as a low pulmonary compliance or high airway resistance) are operative. When this is the case, the required minute volume is made up by a judicious mix of respiratory rate and tidal volume to achieve a balance to optimize gas exchange on the one hand, and pulmonary mechanics and hemodynamics on the other.

5.1.2 Pressure-Targeted Ventilation

In pressure-targeted ventilation, the tidal volumes are influenced by the preset pressure levels. Thus, any factor (such as a change in compliance or resistance of the respiratory system) that causes the targeted airway pressures to be reached at an earlier point of time will decrease the tidal volumes.

5.2 Setting the Respiratory Rate

In the control modes of ventilation (e.g., assist-control mode and pressure control mode) as also in the intermittent mandatory ventilation mode, a minimum backup respiratory rate is set. The patient is allowed to breathe above this rate if he or she chooses.

In the PSV mode, the patient is allowed to choose his or her own respiratory rate and control the inspiratory flow as well as the volume of the tidal breath.

The size of the tidal volumes has a direct bearing on respiratory rate. If the tidal volume is increased, the respiratory rate must necessarily fall for the minute volume to remain the same, and vice versa. Factors that determine $PaCO_2$ (such as the body's metabolic rate and dead-space ventilation), by directly influencing the required minute volume, can impact upon the respiratory rate. Hypoxia is also a potent stimulus of the respiratory drive. With complex inputs from the CNS, lung parenchyma, muscles of respiration, and the chest wall, all these factors influence the respiratory frequency.

Most adults who are in a relatively stable clinical state require 8–12 mandatory breaths/min. Patients with hypoxemic respiratory failure frequently require twice this or more. In restrictive lung disease the lung capacity is small, and much smaller tidal volumes can be accommodated within the lungs. In such cases a higher respiratory rate is necessary to compensate for the low tidal volumes in order to achieve the target minute ventilation: a respiratory rate in excess of 20 breaths/min is frequently required to fulfill the minute volume requirements of restricted patients.

Each respiratory cycle consists of an inspiration followed by expiration. Sometimes, a pause is added just after inspiration to hold the lungs open for a little longer and to, thus, improve oxygenation. When a pause is used, it is considered as a part of the inspiratory time.

A high respiratory rate will shorten the respiratory cycle as a whole. Both inspiratory and expiratory times then decrease. If the inspiratory time is short, diseased alveoli will fail to fill properly (see discussion under Sect. 5.5, below). Also, importantly, if the expiratory time is too short, the inspired gas may not be exhaled within this time leading to air trapping within the lung.

5.3 Setting the Flow Rate

The peak inspiratory flow rate, as set by the physician during volume-targeted ventilation, is an important determinant of patient comfort. The inspiratory flow rate should be set to match the patient's inspiratory demands. When the patient's inspiratory flow demands are in excess of the set inspiratory flow rate, patient-ventilator asynchrony is likely to result.

Generally, the inspiratory flow rate needs to be set in the range of 40–100 L/min. Lower inspiratory flows are sometimes deliberately set, in order to increase the inspiratory time (see Fig. 5.2).

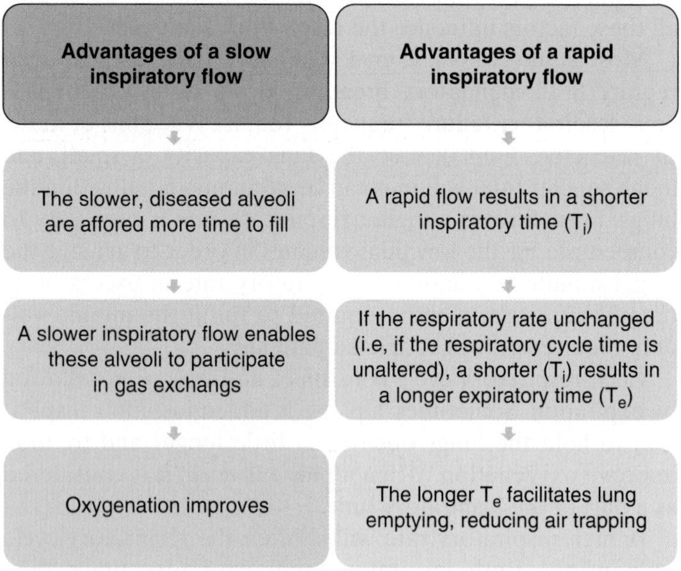
Advantages of a slow inspiratory flow
The slower, diseased alveoli are afforded more time to fill
A slower inspiratory flow enables these alveoli to participate in gas exchangs
Oxygenation improves
Advantages of a rapid inspiratory flow
A rapid flow results in a shorter inspiratory time (T_i)
If the respiratory rate unchanged (i.e, if the respiratory cycle time is unaltered), a shorter (T_i) results in a longer expiratory time (T_e)
The longer T_e facilitates lung emptying, reducing air trapping

FIGURE 5.2. The physiological advantages of different inspiratory flow rates.

Diseased alveoli have longer time constants. This means that they take longer to fill and to empty. If the inspiratory time is too short, these alveoli, may not fill properly in the time available. A slow inspiratory flow rate results in a longer inspiratory time. The longer inspiratory time enables the slower alveoli to cope.

When airway resistance is high such as in bronchospasm, the expiratory time is at a premium and the lungs may not be able to empty completely during expiration. Air trapping increases the risk of barotrauma and hypotension. In such cases, increasing the inspiratory flow rate will enable the set tidal volume to be delivered to the lungs more rapidly, thereby abbreviating the inspiratory time. Within a given respiratory cycle time, the shortened inspiratory time will make available a longer time for expiration; this will facilitate lung emptying.

On the other hand, increasing the inspiratory flow rate will also increase the peak airway pressure. A higher peak airway pressure can increase the risk for barotrauma. Care should be taken to see that the peak airway pressure does not exceed about 30–35 cm H_2O. However, higher inspiratory flows by faster emptying the lungs will decrease the *pause* pressures. Since mean airway pressure (MAP) is probably more important in the genesis of barotrauma than the peak airway pressure, the risk of barotrauma may actually decrease (despite a modest elevation in the peak airway pressure) when the flow rate is increased (Fig. 5.3).

When ventilation is pressure targeted, the cumulative result of the interaction of several factors determines inspiratory flow; for example, the set pressure, airway resistance, and patient effort.

5.4 Setting the Ratio of Inspiration to Expiration (I:E Ratio)

The normal ratio of the inspiratory time to the expiratory time (I:E ratio) is 1:1.5–1:2; that is, the expiratory time is almost twice as long as inspiratory time. The I:E ratio can be manipulated in

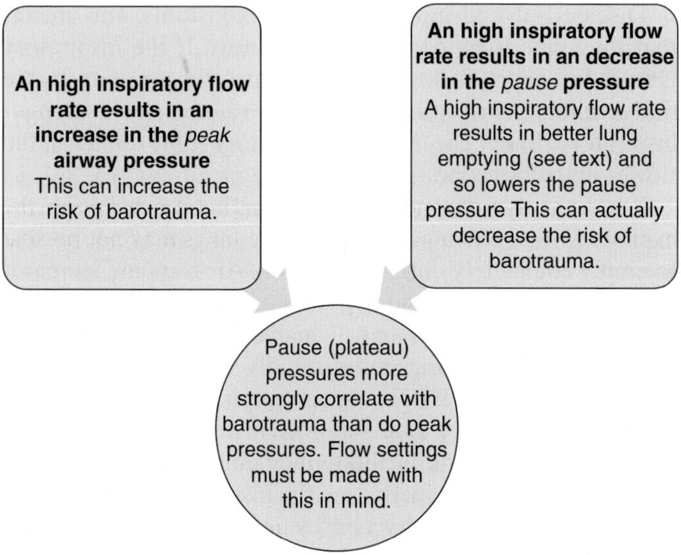
An high inspiratory flow rate results in an increase in the peak airway pressure
This can increase the risk of barotrauma.
An high inspiratory flow rate results in an decrease in the pause pressure
A high inspiratory flow rate results in better lung emptying (see text) and so lowers the pause pressure This can actually decrease the risk of barotrauma.
Pause (plateau) pressures more strongly correlate with barotrauma than do peak pressures. Flow settings must be made with this in mind.

FIGURE 5.3. Physiological effects of high inspiratory flow rates.

ventilated patients to serve specific goals. A shorter inspiratory time encourages lung emptying and a longer inspiratory time improves oxygenation. Thus, adjustments in I:E ratios are goal oriented. Patients with high inspiratory demands demonstrate greater comfort levels with high inspiratory flows; high inspiratory flows translate into shorter inspiratory times.

As mentioned above, longer inspiratory times are sometimes used with the intention of improving oxygenation. When the inspiratory time is lengthened so that it is at least as long as the expiratory time (an I:E ratio of 1:1), the physiological I:E ratio is said to have become inverted.

Inverse ratio ventilation (IRV) appears to increase oxygenation principally by increasing the MAP. Recall that MAP is the area under the pressure-time scalar(see section 4.4) – MAP will rise if inspiratory time is prolonged. IRV appears to improve V/Q matching, decrease shunting, and reduce dead-space – presumably by recruiting collapsed alveoli – but that this is the mechanism by which IRV improves oxygenation is by no means clear. Whether these benefits accrue from the prolonged inspiratory time used, or are a consequence of the increased end-expiratory alveolar pressure, is also uncertain. Indeed, similar benefits have been achieved without IRV by the application of an equivalent level of positive end-expiratory pressure (PEEP) alone.

When inverse ratios (e.g., I:E ratios of 1:1, 2:1, 3:1, and so forth) are used, the pattern of breathing is in discordance with the physiological respiratory pattern, and can be extremely uncomfortable for the patient. Patients will generally need deep sedation or pharmacological paralysis.

By shortening the expiratory time, IRV is likely to result in air trapping, especially when the patient is being ventilated with high minute volumes: a raised intrathoracic pressure can lead to barotrauma. In fact, however, IRV is seen to be better tolerated hemodynamically than one would expect (Fig. 5.4).

In pressure-controlled ventilation (see section 4.8 modes), the inspiratory time is one of the determinants of the tidal volume. The area under the inspiratory flow-time scalar represents the inspiratory tidal volume (Fig. 5.4 Chap. Waveforms). As a result of a relatively short inspiratory time (panel A Fig. 5.4), flow is seen to cease at a point well above the baseline. As the preset inspiratory time is lengthened, flow is seen to extend all the way up the baseline (panel B Fig. 5.4), increasing tidal volume (the area under the curve). Further increasing

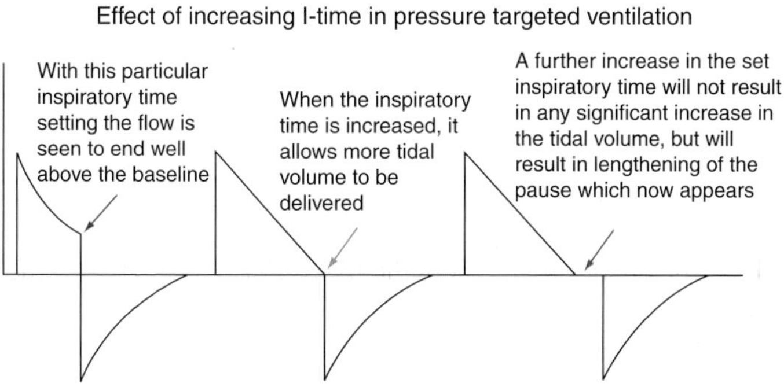
Effect of increasing I-time in pressure targeted ventilation
With this particular inspiratory time setting the flow is seen to end well above the baseline
When the inspiratory time is increased, it allows more tidal volume to be delivered
A further increase in the set inspiratory time will not result in any significant increase in the tidal volume, but will result in lengthening of the pause which now appears

FIGURE 5.4. Effect of prolonging inspiratory time in pressure control ventilation.

the inspiratory time beyond this point will have a trivial effect on the tidal volume: with increasing inspiratory time, a pause will be seen to appear and lengthen (Panel C Fig. 5.4).

5.5 Setting the Flow Profile

Flow is defined as volume per unit time. For a given tidal volume and I:E ratio, the inspiratory flow can be profiled differently to realize different clinical goals.

5.5.1 The Square Waveform

When the inspiratory flow is constant and unvarying through the delivery of the entire tidal volume, the flow pattern is referred to as a square wave pattern (syn, rectilinear waveform). In the rectilinear wave pattern, the inspiratory flow rises rapidly to the preset peak inspiratory flow level and then remains constant until the preset tidal volume has been delivered; at this point, inspiration abruptly ceases (Fig. 5.5).

Because of its similarity to that distinctive British headgear, the square wave flow pattern has also been described as the top-hat waveform. Although this waveform should theoretically ensure a constant flow throughout inspiration, the inspiratory flow rate often tends to decline somewhat toward the end, owing to the increasing impedance offered by the distending lungs.

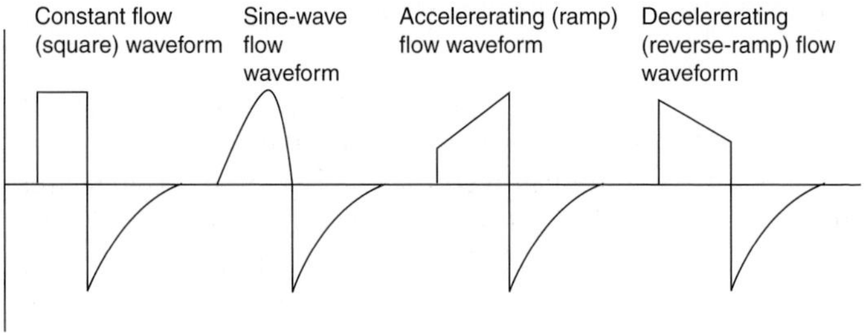
Constant flow (square) waveform
Sine-wave flow waveform
Accelererating (ramp) flow waveform
Decelererating (reverse-ramp) flow waveform

FIGURE 5.5. Types of flow waveforms.

5.5.2 *The Decelerating Waveform*

In the decelerating pattern of flow (also called the reverse-ramp pattern), the inspiratory flow rate exponentially decreases with time (Fig. 5.5). This flow pattern has the advantage of reducing the steep rise in airway pressures that occur as the lung is progressively inflated during a tidal breath.

5.5.3 *The Accelerating Waveform*

In the accelerating flow waveform ("the ramp"), there is a progressive increase in the rate of airflow with time. At a predetermined pressure limit, the airflow plateaus to a rectilinear pattern, and constancy in the flow rate is maintained till the end of inspiration.

5.5.4 *The Sine Waveform*

In the sine waveform, the inspiratory flow increases smoothly to a peak, and then decreases again toward the culmination of the tidal breath (Fig 5.5).

Only volume-targeted modes of ventilation offer a choice in terms of flow wave patterns. In pressure-targeted ventilation, to maintain the constancy of pressure, the inspiratory waveform is necessarily decelerating.

5.6 Setting the Trigger Sensitivity

Trigger sensitivity is the negative airway pressure that the patient must generate before ventilator delivers a tidal breath. Contemporary ventilator technology uses either flow or pressure transducers within its circuitry to detect patient effort.

Setting the trigger sensitivity is essentially determining how much of a negative change must occur in flow or pressure within the circuit before the ventilator delivers a tidal breath. The ventilator senses any significant flow or pressure change within the circuit as the patient attempts to inhale and thereupon promptly delivers a breath. The purpose of trigger sensitivity is to coordinate the delivery of the inspiratory breath with patient's own inspiratory effort.

Ideally, the trigger sensitivity should be low so that minimal energy is spent by the patient in triggering the ventilator, but not so low as to cause spontaneous triggering of the ventilator by miniscule changes in airway conditions that are not in fact the patient's efforts at inspiration.

In the conventional *pressure* trigger systems, appropriate trigger sensitivity in most situations is –0.5 to –1.5 cm H_2O; the newer (and possibly more efficient) *flow* cycling systems should also be set to a maximum sensitivity.

5.7 Setting PEEP

The application of a small amount of PEEP has been considered physiological. It is generally thought that a PEEP level of 3–5 cm of H_2O reproduces the "back pressures" generated by a normal glottis in nonintubated subjects. This level of "physiological" PEEP can theoretically prevent the airway closure that might be anticipated in a situation where a functioning glottis is absent – as in the intubated patient. In actual fact, a low level of PEEP has not been shown to prevent postsurgical atelectasis in the setting of cardiac surgery.

The application of PEEP can serve several clinical ends (Fig. 5.6)

5.7.1 Improvement in Oxygenation

PEEP serves as a splint for unstable alveoli, preventing their collapse. By opening and holding open diseased alveoli, PEEP recruits these lung units into the population of alveoli participating in gas exchange, especially in lower lung zones, and as a result of this, oxygenation improves. Once all the potentially salvageable alveolar units are opened up, any further increase in PEEP beyond this point is likely to be deleterious.

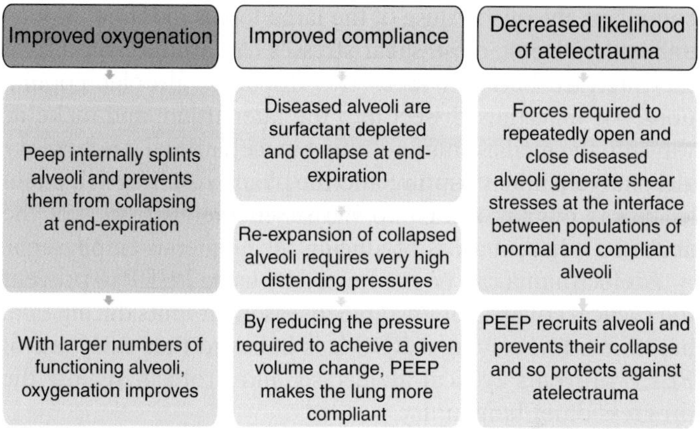
Improved oxygenation
Peep internally splints alveoli and prevents them from collapsing at end-expiration
With larger numbers of functioning alveoli, oxygenation improves
Improved compliance
Diseased alveoli are surfactant depleted and collapse at end-expiration
Re-expansion of collapsed alveoli requires very high distending pressures
By reducing the pressure required to acheive a given volume change, PEEP makes the lung more compliant
Decreased likelihood of atelectrauma
Forces required to repeatedly open and close diseased alveoli generate shear stresses at the interface between populations of normal and compliant alveoli
PEEP recruits alveoli and prevents their collapse and so protects against atelectrauma

FIGURE 5.6. Physiological effects of positive end-expiratory pressure (PEEP).

Recruitment of alveoli also increases the functional residual capacity of the lung. Normal alveoli do not close completely even at the very end of expiration. This is principally on account of their surfactant content (see section17.1). When alveoli are diseased, they are depleted of surfactant and become unstable. Unstable alveoli tend to collapse at the end of expiration when the lung volume is low and the distending pressure minimal. Reexpansion of collapsed alveoli requires a much greater distending pressure than the pressure required to inflate patent healthy alveoli. When a high pressure is required to bring about a given degree of lung inflation, it means that the compliance is low (compliance is change in pressure over change in volume) and the lung is stiff.

5.7.2 Protection Against Barotrauma and Lung Injury

PEEP protects against atelectrauma, a form of barotrauma. When diseased alveoli repeatedly open and close, shear stresses are generated at their interface with normal and compliant alveoli; because of the large forces required to open unhealthy alveoli, these shear stresses can produce rupture at the interface between these two disparate alveolar populations. Air may, thus, dissect into the interstitium and make its way into the mediastinum resulting in mediastinal emphysema; alternatively, it may rupture into the pleura resulting in a pneumothorax or may track into the subcutaneous tissues of the neck and adjacent areas producing subcutaneous emphysema.

Atelectrauma can be minimized by using PEEP to prevent the cyclical collapse of unstable diseased air units during tidal breathing. In evolving ARDS it is believed that early use of PEEP prevents cyclical atelectasis and protects against the progression of lung injury.

5.7.3 Overcoming Auto-PEEP

The benefits of PEEP have been proven in dynamic hyperinflation.

Airflow across a tube is dependent on the pressure gradient between its ends. Air will flow, from a region of higher pressure to the region of lower pressure. At end-expiration, normally, the pressure at the mouth should equate with alveolar pressure since a state of no-flow is present.

If, due to dynamic hyperinflation, auto-PEEP is present, the alveolar pressure at end-expiration will be higher than the pressure at the mouth. For air to flow toward the alveoli during inspiration, the pressure in the central airway would require to be higher than the alveolar pressure. Therefore, to create a pressure gradient for airflow during inspiration, the pressure in proximal airway would need to exceed auto-PEEP.

The spontaneously breathing subject would now have to generate a negative intrathoracic pressure in excess of the auto-PEEP for air to flow into the alveoli. The extra respiratory effort required to do this can severely challenge the patient with a poor respiratory reserve, and this can hasten the onset of respiratory failure.

Employing a small amount of external PEEP in this setting can help. The gradient now would be reduced to the equivalent of the auto-PEEP minus the applied PEEP; the reduced gradient will considerably unload the respiratory muscles and reduce the work of breathing. It has been shown that an applied PEEP of at least 50% of the auto-PEEP is required to obtain clinical benefit. The magnitude of applied PEEP should therefore be two-thirds to three-fourths of the measured auto-PEEP. Excessive applied PEEP can actually increase air trapping and worsen dynamic hyperinflation. An applied PEEP that exceeds 85% of the auto-PEEP can be expected to increase intrathoracic pressure (with consequent adverse impact on circulation).

5.8 Indications for PEEP

PEEP is indicated for lung diseases like ARDS or cardiogenic pulmonary edema where the pattern of the lung injury is more or less uniform. In ARDS, PEEP increases the functional residual capacity by opening up closed alveoli. It also increases ventilation in those poorly ventilated areas which have an intact perfusion, thereby decreasing the shunt fraction. It thereby enables lower levels of FIO_2 to be given, thereby minimizing the risk of O_2 toxicity.

5.9 Forms of PEEP

In the mid-1970s, the term "best PEEP" was used by Suter to describe the level of PEEP at which the O_2 content of arterial blood (CaO_2) was maximized; at this level of PEEP, it was shown that lung compliance had the highest value. The term "Optimal PEEP" was used by Kirby to describe the value of PEEP that achieved the greatest reduction in the shunt fraction without compromising cardiac output.

5.10 Titrating PEEP

The top and the bottom parts of the pressure–volume curve are flat. On these sections, for a given amount of applied pressure there is a relatively small change in volume. In other words, on these sections of the pressure–volume curve, the lung is stiff and noncompliant. The goal therefore is to apply enough PEEP to make the lung operate on the steep middle part of the pressure–volume curve where lung compliance is good and the mechanics favorable.

The region at which the upper steep portion of the pressure–volume curve merges into the top flat portion of the curve is called the (upper) deflection point. If the level of PEEP is set high enough for the system to operate on the upper flat portion of the pressure–volume curve, alveolar distention occurs and the lung is relatively noncompliant.

The bottom of the steep vertical section of the pressure–volume curve, where it merges with the flat lower part, is called the lower inflection point (P_{flex}); P_{flex} is thought to represent the point where alveolar recruitment occurs. Operating at a lower level of PEEP just above the P_{flex} intuitively seems safer than operating at a higher level on the steep portion. Although this strategy may be safer, alveolar overdistension is still possible especially in the upper zones of the lung. Thus, PEEP should be applied carefully, in graded increments and the compliance calculated after every change. When the compliance begins to improve rapidly after increasing the level of PEEP, it means that the P_{flex} or the inflection point has been passed and the lung is now operating on the steep part of the pressure–volume curve. With further increments in PEEP, compliance will again begin to fall. This means that the upper deflection point has been reached (Fig. 5.7).

With charting of the upper deflection and the lower inflection points, it is easier to set the desired level of PEEP between these two points (preferably closer to the inflection than to the deflection point) and this would be expected to assure the most compliant lung possible under the circumstances.

All the alveolar units in the lung do not behave in the same way, and in patients with ARDS, the P_{flex} may vary between different alveolar populations. At the bedside, pressure–volume curves can be constructed by inflating the chest of a pharmacologically paralyzed patient with a super syringe,

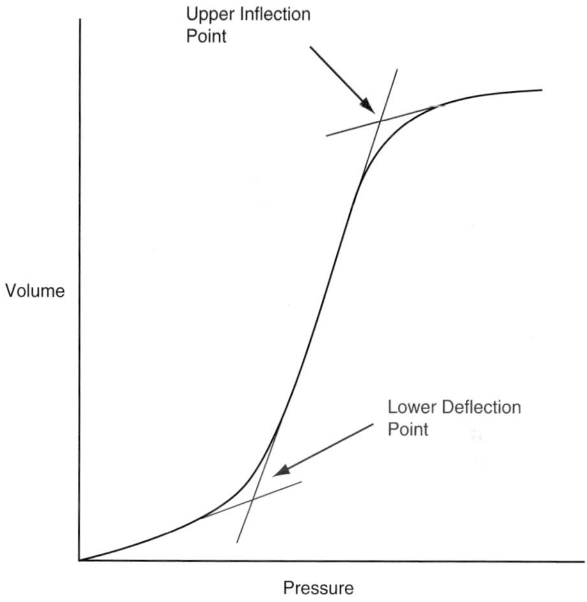
Upper Inflection
Point
Volume
Lower Deflection
Point
Pressure

FIGURE 5.7. Titration of PEEP.

though newer ventilators do offer more convenient ways of measurement (Fig. 5.8).

Lung compliance can be calculated by the formula:

$$V_t / P_{pl} - PEEP,$$

Estimates of lung compliance made this way are not very accurate. It also appears that there is a substantial element of interobserver variability in the determination of P_{flex} (this may be as much as 9–15 cm H_2O).

The mean alveolar pressure (which determines alveolar volume) is paralleled by the plateau pressure; plateau pressures of less than 30 cm H_2O are considered safe, though these should probably be kept down to less than 25 cm if possible.

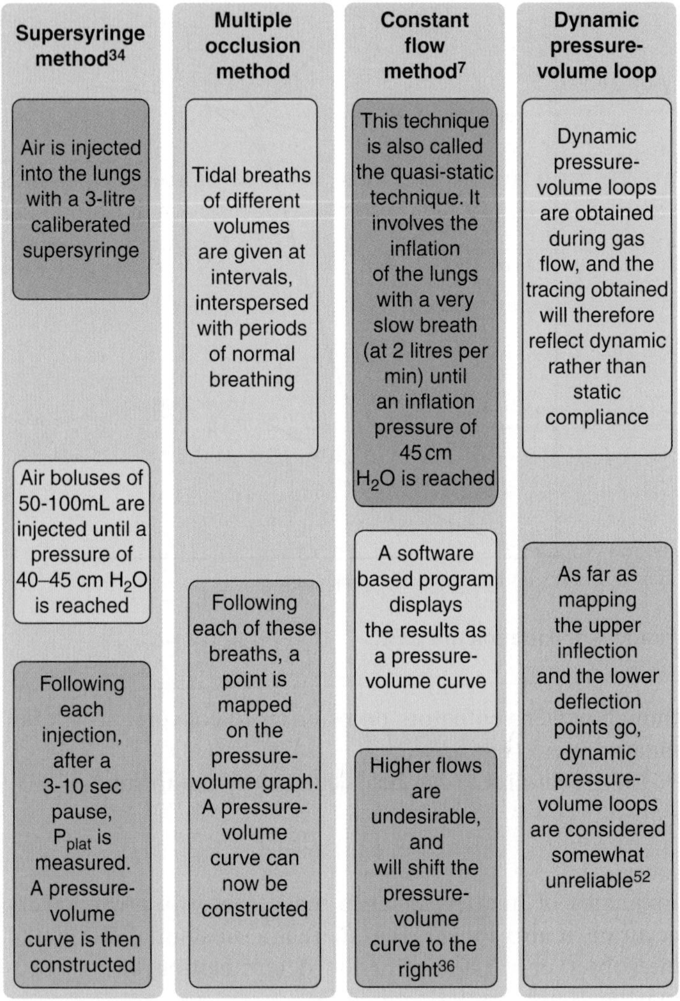

Supersyringe method[34]
Air is injected into the lungs with a 3-litre caliberated supersyringe
Air boluses of 50-100mL are injected until a pressure of 40–45 cm H_2O is reached
Following each injection, after a 3-10 sec pause, P_{plat} is measured. A pressure-volume curve is then constructed
Multiple occlusion method
Tidal breaths of different volumes are given at intervals, interspersed with periods of normal breathing
Following each of these breaths, a point is mapped on the pressure-volume graph. A pressure-volume curve can now be constructed
Constant flow method[7]
This technique is also called the quasi-static technique. It involves the inflation of the lungs with a very slow breath (at 2 litres per min) until an inflation pressure of 45 cm H_2O is reached
A software based program displays the results as a pressure-volume curve
Higher flows are undesirable, and will shift the pressure-volume curve to the right[36]
Dynamic pressure-volume loop
Dynamic pressure-volume loops are obtained during gas flow, and the tracing obtained will therefore reflect dynamic rather than static compliance
As far as mapping the upper inflection and the lower deflection points go, dynamic pressure-volume loops are considered somewhat unreliable[52]

FIGURE 5.8. Methods of charting the upper inflection and the lower deflection point.

5.10.1 Other Advantages of PEEP

There are other issues that need to be taken into consideration when deciding what level of PEEP will best serve the patient.

Patients with diffuse lung disease often have serious deficiencies in their capacity to oxygenate the blood. The high levels of supplementary oxygen that are used in an attempt to avert hypoxemia may in themselves be detrimental. If a fraction of inspired oxygen (FIO_2) of >0.6 is used for protracted periods, lung injury may be worsened. PEEP is made use of to improve the patient's oxygenation, and thus, to accomplish a reduction in FIO_2 to the lowest possible level – or at the very least, to avoid the administration of an FIO_2 of >0.6 for prolonged intervals of time.

5.10.2 Disadvantages of PEEP

PEEP itself is not without harmful effects. A level of PEEP that will near-saturate the hemoglobin may sometimes impair the circulation significantly. Thus, what is gained in terms of arterial oxygenation may be lost in terms of the decrease in cardiac output; the latter by itself can reduce O_2 delivery to the tissues.

5.11 Optimizing Ventilator Settings for Better Oxygenation

Hypoxemia can either result from a low alveolar tension of oxygen, or from the processes limiting the transport of O_2 from the air to the blood. The two fundamental approaches exist by which the alveolar tension of oxygen can be theoritically increased:

1. Increasing the fraction of inspired oxygen.
2. Increasing the alveolar ventilation (VA).

5.11.1 Increasing the FIO_2

Manipulation of the fraction of inspired oxygen (FIO_2) has the most direct effect on the arterial oxygen tension (PaO_2). The relationship between FIO_2 and PaO_2 is linear, and provided other mechanisms of hypoxemia (e.g., a raised shunt fraction) are not operative, the effect of increasing the fraction of inspired oxygen has a salutary effect on arterial oxygen tensions.

5.11.2 Increasing the Alveolar Ventilation

A smaller increase in PaO_2 can be achieved by increasing the VA. However, this method is not used for increasing PaO_2 for two reasons. First, the relationship between the VA and PaO_2 is curvilinear; progressively greater changes in VA achieve correspondingly lower changes in PaO_2. Second, changes in VA have a profound effect on CO_2, and so changes in VA designed primarily at influencing PaO_2 produce extremely large and unwanted changes in $PaCO_2$.

While administering high concentrations of O_2, the possibility of oxygen toxicity must always be kept in mind (see Chap. 9).

The other techniques directed at increasing PaO_2 are aimed at reversing the pathological processes involving gas exchange mechanisms at the alveolar level (see below).

5.12 PEEP

The various mechanisms that produce hypoxemia through mismatching of ventilation and perfusion have been dealt with in Chap. 6. Where there is low-V/Q mismatch – i.e., where ventilation is reduced relative to perfusion – strategies directed at opening (and holding open) closed alveoli can help in reducing the hypoxemia.

The techniques commonly used to this end are PEEP and continuous positive airway pressure (CPAP). When unstable alveolar units are kept from collapsing, this better exposes the capillary bed to the ventilated air, thereby improving the oxygenation.

5.12.1 Flow Waveforms

Oxygenation can also be improved by manipulating the "shape" of the inspired breath. When a high inspiratory flow rate is set, alveoli fill up rapidly. Although rapid inspiratory flows are generally more comfortable, diseased alveoli (which are slower to cycle) will not be ventilated adequately in the available time. A decelerating waveform, by providing a gradually slowing flow during lung inflation, may have some advantage in this respect.

5.12.2 *Inspiratory Time*

A prolonged inspiratory time has a similar splinting effect to that of PEEP. This stabilizing effect on alveoli lasts for the duration of inspiration, as long as the pressures in the airway are sustained. A long inspiratory time keeps such vulnerable alveoli open for a longer period than does a short inspiratory time. Within a given respiratory cycle time (inspiratory time + expiratory time), increasing the inspiratory time correspondingly shortens the expiratory time. A short expiratory time, as discussed earlier, will often results in incomplete emptying of the lungs, especially when the administered minute volume is relatively large: dynamic hyperinflation and intrinsic PEEP can result.

As long as the intrinsic PEEP level is not too high, it may actually have a favorable impact on oxygenation by acting in much the same manner as does applied PEEP. When high, intrinsic PEEP can have a detrimental effect upon the circulation.

5.12.3 *Inverse Ratio Ventilation*

IRV entails the employment of an inspiratory time that is at least as long as the expiratory time. Although the use of IRV appears rational in situations of severe hypoxemia, it has not yet been shown to improve outcomes or to reduce complications when compared to PEEP. The "inverted" pattern of breathing can be extremely uncomfortable for the patient, and may require considerable sedation and pharmacological paralysis.

5.12.4 Prone Ventilation

Prone ventilation, in which positional changes of the patient are used to an advantage in improving oxygenation, has been discussed in Chap. 8.

5.12.5 Reducing Oxygen Consumption

Oxygen demands can be very high in febrile or agitated patients, or when patient-ventilator asynchrony occurs. Judicious regulation of ventilatory parameters can reduce the asynchrony, but patients may on occasion require sedation or paralysis to ensure a smoother pattern of breathing so as to decrease oxygen consumption.

5.12.6 Increasing Oxygen Carrying Capacity

The delivery of oxygen to the tissues depends not merely on the saturation of hemoglobin by oxygen, but also upon the hemoglobin level of the blood itself and upon the cardiac output. These factors can be summarized in the equation:

$$DO_2 = \text{Hb} \times \text{Saturation of Hb with } O_2 \times \text{Cardiac output.}$$

In the equation above, dissolved O_2 which is not a major factor at atmospheric pressures has not been taken into consideration.

Since hemoglobin concentration and cardiac output are crucial to oxygen delivery to the tissues, a deficiency of either will seriously impair oxygen delivery, no matter how effective the other measures to improve PaO_2 may be. Efforts therefore must be as much directed toward correcting anemia or a poor cardiac output as in trying to improve blood oxygenation.

5.12.7 Footnote

Whenever ventilator settings are changed, it is useful to keep a couple of generalizations in mind. The effect of a change in settings designed to serve a specific purpose may influence a different ventilatory parameter. The change made may achieve its purpose in part or full: unfortunately, the degree of response of an individual patient to a specific manipulation can be difficult to predict.

Box 5.1 The Open Lung Concept

The pressures required to open collapsed alveoli can be considerable.

Lung involvement is almost always inhomogeneous. Healthy and compliant alveoli lie interspersed with diseased units. The high airway pressures required to ventilate a diseased lung may overdistend and injure these normal alveoli. When a large force is required to distend a lung (that is composed of a relatively large number of diseased units), it means that the lung is poorly compliant (higher pressures are required to achieve a given change in volume).

The application of PEEP (or CPAP) helps in splinting the alveoli, preventing their collapse during expiration. The restoration and maintenance of alveolar patency improve lung compliance. A pliant and yielding lung can now be easily inflated by smaller inflation pressures, leading to a decrease in work of breathing and a decline in the oxygen consumption.

The lower inflation pressures also diminish the risk of barotrauma by minimizing shear stresses at the interface between normal and diseased alveoli (see Chap. 10).

References

1. Abraham E, Yoshihara G. Cardiopulmonary effects of pressure controlled inverse ratio ventilation in severe respiratory failure. *Chest*. 1989;96:1356
2. Albert RK. Least PEEP: primum non-nocere. *Chest*. 1985;87:2
3. Albert RK, Hubmayr RD. The prone position eliminates compression of the lungs by the heart. *Am J Respir Crit Care Med*. 2000;161:1660
4. Al-Saady N, Bennett ED. Decelerating inspiratory flow wave-form improves lung mechanics and gas exchange in patients on intermittent positive pressure ventilation. *Inten Care Med*. 1985;11:68–75
5. Armstrong BW Jr, MacIntyre NR. Pressure-controlled, inverse ratio ventilation that avoids air trapping in the adult respiratory distress syndrome. *Crit Care Med*. 1995;23:279
6. Baker AB, Restall R, Clark BW. Effects of varying inspiratory flow waveform and time in intermittent positive pressure ventilation: emphysema. *Br J Anaesth*. 1982;54:547–554
7. Branson R. Understanding and implementing advances in ventilator capabilities. *Curr Opinion Crit Care*. 2004;10:23
8. Brochard L. Intrinsic (or auto-) positive end-expiratory pressure during spontaneous or assisted ventilation. *Intensive Care Med*. 2002;28:1552–1554
9. Brower R. Should inverse ratio ventilation be used in adult respiratory distress syndrome? *Am J Respir Crit Care Med*. 1994; 149:1354
10. Casetti AV, Bartlett RH, Hirschl RB. Increasing inspiratory time exacerbates ventilator-induced lung injury during high pressure/high-volume mechanical ventilation. *Crit Care Med*. 2002;30:2295–2299
11. Cereda M, Foti G, Musch G, et al Positive end-expiratory pressure prevents the loss of respiratory compliance during low tidal volume ventilation in acute lung injury patients. *Chest*. 1996;109:480
12. Chatte G, Sab J-M, Dubois J-M, et al Prone position in mechanically ventilated patients with severe acute respiratory failure. *Am J Respir Crit Care Med*. 1997;155:473
13. Consensus Conference on the Essentials of Mechanical Ventilation. *Respir Care* 37:999–1130 [special issue] 1992
14. Dambrosio M, Roupie E, Mollet JJ, et al Effects of positive end-expiratory pressure and different tidal volumes on alveolar recruitment and hyperinflation. *Anesthesiology*. 1997;87:495

15. Duncan SR, Rizk NW, Raffin TA. Inverse ratio ventilation: PEEP in disguise? *Chest*. 1987;92:39
16. Feihl F, Perret C. Premissive hypercapnia: how permissive should we be? *Am J Respir Crit Care Med*. 1994;150:1722–1737
17. Fellahi J-L, Valtier B, Bourdarias J-P, et al Does positive end-expiratory pressure ventilation improve left ventricular performance: a comparative study by transesophageal echocardiography in cardiac and noncardiac patients. *Chest*. 1998;114:556
18. Fernandez-Mondejar E, Vazquez-Mata G. PEEP: more than just support? *Inten Care Med*. 1998;24:1
19. Gattinoni L, Pesenti A, Bombino M, et al Relationships between lung computed tomographic density, gas exchange, and PEEP in acute respiratory failure. *Anesthesiology*. 1988;69:824–832
20. Gattinoni L, Pelosi P, Crotti S, et al Effects of positive end-expiratory pressure on regional distribution of tidal volume and recruitment in adult respiratory distress syndrome. *Am J Respir Crit Care Med*. 1995;151:1807
21. Gurevich MJ, Gelmont D. The importance of trigger sensitivity to ventilator response delay in advanced chronic obstructive pulmonary disease with respiratory failure. *Crit Care Med*. 1989;17:354
22. Gurevitch MJ, Van Dyke J, Young ES, et al Improved oxygenation and lower peak airway pressure in severe adult respiratory distress syndrome: treatment with inverse ratio ventilation. *Chest*. 1986;89:211
23. Hickling KG. Premissive hypercapnia. *Respir Care Clin North Am*. 2002;8:155–169
24. Hickling KG, Henderson SJ, Jackson R. Low mortality associated with low volume, pressure limited ventilation with permissive hypercapnia in severe adult respiratory distress syndrome. *Inten Care Med*. 1990;16:372–377
25. Huang CC, Shih MJ, Tsai YH, et al Effects of inverse ratio ventilation versus positive end-expiratory pressure on gas exchange and gastric intramucosal Paco2 and pH under constant mean airway pressure in acute respiratory distress syndrome. *Anesthesiology*. 2001;95(5):1182–1188
26. Hubmayr RD, Abel MD, Rehder K. Physiologic approach to mechanical ventilation. *Crit Care Med*. 1990;18:103–113
27. Kacmarek RM. Management of the patient-mechanical ventilator system. In: Pierson DJ, Kacmarek RM, eds. *Foundations of respiratory care*. New York: Churchill Livingstone; 1992:973–997
28. Kacmarek RM, Venegas J. Mechanical ventilatory rates and tidal volumes. *Respir Care*. 1978;32:466–478

29. Kirby RR, Downs JB, Civetta JM, et al High level positive end expiratory pressure in acute respiratory insufficiency. *Chest.* 1975;67:156
30. Lachmann B. Open the lung and keep it open. *Inten Care Med.* 1992;18:319
31. Laffey JG, O'Croinin D, McLoughlin P, Kavanagh BP. Permissive hypercapnia: role in protective lung ventilatory strategies. *Intensive Care Med.* 2004;30:347–356
32. Laghi F. Effect of inspiratory time and flow settings during assist- control ventilation. *Curr Opin Crit Care.* 2003;9:39–44
33. Lamm WJE, Graham MM, Albert RK. Mechanism by which the prone positioning improves oxygenation in acute lung injury. *Am J Respir Crit Care Med.* 1994;150:184
34. Lee WL, Stewart TE, MacDonald R, et al Safety of pressure-volume curve measurement in acute lung injury and ARDS using a syringe technique. *Chest.* 2002;121:1595
35. Levy P, Similowski T, Corbeil C, et al A method for studying the static volume-pressure curves of the respiratory system during mechanical ventilation. *J Crit Care.* 1989;4:83
36. Lu Q, Vieira SR, Richcouer J, et al A simple automated method for measuring pressure-volume curves during mechanical ventilation. *Am J Respir Crit Care Med.* 1999;159:275
37. Mancebo J. PEEP, ARDS and alveolar recruitment. *Intensive Care Med.* 1992;18:383
38. Manning HL. Peak airway pressure: why the fuss? *Chest.* 1994;105:242.
39. Manning HL, Molinary EJ, Leiter JC. Effect of inspiratory flow rate on respiratory sensation and pattern of breathing. *Am J Respir Crit Care Med.* 1995;151:751–757
40. Manthous CA, Schmidt GA. Inverse ratio ventilation in ARDS. Improved oxygenation without autoPEEP. *Chest.* 1993;103:953
41. Marcy TW, Marini JJ. Inverse ratio ventilation: Rationale and implementation. *Chest.* 1991;100:4494
42. Marini JJ. Should PEEP be used in airflow obstruction? *Am Rev Respir Dis.* 1989;140:141
43. Marini JJ. New approaches to the ventilatory management of the adult respiratory distress syndrome. *J Crit Care.* 1992;87:256–257
44. Marini JJ, Ravenscraft SA. Mean airway pressure: physiologic determinants and clinical importance – Part 2: clinical implications. *Crit Care Med.* 1992;20:1604–1616
45. Martinez M, Diaz E, Joseph D, et al Improvement in oxygenation by prone positioning and nitric oxide in patients with acute respiratory distress syndrome. *Intensive Care Med.* 1999;25:25

46. Mercat A, Graini L, Teboul J-L, et al Cardiorespiratory effects of pressure-controlled ventilation with and without inverse ratio in the adult respiratory distress syndrome. *Chest*. 1993; 104:871
47. Mercat A, Titiriga M, Anguel N, et al Inverse ratio ventilation (I/E – 2/1) in acute respiratory distress syndrome. *Am J Respir Crit Care Med*. 1997;155:1637
48. Munoz J, Guerrero JE, Escalante JL, et al Pressure-controlled ventilation versus controlled mechanical ventilation with decelerating inspiratory flow. *Crit Care Med*. 1993;21:1143
49. O'Keefe GE, Gentilello LM, Erford S, et al Imprecision in lower "inflection point" estimation from static pressure-volume curves in patients at risk for acute respiratory distress syndrome. *J Trauma*. 1998;44:1064
50. Pelosi P, Tubiolo D, Mascheroni D, et al Effects of the prone position on respiratory mechanics and gas exchange during acute lung injury. *Am J Respir Crit Care Med*. 1998;157:387
51. Pepe PE, Hudson LE, Carrico HJ. Early application of positive end-expiratory pressure in patients at risk for the adult respiratory distress syndrome. *N Engl J Med*. 1984;311:281
52. Ranieri GM, Giuiliani R, Fiore T, et al Volume-pressure curve of the respiratory system predicts effects of PEEP in ARDS: "occlusion" versus "constant flow" technique. *Am J Respir Crit Care Med*. 1994;199:19
53. Rossi A, Santos C, Roca J, et al Effects of PEEP on V/Q mismatching in ventilated patients with chronic airflow obstruction. *Am J Respir Crit Care Med*. 1994;149:1077
54. Sassoon CSH, Lodia R, Rheeman CH, et al Inspiratory muscle work of breathing during flow-by, demand-flow, and continuous-flow systems in patients with chronic obstructive pulmonary disease. *Am Rev Respir Dis*. 1992;145:1219–1222
55. Scott LR, Benson MS, Pierson DJ. Effect of inspiratory flow-rate and circuit compressible volume on auto-PEEP during mechanical ventilation. *Respir Care*. 1986;31:1075–1079
56. Slutsky AS. Mechanical ventilation. American College of Chest Physicians' Consensus Conference. *Chest*. 1993;104:1833
57. Smith RA. Physiologic PEEP. *Respir Care*. 1988;33:620
58. Standiford TJ, Morganroth ML. High-frequency ventilation. *Chest*. 1989;96:1380
59. Suter PM, Fairley HB, Isenberg MD. Optimum end-expiratory airway pressure in patients with acute pulmonary failure. *N Engl J Med*. 1975;292:284

60. Sydow M, Burchardi H. Ephraim, et al: Long-term effects of two different ventilatory modes on oxygenation in acute lung injury. *Am J Respir Crit Care Med*. 1994;149:1550
61. Tocker R, Neff T, Stein S, et al Prone positioning and low-volume pressure-limited ventilation improve survival in patients with severe ARDS. *Chest*. 1997;111:1008
62. Tuxen DV. Detrimental effects of positive end-expiratory pressure during controlled mechanical ventilation of patients with severe airflow obstruction. *Am Respir Dis*. 1989;140:5
63. Vitacca M, Lanini B, Nava S, et al Inspiratory muscle workload due to dynamic intrinsic PEEP in stable COPD patients: effects of two different settings of non-invasive pressure-support ventilation. *Monaldi Arch Chest Dis*. 2004;61:81–85

Chapter 6
Ventilator Alarms

Sophisticated alarms built into modern ventilators ensure that the physician is alerted whenever there is a significant change in specific parameters. If the patient or the ventilator operates outside the limits considered appropriate by the physician, or if any malfunction develops in the ventilator, gas source, or ventilator tubing and circuitry, in-built alarms will warn the physician to the problem at hand and help forestall the development of complications.

6.1 Low Expired Minute Volume Alarm

This alarm is activated when the expired minute volume falls to a level below the minimum operational minute volume preset by the physician. A low expired minute volume usually means that there is a leak in the system. Such a leak can occur when the ET (or TT) cuff is inadequately inflated or if it has ruptured. An upward migration of the endotracheal tube out of the larynx will also result in a leak.

The development of a pneumothorax usually leads to a concomitant activation of the high pressure alarm, but when an intercostal drain has been placed, a persistent air leak from a bronchopleural fistula can occasionally be large enough to cause the expired minute volume to fall (Fig. 6.1).

When there is an obstruction in the ventilatory circuit such as a blocked endotracheal tube or a clogged HME, the upper pressure limit will be exceeded, resulting in the premature

A. Hasan, *Understanding Mechanical Ventilation*,
DOI: 10.1007/978-1-84882-869-8_6,

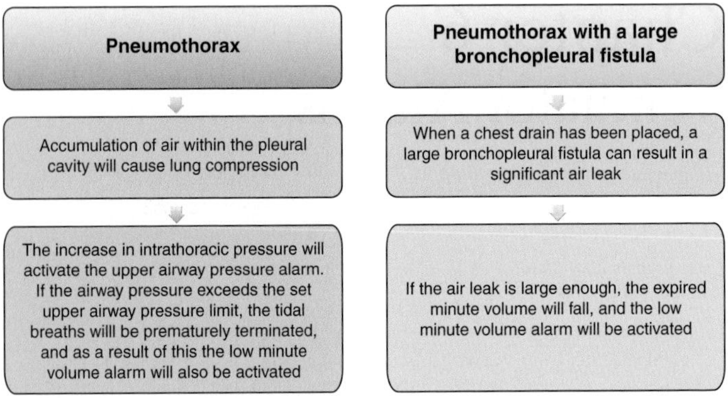
Pneumothorax
Accumulation of air within the pleural cavity will cause lung compression
The increase in intrathoracic pressure will activate the upper airway pressure alarm. If the airway pressure exceeds the set upper airway pressure limit, the tidal breaths willl be prematurely terminated, and as a result of this the low minute volume alarm will also be activated
Pneumothorax with a large bronchopleural fistula
When a chest drain has been placed, a large bronchopleural fistula can result in a significant air leak
If the air leak is large enough, the expired minute volume will fall, and the low minute volume alarm will be activated

FIGURE 6.1. Airway alarm activation in pneumothorax with and without a bronchopleural fistula.

termination of the inspiratory breath; the curtailment of tidal volumes will cause the delivered minute volume to fall (see Fig. 6.3 & 6.4). A downward migration of endotracheal tube can lead to the tidal volume intended for both lungs, to be delivered to only the right lung or even the right middle and lower lobes. A rise in the airway pressure then prematurely terminates the inspiration when the upper pressure limit has been reached, simultaneously activating the lower exhaled minute volume alarm.

When on spontaneous breathing modes such as the pressure support or CPAP, if the patient is not breathing often enough or deeply enough, the low exhaled minute volume will be triggered (Fig.).

Troubleshooting entails a systematic search for all the possibilities described in Fig. 6.2. The endotracheal/tracheotomy tube tip position should be verified. Palpation of the pilot bulb and auscultation over the patient's larynx may reveal a leaking endotracheal/tracheotomy cuff. The Y-connector, patient tube, HME, and humidifier circuits should be checked to exclude any loose connection responsible for the leak. The adequacy of the patient's respiratory effort should be assessed (on a spontaneous mode of ventilation) to rule out insufficiency of effort as the cause of the low minute volume. Finally,

Conditions leading to activation of the low expiratory minute volume alarm	Conditions leading to the activation of the high expiratory minute volume alarm

• Disconnection from the ventilator
• Leak in connections:
  • Y-connector
  • HME
  • Humidifier circuit
• Cuff deflation, leak or rupture
• Upward migration of endotracheal tube out of the larynx
• Hypoventilation (see also Box 6.1)
• Large bronchopleural fistula with chest drain in-situ
• Ventilator malfunction
	• Pain
	• Anxiety
	• Hypoxemia
	• Metabolic acidosis
	• Excessive CO_2 production
	• Fever
	• Hypercatabolic states (excessive CO_2 production)
	• Calorie loading (excessive CO_2 production)
	• Ventilator malfunction

FIGURE 6.2. Conditions that can activate the minute volume alarm.

if the upper airway pressure alarm has been activated as well, any cause of obstruction within the ventilator tubings or within the breathing tube, clogging of the HME, or even a pneumothorax can be anticipated.

6.2 High Expired Minute Volume Alarm

Hyperventilation by the patient due to any reason can trigger the alarm for high expired minute volume. A variety of causes such as pain, anxiety, hypoxemia, and a physiologic response to metabolic acidosis can result in hyperventilation.

Troubleshooting entails clinical assessment to seek out the cause for hyperventilation. If required, raising the upper airway pressure limit to a higher level will allow the patient to continue breathing at an increased rate without triggering the alarm. Needless to say, setting the alarm limit at an inappropriately low level in the first place will result in its activation by a patient who is breathing at a minute volume that is appropriate to his needs.

When hyperventilation does not appear to be the cause for alarm activation, a faulty flow transducer may be responsible for the alarm signal.

6.3 Upper Airway Pressure Limit Alarm

Whenever the airway pressure exceeds the set upper airway pressure limit, the alarm is activated. When the alarm is triggered, the ventilator immediately cycles to expiration, terminating the inspiration (see Fig. 6.3). The upper airway pressure limit is typically set at 10–15 cm H_2O above the observed peak inspiratory pressure. Secretions and encrustation within the breathing tube, or its kinking or biting by the patient, can raise the airway pressure and activate the alarm. Clogging of the heat-moisture exchanger by expectorated secretions can have the same effect. Slipping of endotracheal tube into the right main bronchus or the intermediate bronchus will lead to the activation of the alarm by the mechanisms discussed earlier. Patient-related events such as a coughing or clashing with a ventilator-delivered

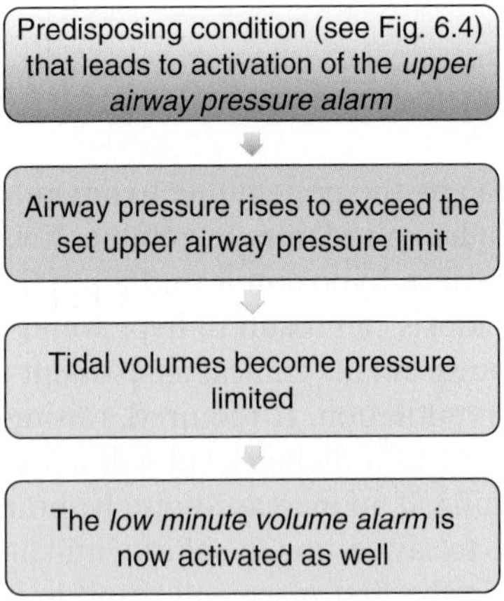
Predisposing condition (see Fig. 6.4) that leads to activation of the *upper airway pressure alarm*
Airway pressure rises to exceed the set upper airway pressure limit
Tidal volumes become pressure limited
The *low minute volume alarm* is now activated as well

FIGURE 6.3. Conditions that lead to activation of the upper airway pressure alarm will often activate the low minute volume alarm as well.

breath can momentarily trigger the alarm, but bronchospasm and pneumothorax will result in a sustained rise in the airway pressure leading to persistent alarm activation. A fall in static compliance of the lung due to lobar collapse, pneumonia, and pulmonary edema is also capable of raising the airway pressure and triggering the alarm (Figs. 6.3 and 6.4).

Troubleshooting involves the restoration of the patency of the patient tube by suctioning, or even replacing the endotracheal or tracheotomy tube when blockage is significant, or repositioning a migrated endotracheal tube to its intended location. Careful auscultation may reveal a difference in breath entry on the two sides suggesting lobar collapse or a pneumothorax. A symmetric increase in crepitations bilaterally in a situation against a background of cardiac insuffiency may suggest pulmonary edema; the

Upper airway pressure alarm

- Coughing
- Endotracheal/tracheostomy tube obstruction
- Kinking of endotracheal tube
- Biting of endotracheal tube
- Increased airway secretions
- Clogging of HME
- Excessive condensation ("raining out") into the ventilator circuit
- Downward migration of endotracheal tube into a mainstem bronchus
- Herniation of the endotracheal tube cuff
- Bronchospasm
- 'Clashing' with the ventilator
- Low lung compliance (pulmonary edema, pneumothorax, collapse of a lobe or lung, consolidation)
- Inspiratory/expiratory valve malfunction

Lower airway pressure alarm

- Disconnection
- Upward migration of ET
- Circuit leak at connection points
  - HME
  - Humidifier
  - Water trap
  - Closed suction catheter
  - Temperature sensors
  - In-line nebulizers
  - Exhalation valve
- ET Cuff
  - Inadequately inflated ET cuff
  - ET cuff deliberately under-inflated to provide a "minimal leak" (section 10.3.2 & 10.3.2.1)
- Pilot bulb leakage
- Bronchopleural fistula with chest drain in situ

FIGURE 6.4. Conditions that can lead to activation of the airway pressure alarms.

presence of wheeze points to airways obstruction as a cause of raised airway pressures. A chest film may be valuable in this setting, helping to confirm the presence or absence of pneumothorax, lobar or unilateral lung collapse, pulmonary edema or a worsening pneumonia. Treatment of bronchospasm and regulation of ventilator settings to ensure better patient-ventilator synchrony may be necessary in the relevant circumstance. When a pneumothorax is responsible for the problem, it must be tackled urgently, and a chest drain inserted forthwith.

6.4 Low Airway Pressure Limit Alarm

The low airway pressure limit is typically set at 10–15 cm H_2O below the observed peak inspiratory pressure. The alarm is activated if the airway pressure falls, such as in leaks or disconnections (see Fig. 6.4).

6.5 Oxygen Concentration Alarms

The upper and lower FIO_2 alarms are meant to monitor the FIO_2 being delivered to the patient. When a particular FIO_2 is chosen for the patient, the upper and lower FIO_2 limits are set approximately 5–10% above and below the chosen FIO_2, respectively. This allows monitoring the delivered FIO_2 within narrow limits.

6.6 Low Oxygen Concentration (FIO_2) Alarm

A fall in the FIO_2 as a result of a decrease in the central piped oxygen supply to the ventilator will result in a lower than intended FIO_2 being supplied to the patient, and the alarm will be triggered.

Resetting the FIO_2 to a lower level without making a compensatory adjustment in the lower FIO_2 limit will also cause the alarm to be activated.

6.7 Upper Oxygen Concentration (FIO_2) Alarm

A drop in the central piped air supply will cause a rise in the proportion of oxygen in the gas mixture being delivered to the patient. The FIO_2 then rises, and if it does so beyond the upper oxygen concentration limit, this alarm is activated.

Deliberately increasing the FIO_2 to a higher level (to compensate for a falling PaO_2) will also result in alarm activation, if the new FIO_2 has exceeded the set upper O_2 concentration limit. Corrective action is taken by making an upward adjustment in the upper O_2 concentration alarm limit such that it once again exceeds the delivered FIO_2.

6.8 Power Failure

The power failure alarm is activated when the electrical supply to the ventilator is interrupted.

6.9 Apnea Alarm

The apnea alarm should be set such that it is activated if the patient makes no attempt to breathe for at least 15–20 s, on a spontaneous mode of breathing. Many ventilators automatically switch over to a backup mode that ensures full mechanical support until spontaneous breaths are resumed.

Box 6.1 Lack of Triggering

Drugs (sedatives, paralyzing agents)
CNS injury or disease
Hyperoxic hyperventilation
Hypocapnia
Metabolic alkalosis
Central sleep apneas (lack of triggering during sleep)
Uremia
Hypothermia
Respiratory muscle weakness

6.10 Two-Minute Button

When the 2-min button on the ventilator is pressed in response to an alarm, the relevant alarm is silenced for a period of 2 min. Since pressing the 2-min button will silence the alarm without rectifying the problem responsible for its activation, efforts should be directed at uncovering the underlying derangement rather than merely silencing the alarm.

References

1. Black JW, Grover BS. A hazard of pressure support ventilation. *Chest*. 1998;93(2):333
2. Blanch PB. Mechanical ventilator malfunctions: a descriptive and comparative study of 6 common ventilator brands. *Respir Care*. 1999;44:1183–1192
3. Bourke AE, et al Failure of a ventilator alarm to detect patient disconnection. *J Med Eng Technol*. 1987;11(2):65–67
4. Brown BR. Understanding mechanical ventilation: indications for and initiation of therapy. *J Okla State Med Assoc*. 1994;87:353–357
5. Brunner JX, et al Prototype ventilator and alarm algorithm for the NASA Space Station. *J Clin Monit*. 1989;5(2):90–99
6. Campbell RS, et al Pressure-controlled versus volume-controlled ventilation: does it matter? *Respir Care*. 2002;47(4):416–424
7. Dupuis YG. *Ventilators: Theory and Clinical Application*. St. Louis: CV Mosby; 1986
8 Feihl F, et al Permissive hypercapnia. How permissive should we be? *Am J Respir Crit Care Med*. 1994;150(6 Pt 1):1722–1737
9. Kallet RH, et al Implementation of a low tidal volume ventilation protocol for patients with acute lung injury or acute respiratory distress syndrome. *Respir care*. 2001;46(10):1024–1037
10. Milligan KA. Disablement of a ventilator disconnects alarm by a heat and moisture exchanger [letter]. *Anaesthesia*. 1992;47(3):279
11. Monaco F, Goettel J. Increased airway pressure in bear 2 and 3 circuits. *Respir Care*. 1999;36(2):132
12. Pottie JC, et al Alarm failure in the oxygen-air mixture. *Ann Fr Anesth Reanim*. 1993;12(6):607–608
13. Pryn SJ, et al Ventilator disconnection alarm failures. The role of ventilator and breathing accessories. *Anaesthesia*. 1989;44(12):978–981
14. Tobin MJ. What should the clinician do when the patient "fights the ventilator?". *Respir Care*. 1991;36(5):395

Chapter 7
Monitoring Gas Exchange in the Mechanically Ventilated Patient

7.1 The Arterial Oxygen Tension

One of the primary goals of mechanical ventilation is to provide enough oxygen to the tissues for aerobic metabolism. Constant monitoring of the adequacy of oxygen therapy is imperative to the ultimate success of mechanical ventilation.

Oxygen is available for inspiration at sea level at a partial pressure of about 160 mmHg, but the tension of oxygen within the oxygen-processing unit of the cell (the mitochondrion) is relatively a tiny fraction of this (see Fig. 7.1). Although the partial pressure at the site of oxygen utilization is not known, the

At sea level, the partial pressure of O_2 is: 160 mmHg
760 mmHg x 0.21 = 160 mmHg

Oxygen is available for inspiration at sea level at a partial pressure of about 160 mm Hg

Within the respiratory tract the partial pressure of O_2 is about 150 mmHg 0.21 x (760–47) x 0.21 = 149 mmHg

As it enters the respiratory system, O_2 is humidified by the addition of water vapour (partial pressure 47 mm Hg). Humidification serves to make the insired air more breathable; it also results in the drop of the partial pressure of oxygen to about 150 mmHg

FIGURE 7.1. The oxygen cascade. (Adapted from Hasan[23])

A. Hasan, *Understanding Mechanical Ventilation*,
DOI: 10.1007/978-1-84882-869-8_7,

In the alveoli the partial pressure of O_2 (PAO_2) is about 100 mmHg
149–(40/0.8) = 99 mmHg

40 is the normal value of $PaCO_2$ in mmHg.

Since CO_2 is easily diffusible across the alveolocapillary membrane, arterial CO_2 ($PaCO_2$) can be assumed to be the same as alveolar CO_2 ($PACO_2$).

0.8 is the respiratory quotient

In the alveoli, oxygen diffuses into the alveolar capillaries and carbon dioxide is added to the alveolar air. The result of a complex interaction between three factors [alveolar ventilation, CO_2 production (VCO_2) and the relative consumption of C_2 (VO_2)] causes the partial pressure of CO_2 in the alveolus to drop to 100 mmHg. this is the pressure of oxygen that equates with the pressure of oxygen in the pulmonary veins, and therefore, with the pressuire of oxygen in the systemic arteries.

VCO_2 = 250 mL of CO_2/min

VO_2 = 300 mL of O_2/min

In the systemic arteries the partial pressure of O_2 (PaO_2) is about 95 mmHg

A small amount of deoxygenated blood is added to the systemic arteries (because of a small physiological shunt that normally exists in the body). This is due to unoxygenated blood emptied by the bronchial and thesbesian veins back into the pulmonary veins and the left side of the heart. This "shunt fraction" which represents about 2–5% of the cardiac output, causes the systemic arterial oxygen to "fall fractionally" from 100 mmHg, to about 95 mmHg or less.
Thus, in spite of normal gas exchange, the PaO_2 may be 5–10 mmHg lower than the PAO_2.

In the mitochondrion the partial pressure of O_2 is unknown

Due to substantial diffusion barriers, the amount of oxygen made available to the oxygen-processing unit of the cell (the mitochondrion) is a relatively tiny amount. The mitochondrion appears to continue in its normal state of aerobic metabolism with minimal oxygen requirements. In hypoxia, a fall in the PaO_2 within mitochondria (to possible less than 1 mmHg), is required to shift the energy producing pathways towards the much less efficient anaerobic metabolism

FIGURE 7.1. (continued)

mitochondrion appears to continue in its normal state of aerobic metabolism with minimal oxygen requirements. In hypoxia, with a fall in the PaO_2 within mitochondria (to possibly less than 1 mmHg), aerobic metabolism is considerably reduced, and there is a shift in the energy producing pathways toward the much less efficient anaerobic metabolism (Fig. 7.1).

PaO_2: The measurement of oxygen in the blood serves as a surrogate for the measurement of oxygen in the tissues, there being no practical way to reliably assess the state of tissue oxygenation. Several methods exist for the estimation of the state of oxygenation of the blood, the most direct of these being the measurement of the arterial oxygen tension (PaO_2), which can readily be done by sampling of the arterial blood gases (ABGs).

As a rule of the thumb, when the lungs are normal, multiplying the fraction of inspired oxygen into 5 gives the approximate expected PaO_2 for that FIO_2. For instance, if the FIO_2 is 21% (which is the case when a person is breathing room air), the expected PaO_2 for this FIO_2 would be $21 \times 5 = 105$ (this is an approximation). Similarly, breathing 50% O_2 (FIO_2 0.5) would result in a PaO_2 of roughly $50 \times 5 = 250$. If the measured PaO_2 is significantly lower than the expected PaO_2, a problem with the gas exchange mechanisms of the lungs can be anticipated, and a reason for the hypoxemia must be sought.

PaO_2/FIO_2 ratio: The PaO_2/FIO_2 ratio is derived from this line of reasoning. This ratio makes it possible to compare the arterial oxygenation in patients breathing different fractions of inspired oxygen. A patient who has a normal PaO_2 of approximately 100 mmHg while breathing room air, would have a PaO_2/FIO_2 of $100/0.21 = 500$. The normal range for the PaO_2/FIO_2 ratio is 300–500. Values of less than 250 imply a significant problem in the gas exchange mechanisms of the lung. In the context of acute lung injury (ALI), values less than 300 suggest ALI, and values less than 200 are diagnostic of ARDS in the appropriate clinical setting. Though this formula serves well as a rough guide in most situations, it is not very reliable over the extremes of FIO_2.

PaO_2/PAO_2: A better estimate of oxygenation is the PaO_2/PAO_2 ratio. The PaO_2/PAO_2 ratio is the proportion of oxygen in the alveolus that eventually gains entry into the pulmonary capillary blood. To employ this formula, the oxygen tension of the arterial blood (PaO_2) as well as the partial pressure of

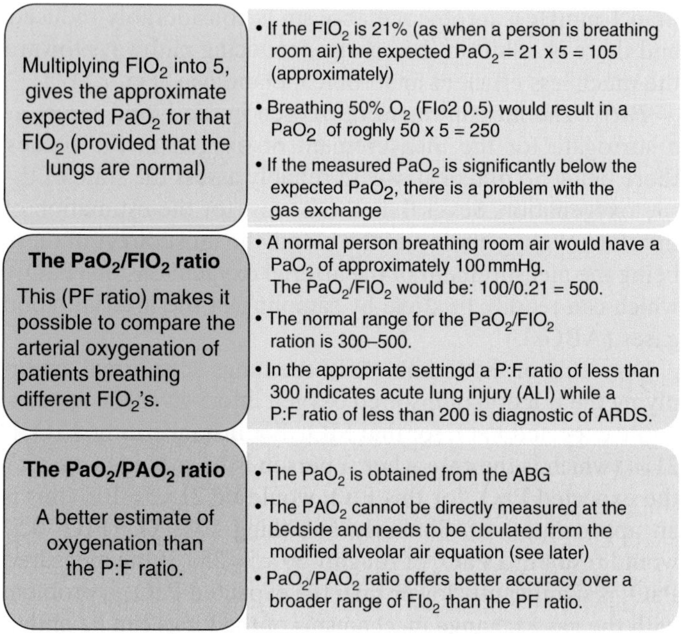
Multiplying FIO_2 into 5, gives the approximate expected PaO_2 for that FIO_2 (provided that the lungs are normal)
• If the FIO_2 is 21% (as when a person is breathing room air) the expected PaO_2 = 21 x 5 = 105 (approximately)
• Breathing 50% O_2 (Flo2 0.5) would result in a PaO_2 of roghly 50 x 5 = 250
• If the measured PaO_2 is significantly below the expected PaO_2, there is a problem with the gas exchange
The PaO_2/FIO_2 ratio
This (PF ratio) makes it possible to compare the arterial oxygenation of patients breathing different FIO_2's.
• A normal person breathing room air would have a PaO_2 of approximately 100 mmHg.
The PaO_2/FIO_2 would be: 100/0.21 = 500.
• The normal range for the PaO_2/FIO_2 ration is 300–500.
• In the appropriate settingd a P:F ratio of less than 300 indicates acute lung injury (ALI) while a P:F ratio of less than 200 is diagnostic of ARDS.
The PaO_2/PAO_2 ratio
A better estimate of oxygenation than the P:F ratio.
• The PaO_2 is obtained from the ABG
• The PAO_2 cannot be directly measured at the bedside and needs to be clculated from the modified alveolar air equation (see later)
• PaO_2/PAO_2 ratio offers better accuracy over a broader range of FIo_2 than the PF ratio.

FIGURE 7.2. Assessing arterial oxygenation at the bedside. (Adapted from Hasan[23])

oxygen in the alveoli (PAO_2) must be known. Although the PaO_2 is easily read out from the ABG, the PAO_2 cannot be directly measured at the bedside and needs to be calculated (see A–a DO_2 below). The PaO_2/PAO_2 ratio offers better accuracy over a broader range of FIO_2 than the PF ratio. When the PaO_2/PAO_2 ratio is very low, it is obvious that high fractions of inspired oxygen do not translate into improved blood oxygenation: in such situations a high shunt fraction can be expected.

A–a DO_2: The alveoloarterial diffusion of oxygen (A–a DO_2) is another way of looking at the ease with which the administered oxygen diffuses into the blood; it is another measure of the efficiency of the lungs to oxygenate the blood. The A–a DO_2 is the difference between the alveolar O_2 tension (PAO_2) and the arterial oxygen tension (PaO_2). Calculation of both, the A–a DO_2 as well as the PaO_2/PAO_2 ratio, requires knowledge of the PAO_2. PAO_2 is calculated from the simplified form of the alveolar gas equation (see Fig. 7.3).

The partial pressure of the O_2 in the inspired air depends on the fraction of O_2 in the inspired air in relation to the barometric pressure at that altitude, and also upon the water vapour pressure (the upper airways completely saturate the inhaled air with water).

$$PIO_2 = FIO_2\,(Pb - Pw)$$

Where,
PIO_2 = Inspired PO_2
Pb = Barometric pressure
Pw = Water vapour pressure, 47 mmHg at the normal body temperature

$$PAO_2 = PIO_2 - 1.2\,(PaCO_2)$$

Where,
PAO_2 = Partial pressure of O_2 in the alveolus
$PaCO_2$ = Partial pressure of CO_2 in the arterial blood. Because of the excellent diffusibility of CO_2 across biological membranes, the value of $PaCO_2$ is taken to be the same as the $PACO_2$ (the partial pressure of CO_2 in the alveolus). Multiplying $PaCO_2$ by 1.2 is the same as dividing $PaCO_2$ by 0.8 (0.8 is the respiratory quotient)

Substituting the value of PIO_2 into the above equation,

$$PAO_2 = [FIO_2\,(Pb-Pw)] - [1.2 \times PaCO_2]$$

The above abbreviated form of the equation serves well for clinical use, in place of the alveolar air equation proper[31] which is:

$$PAO_2 = PIO_2 - (PACO_2) \times [FIO_2 + [(1-FIO_2)/R]$$

FIGURE 7.3. The modified alveolar air equation. (Adapted from Hasan[23])

The simplified formula is much less labor intensive and easier to apply, but may have a significant margin of error especially when higher FIO_2 is used. Another drawback of this equation is that the respiratory quotient is often assumed to be 0.8, which may not always be the case in a critically ill patient with an altered body metabolism and on complex nutritive supplementation. Furthermore, estimates of FIO_2 are often misleading if a patient on conventional oxygen devices has an irregular pattern of breathing.

The factors determining PAO_2 and PaO_2 have been listed in Fig. 7.4.

The determinants of PAO_2 are	The determinants of PaO_2 are:
• The fractional concentration of oxygen in the inhaled air (FIO_2) • The partial pressure of CO2in the arterial blood ($PaCO_2$) • Barometric pressure (PB). PB is constant for a given altitude	• Lung pathology • Mixed venous O_2 content

FIGURE 7.4. Determinants of PAO_2 and PaO_2. (Adapted from Hasan[23]).

Normally, the A–a DO_2 ranges from 7 to 14 mmHg on room air. A–a DO_2 is less than 70 mmHg while breathing 100% oxygen. Notice that the normal A–a DO_2 gradient widens with higher fractions of inspired O_2. This A–a difference reaches a maximum when the PAO_2 exceeds 350–450 mmHg and then again decreases at a higher PO_2, thus describing a bell shaped curve. Thus, between the two extremes of inhaled FIO_2 (0.21 and 1.0), the expected A-a DO_2 level even in the normal subject is difficult to predict. There exists no reliable reference value for the A–a DO_2 when a patient is on intermediate levels of FIO_2.

The A–a DO_2 normally increases with age. The predicted value of A–a DO_2 can be calculated by the following equation (see also Fig. 7.5):

$$A-a\ DO_2 = 2.5 + (0.25 \times \text{Age in years}).$$

The A–a DO_2 is widened when a *V*/*Q* mismatch, right to left shunt, or diffusion defect is the mechanism producing the hypoxemia. It is not widened in disorders causing hypoventilation – here, the problem lies with the deficient bulk flow of air into the lungs and not with the problems concerning alveoli, the alveolar capillary interface, or the alveolar capillary bed. The A–a DO_2 is prone to errors in its calculation (Fig. 7.6) and this must be kept in mind.

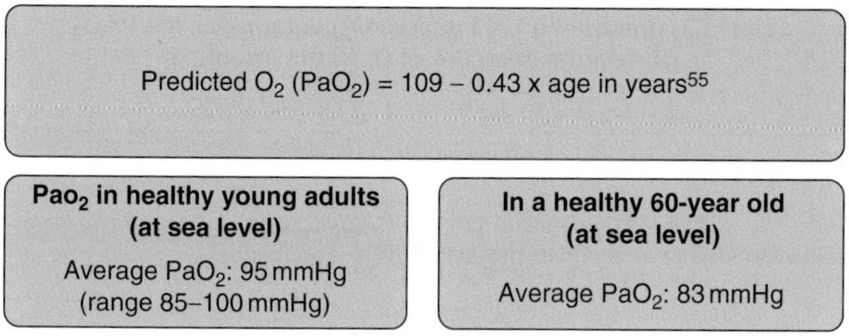
Predicted O2 (PaO2) = 109 – 0.43 x age in years55
Pao2 in healthy young adults (at sea level)
Average PaO2: 95 mmHg (range 85–100 mmHg)
In a healthy 60-year old (at sea level)
Average PaO2: 83 mmHg

FIGURE 7.5. Predictive equation for the estimation of PaO_2 at (sea level) in different age groups.

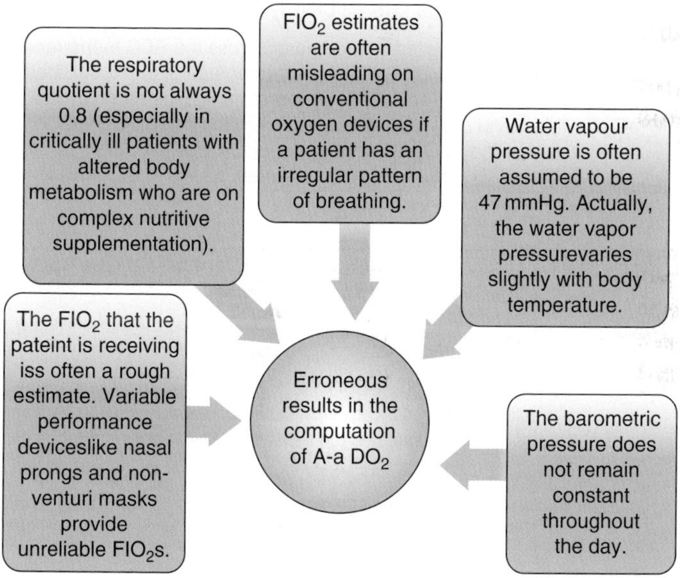
The respiratory quotient is not always 0.8 (especially in critically ill patients with altered body metabolism who are on complex nutritive supplementation).
FIO2 estimates are often misleading on conventional oxygen devices if a patient has an irregular pattern of breathing.
Water vapour pressure is often assumed to be 47 mmHg. Actually, the water vapor pressurevaries slightly with body temperature.
The FIO2 that the pateint is receiving iss often a rough estimate. Variable performance deviceslike nasal prongs and non-venturi masks provide unreliable FIO2s.
Erroneous results in the computation of A-a DO2
The barometric pressure does not remain constant throughout the day.

FIGURE 7.6. Sources of error in the A-aDO_2 calculation. (Adapted from Hasan[23])

The relationship between FIO_2, PAO_2, PaO_2, and SpO_2 (the oxygen saturation of the blood) has been summarized in Fig. 7.7.

The FIO_2 (the fraction of inspired O_2) determines the PAO_2 (the partial pressure of O_2 in the alveolus)

PAO_2 is also determined by PB and PCO_2.

↓

The PAO_2 determines the PAO_2 (partial pressure of O_2 in the pulmonary capillaries)

O_2 molecules diffuse across the alveolus-capillary membrane into the pulmonary cappillaries, and equilibriate with the O_2 in the arterial blood. Thus, PAO_2 determines the PaO_2 (or how much O_2 is dissolved in the plasma)

↓

SpO_2 (O_2 saturation of the arterial blood) is determined by the PaO_2

The O_2 molecules in the arterial blood pass across the RBC membrane and bind to hemoglobin(Hb). SpO_2 is the percentage of the heme sites that are bound to O_2 molecules. SpO_2 therefore is determined by the PaO_2 (or the partial pressure that O_2 exerts in the blood). Generally. the higher the PaO_2, the higher the SpO_2. However this relationship is not linear

↓

CaO_2 (the O_2 content of arterial blood) is determined by the SpO_2 and the Hb concentration

SpO_2 along with the amount of Hb available in the blood determines the CaO_2 (or the content of O_2 in the arterial blood)

$CaO_2 = [1.34 \times \text{Hb (in gm/dl)}^* \times SpO_2] + [PaO_2 \times 0.003 \text{ m L } O_2/\text{mmHg}]$
(*1.34 mL of oxygen combine with each gram of Hb
0.003 mL is the solubility of O_2 in each dl of blood per mmHg)

The maximum amount of O_2 that can combine with the available Hb is termed the ***oxygen capacity****. For a normal Hb of 15 gm/dL, the O_2 capacity is = 1.34x15 = 20 mL/dL*

FIGURE 7.7. The relationship between FIO_2, PAO_2, PaO_2, and SpO_2. (Adapted from Hasan[23])

7.2 Pulse Oximetry

Hemoglobin possesses a unique structure (Fig. 7.8).

The function of hemoglobin, of course, is to carry oxygen, to which its structure is wonderfully adapted (Fig. 7.9). Hemoglobin also helps in the carriage of CO_2. Only about

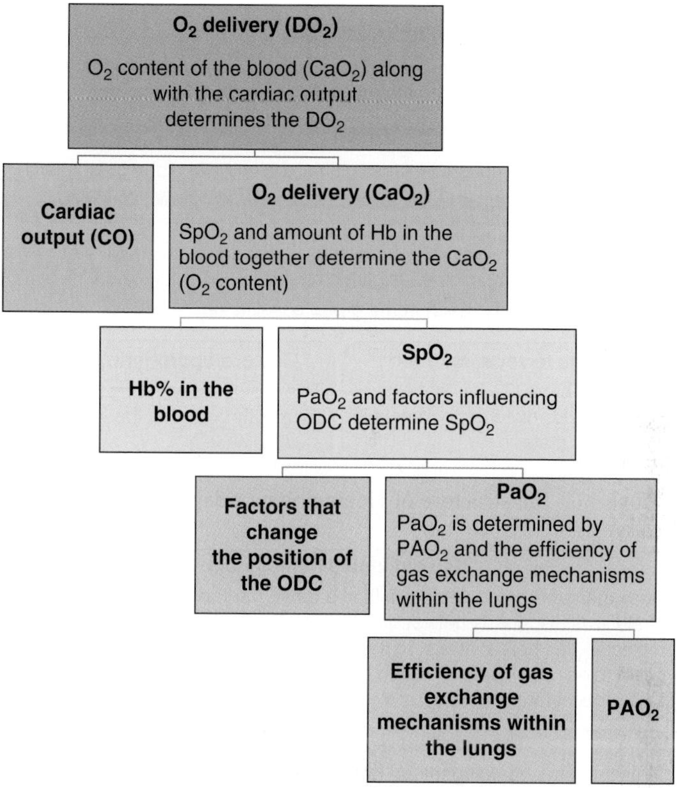
O2 delivery (DO2)
O2 content of the blood (CaO2) along with the cardiac output determines the DO2
Cardiac output (CO)
O2 delivery (CaO2)
SpO2 and amount of Hb in the blood together determine the CaO2 (O2 content)
Hb% in the blood
SpO2
PaO2 and factors influencing ODC determine SpO2
Factors that change the position of the ODC
PaO2
PaO2 is determined by PAO2 and the efficiency of gas exchange mechanisms within the lungs
Efficiency of gas exchange mechanisms within the lungs
PAO2

FIGURE 7.8. The relationship between PAO_2, PaO_2, SpO_2, CaO_2, and DO_2. (Adapted from Hasan[23])

5% of all the CO_2 transported in the blood is in the form of carbamino compounds (viz., bound to hemoglobin), but carbamino compounds account for 30% of the CO_2 that evolves in the lungs, from the red blood cells circulating within the pulmonary capillaries (About 5% of CO_2 that is carried is dissolved in plasma. The bulk of the CO_2 is carried in the form of bicarbonate).

Hemoglobin also serves indirectly, as a regulator of vasomotor tone. Nitric oxide (NO) is capable of reacting with the cysteine residue at position 93 of the β-chain of hemoglobin. The resulting nitrosothiol, *S*-nitrosylated hemoglobin is a

The structure of hemoglobin

The special ability of hemoglobin to imbibe O_2 from the pulmonary capillaries and release it to the tissues derives from its unique quartenary structure.

Globin

The Hb molecule consists of four globin chains (two alpha chains each of 141 amino acids, and two beta chains each of 146 amino acids)

Heme

One heme group binds *each* globin chain.

Each heme group consists of:

One ferrous ion (Fe^{++})

In order to carry O_2, it is necessary for heme's ferrous iron to remain in the ferrous state.

One protoporphyrin IX ring

This protoporphyrin ring is covalently bound to the ferrous ion.

FIGURE 7.9. The structure of Hemoglobin (Adapted from Hasan[23])

Deoxygenated hemoglobin

Deoxygenated hemoglobin exists in a tense (taut) configuration because of electrostatic bonds between its beta globin chains. The hemoglobin molecule has helical twists. In the nonhelical sections the polypeptide chain folds upon itself, creating clefts within which the four heme groups lie at equidistant intervals

The attachment of the first O_2 molecule

In its taut state, deoxygenated hemoglobin has little affinity for O_2. The attachment of the first O_2 molecule to one of the globin chains generates chemical and mechanical stresses resulting in the severing of electrostatic bonds. This allows the hemoglobinmolecule to unfold slightly

The attachment of the second O_2 molecule

As the hemoglobin molecule relaxes and unfolds it exposes the other O_2 binding sites within its clefts; this facilitates the addition of another molecule of O_2 to the hemoglobin, more rapidly than the first

The attachment of the third and fourth O_2 molecules

The binding of the second molecule of O_2 results in further relaxation of the coils of the hemoglobing molecule, accelerating the uptake of the third and the fourth O_2 molecules

FIGURE 7.10. Cooperativity. (Adapted from Hasan[23])

vasodilator. The unique and recently recognized vasodilator property of hemoglobin is dependent on its complex and ill understood reactions with NO.[55]

Although the direct measurement of arterial O_2 tension by ABG sampling is a very accurate way of assessing oxygenation, it has its disadvantages. Intermittent sampling of ABGs is likely to be inconvenient and painful for the patient, and has the potential for bleeding, infection, arterial thrombosis, and even gangrene in an extremity. Continuous ABG sampling by means of an indwelling arterial cannula obviates the need for frequent arterial punctures and is generally used in unstable clinical situations. Real-time monitoring of ABGs enables the clinician to carefully monitor the patient's condition. However, continuous sampling is also associated with significant complications, for which the patient needs to be closely watched.

Pulse oximetry is a convenient way of continuously monitoring the oxygen status of the blood. Cyanosis is the clinical hallmark of hemoglobin desaturation, but is not always easy to assess at the bedside and may be notoriously difficult to appreciate in an anemic patient. Frank cyanosis is not usually apparent until the deoxygenated hemoglobin falls to 5 g/dL. In severe anemia, enough hemoglobin may not be available for cyanosis to be apparent, even when severe hypoxemia exists.

The invention of nonpulsatile oximetry by Carl Matthes in 1935, and its later modification to the present pulsatile form by Takuo Aoyagi in 1974, provided a vital tool for the assessment of the oxygen saturation of hemoglobin.[35] Such is the dependency on pulse oximetry in modern critical care units that it has often been described as the fifth vital sign in clinical medicine.

Two types of pulse oximeters are in contemporary use: transmission pulse oximeters and reflectance pulse oximeters.

Transmission pulse oximeters, which are extensively used, involve a pair of light emitting diodes (LEDs) with a photodetector placed on opposite sides of the interposed tissue, typically a finger (usually the index finger), or a toe (usually the great toe), or the earlobe; the foot of a neonate and the adult nose bridge have also on occasion been used.

Reflectance pulse oximeters, not so popular, involve a technique in which photowaves from LEDs are bounced off an appropriate surface (e.g., the skull bone). The reflected beam of light passes back through the tissue (e.g., the skin of the forehead) to reach a photodetector placed adjacent to the LEDs.

7.2.1 Principle of Pulse Oximetry

For the analysis of oxyhemoglobin and deoxyhemoglobin percentages in the blood, the principle of spectrophotometry is applied. This principle relies on the Beer–Lambert law, which states that the concentration of light-absorbing species within a sample is a logarithmic function of the amount of light absorbed by that sample. In the case of oximetry, the light-absorbing species are oxyhemoglobin and deoxyhemoglobin (see Fig. 7.11).

Light at two different wavelengths is passed through an interposed part of the body, and the absorbance of light at these two wavelengths is measured by a photodetector placed at the opposite side.[32] Since hemoglobin and deoxygenated hemoglobin absorb light at different wavelengths, two separate diodes – one emitting light at a wavelength of 660 nm (in the red band of the spectrum) and the other at a wavelength of 940 nm (in the infrared band of the spectrum) – are used. The shorter wavelength is better absorbed by the saturated (oxygenated) hemoglobin; the longer wavelength of the two is preferentially absorbed by the reduced (deoxygenated) hemoglobin.

The photodiodes emit the light physically at several hundred times per second. This technical innovation is designed to differentiate the light absorbance of the arterial blood from that of the venous blood and the surrounding tissue.[40]

Additionally, the principle of optical plethysmography is made use of to display the amplitude of pulse and the heart rate. During ventricular systole and diastole, there is a phasic increase and decrease respectively, of blood volume in the perfused organs. Transmission of light across the sampling site decreases during systole, since the light has to travel a

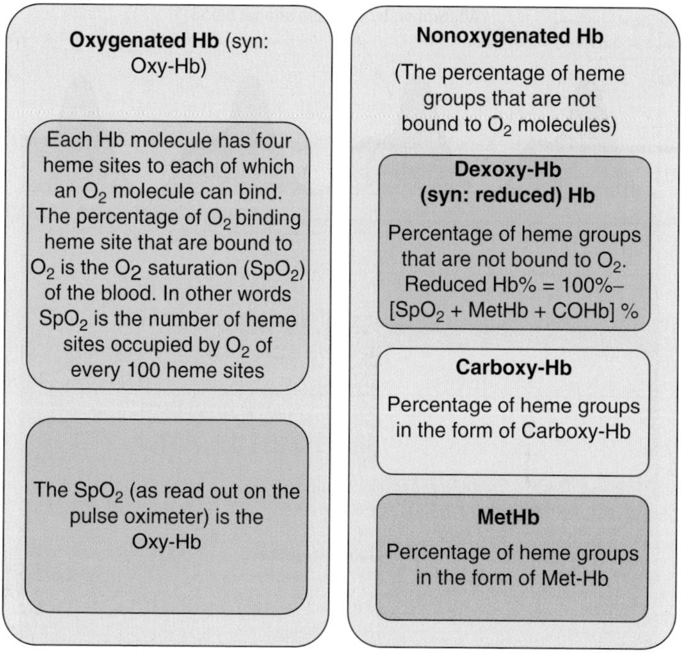
Oxygenated Hb (syn: Oxy-Hb)
Each Hb molecule has four heme sites to each of which an O2 molecule can bind. The percentage of O2 binding heme site that are bound to O2 is the O2 saturation (SpO2) of the blood. In other words SpO2 is the number of heme sites occupied by O2 of every 100 heme sites
The SpO2 (as read out on the pulse oximeter) is the Oxy-Hb
Nonoxygenated Hb
(The percentage of heme groups that are not bound to O2 molecules)
Dexoxy-Hb (syn: reduced) Hb
Percentage of heme groups that are not bound to O2. Reduced Hb% = 100%– [SpO2 + MetHb + COHb] %
Carboxy-Hb
Percentage of heme groups in the form of Carboxy-Hb
MetHb
Percentage of heme groups in the form of Met-Hb

FIGURE 7.11. Oxygenated and non-oxygenated hemoglobin. (Adapted from Hasan[23])

longer distance through the distended finger or ear lobe. On the other hand, light transmission through the sampling site increases during diastole. A phasic signal is presented to the sensor, which calculates the pulse amplitude according to the relative absorbencies during systole and diastole (Figs. 7.12).

One of the principal limitations of oximetry is in the fact that it monitors oxygen saturation (SpO_2) and not the actual oxygen tension in the blood. The top part of the oxygen dissociation curve being relatively flat, it is possible for major changes in the PaO_2 to occur on this segment without perceptible changes in the SpO_2. Thus, a falling PaO_2 in the initial stages of respiratory failure gives no inkling of a worsening hypoxemia (when SpO_2 is used to monitor oxygenation) as long as the PaO_2 continues to lie on the flat segment of the

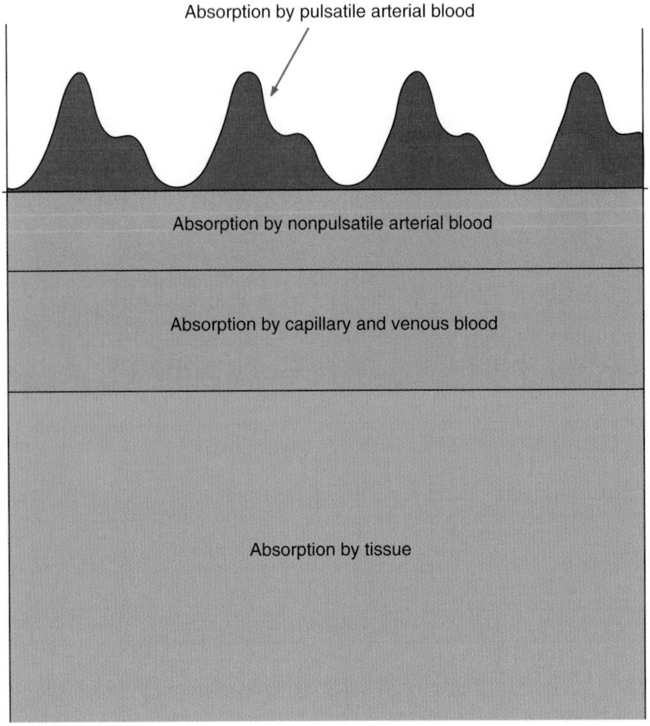
Absorption by pulsatile arterial blood
Absorption by nonpulsatile arterial blood
Absorption by capillary and venous blood
Absorption by tissue

FIGURE 7.12. Light absorbance during pulse oximetry.

oxygen dissociation curve. Once the PaO_2 drops to a point where it lies on the steep part of the oxygen dissociation curve, the saturation begins to drop sharply. Valuable time may be lost due to the failure to appreciate an increasing hypoxemia at an early stage. Thus, a patient on supplementary oxygen who has a PaO_2 of say, 200 mmHg, would have to drop his PaO_2 by 140 mmHg (to a PaO_2 of 60 mmHg) before having an oximetrically detectable fall in the SpO_2 (Fig. 7.14).

The assessment of O_2 saturation can be unreliable in severe hypoxemia. An SpO_2 value of 80% has been proposed as a threshold value, below which the reliability of O_2 measurement by oximetry is undependable.[17,19] On the other hand, it has been argued that the accuracy falls by just 1%

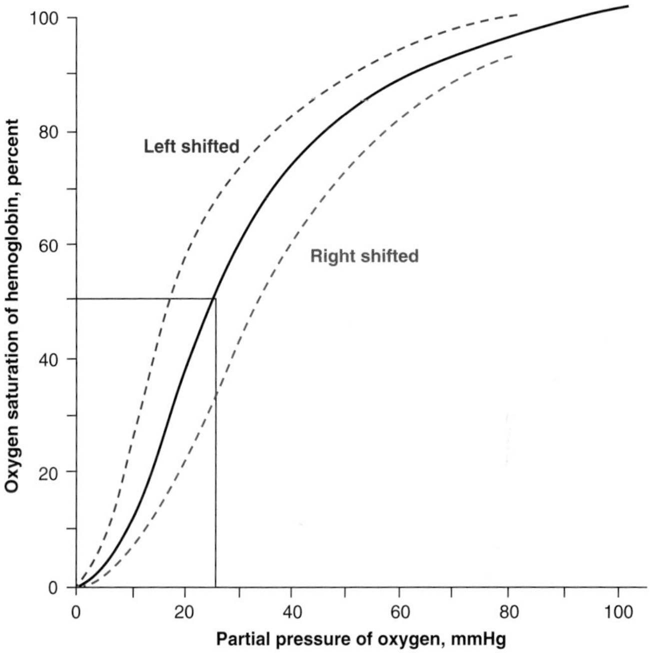

100
80
60
40
20
0
Oxygen saturation of hemoglobin, percent
Left shifted
Right shifted
0
20
40
60
80
100
Partial pressure of oxygen, mmHg

FIGURE 7.13. The oxyhemoglobin dissociation curve.

when saturations between 50 and 70% are encountered, compared to the accuracy measured when saturations are above 70%.

The other obvious disadvantage of oximetry (compared to ABG analysis) is that oximetry does not measure $PaCO_2$: as a result, assessment of the adequacy of ventilation is not possible. Although PaO_2 monitoring may be considered to be advantageous over SpO_2 monitoring (inasmuch as it measures the exact level of oxygen in the arterial blood), it must be realized that while the SpO_2 is a direct measure of the oxyhemoglobin saturation in the blood, the PaO_2 (as exhibited on the ABG sample) measures the tension of the O_2 dissolved in the plasma. The latter has only an indirect correlation with the oxyhemoglobin, with which it is in equilibrium.

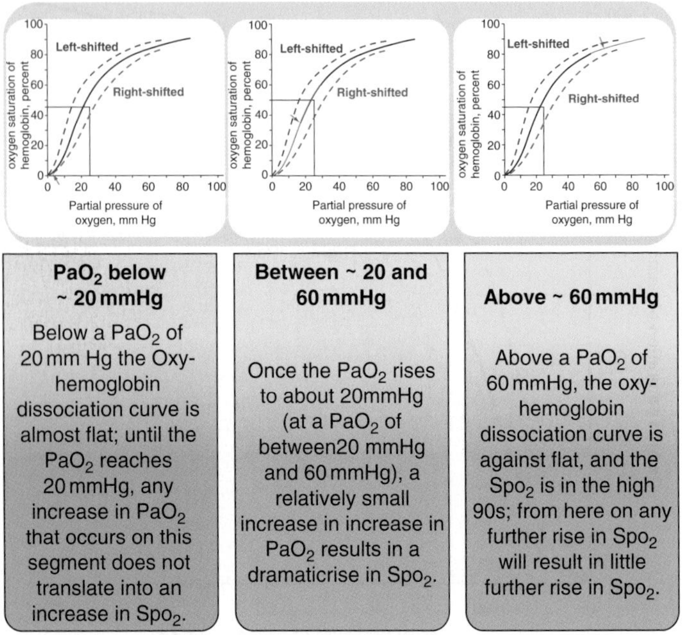
Left-shifted
Right-shifted
oxygen saturation of hemoglobin, percent
Partial pressure of oxygen, mm Hg
PaO2 below ~ 20 mmHg
Below a PaO2 of 20 mm Hg the Oxy-hemoglobin dissociation curve is almost flat; until the PaO2 reaches 20 mmHg, any increase in PaO2 that occurs on this segment does not translate into an increase in Spo2.
Between ~ 20 and 60 mmHg
Once the PaO2 rises to about 20mmHg (at a PaO2 of between20 mmHg and 60 mmHg), a relatively small increase in increase in PaO2 results in a dramaticrise in Spo2.
Above ~ 60 mmHg
Above a PaO2 of 60 mmHg, the oxy-hemoglobin dissociation curve is against flat, and the Spo2 is in the high 90s; from here on any further rise in Spo2 will result in little further rise in Spo2.

FIGURE 7.14. Hypoxemia and the oxyhemoglobin dissociation curve. (Adapted from Hasan[23])

When the oxyhemoglobin dissociation curve is shifted either to the right or to the left, PaO_2 measurement can result in underestimation or overestimation respectively, of the SpO_2.

The rightward shift of the oxyhemoglobin dissociation curve as in acidemia or fever facilitates O_2 release to the tissues; in the right-shifted curve, the hemoglobin is less saturated relative to the PaO_2. In this situation, reliance on the PaO_2 to estimate the SpO_2 would be liable to result in an overestimation of the hemoglobin saturation. Conversely, conditions such as alkalemia or hypothermia, which cause a leftward shift of the oxyhemoglobin dissociation curve, result in high oxyhemoglobin saturation relative to the PaO_2; here the PaO_2 would be liable to underestimate the SpO_2 (Figs. 7.15 and 7.16).

A time lag between a change in O_2 saturation and its detection by the oximeter can occur because signal averaging by the oximeter can take several seconds. This "response time" may be a source of potential problems in a rapidly changing clinical situation (e.g., in the case of a patient who has just been intubated). In general, the response time is shorter when the probe is placed on the earlobe rather than on the finger; the

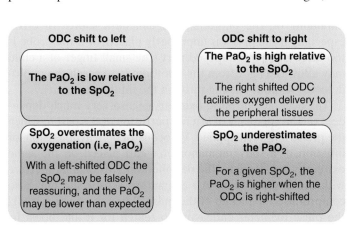

ODC shift to left	ODC shift to right
The PaO_2 is low relative to the SpO_2	**The PaO_2 is high relative to the SpO_2** The right shifted ODC facilities oxygen delivery to the peripheral tissues
SpO_2 overestimates the oxygenation (i.e, PaO_2) With a left-shifted ODC the SpO_2 may be falsely reassuring, and the PaO_2 may be lower than expected	**SpO_2 underestimates the PaO_2** For a given SpO_2, the PaO_2 is higher when the ODC is right-shifted

FIGURE 7.15. Overestimation or underestimation of PaO_2. (Adapted from Hasan[23])

Leftward shift of the ODC occurs in the following conditions:	Rightward shift of the ODC cccurs in the following conditions:
• Alkalemia • Hypothermia • Abnormal hemoglobins, eg., • *Carboxy-hemoglobin* • *Met-hemoglobin* • *Fetal hemoglobin* • Myxedema • Low inorganic phosphates	• Acidemia • Fever • Abnormal hemoglobins, eg., • *Hb kansas* • Thyrotoxicosis • Raised inorganic phosphate • Anemia • Steroid therapy

FIGURE 7.16. Conditions that can shift the oxyhemoglobin dissociation curve. (Adapted from Hasan[23])

response time is the longest when the probe is placed on a toe. With modern pulse oximeters, once the probe is clipped on, output stabilization takes less than 1 min to occur. Subsequent changes in oxygen saturations take less than 10 s to register.

It is also possible for artefactual errors to produce inaccuracies in the SpO_2 displayed. Interference by ambient light impinging on the photodetector can be a source of error, especially if the probe is improperly placed, or if the probe is too large for the interposed part (the small finger of a child may allow the light from the photodiode to reach the photodetector without passing through the interposed digit).[32]

The accuracy of pulse oximetry is also very much dependent on the adequacy of arterial perfusion of the part to which the probe has been applied. Vasoconstriction, hypotension, or inflation of a sphygmomanometer cuff placed on the same extremity can decrease the peripheral perfusion and interfere with the SpO_2 reading. An edematous sensor site may also compromise the pickup of the pulse. When the pulse is weak, the pulse oximeter endeavors to search for it and boost its amplitude, but in doing so, may amplify the background noise. A low signal-to-noise ratio can then lead to errors, but most current devices in vogue have an inbuilt program that warns the clinician of weak pulse strength. In such situations, the oximeter may simply not display the saturation.

One way to verify the accuracy of the SpO_2 in this setting is to check the amplitude of the pulse waveform. In the presence of a satisfactory waveform, the oximetric readings are likely to be correct. Another way is to compare the pulse rate on the display of the oximeter with a manually counted pulse rate. A discrepancy between the two suggests an inaccurate oximetric reading.

Besides this, motion artifact can give misleading results. Shivering, convulsions, or movement of the patient can lead to a poor signal[19,31]; proximity to MRI scanners, cellular phones, electrocautery equipment, or other sources of electromagnetic radiation can also cause interference. Fluorescent, infrared, and xenon lamps may interfere with the photodetector and cause false values to be displayed (Fig. 7.17).

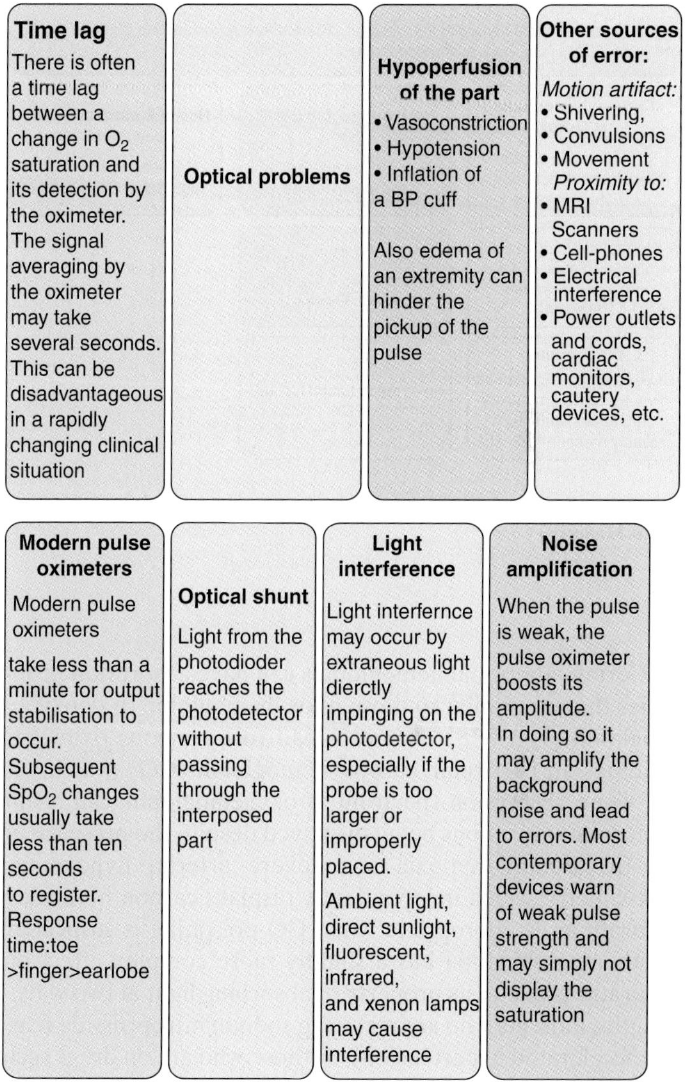
Time lag
There is often a time lag between a change in O_2 saturation and its detection by the oximeter. The signal averaging by the oximeter may take several seconds. This can be disadvantageous in a rapidly changing clinical situation
Optical problems
Hypoperfusion of the part
• Vasoconstriction
• Hypotension
• Inflation of a BP cuff
Also edema of an extremity can hinder the pickup of the pulse
Other sources of error:
Motion artifact:
• Shivering,
• Convulsions
• Movement
Proximity to:
• MRI Scanners
• Cell-phones
• Electrical interference
• Power outlets and cords, cardiac monitors, cautery devices, etc.
Modern pulse oximeters
Modern pulse oximeters
take less than a minute for output stabilisation to occur. Subsequent SpO_2 changes usually take less than ten seconds to register. Response time:toe >finger>earlobe
Optical shunt
Light from the photodioder reaches the photodetector without passing through the interposed part
Light interference
Light interfernce may occur by extraneous light dierctly impinging on the photodetector, especially if the probe is too larger or improperly placed.
Ambient light, direct sunlight, fluorescent, infrared, and xenon lamps may cause interference
Noise amplification
When the pulse is weak, the pulse oximeter boosts its amplitude. In doing so it may amplify the background noise and lead to errors. Most contemporary devices warn of weak pulse strength and may simply not display the saturation

FIGURE 7.17. Sources of error with pulse oximetry. (Adapted from Hasan[23])

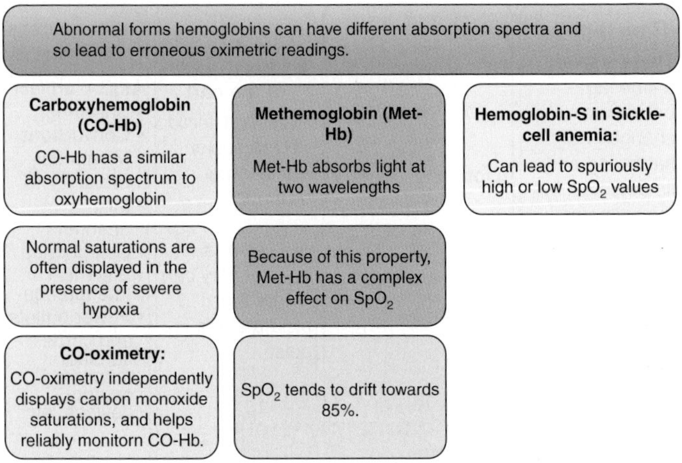
Abnormal forms hemoglobins can have different absorption spectra and so lead to erroneous oximetric readings.
Carboxyhemoglobin (CO-Hb)
CO-Hb has a similar absorption spectrum to oxyhemoglobin
Normal saturations are often displayed in the presence of severe hypoxia
CO-oximetry:
CO-oximetry independently displays carbon monoxide saturations, and helps reliably monitorn CO-Hb.
Methemoglobin (Met-Hb)
Met-Hb absorbs light at two wavelengths
Because of this property, Met-Hb has a complex effect on SpO_2
SpO_2 tends to drift towards 85%.
Hemoglobin-S in Sickle-cell anemia:
Can lead to spuriously high or low SpO_2 values

FIGURE 7.18. Absorption spectra of abnormal hemoglobins. (Adapted from Hasan[23])

Certain abnormal hemoglobins can have absorption properties that are similar to those of oxyhemoglobin or deoxyhemoglobin (Fig. 7.18). This can lead to erroneous oximetric readings. In particular, carboxyhemoglobin (CO), which has the same absorption spectrum as oxyhemoglobin, can result in normal saturations being displayed despite the presence of life-threatening hypoxia and severe arterial hypoxemia. Cooximetry, which independently displays carbon monoxide saturations, is appropriate when CO poisoning is suspected. Methemoglobinemia has a slightly more complex effect on saturations due to its property of absorbing light at two wavelengths. Patients who are receiving sodium nitroprusside (e.g., for accelerated hypertension), or those who are on drugs such as dapsone, may have methemoglobin (Met-Hb) levels that are high enough to interfere with the SpO_2 readings. Due to the special ability of Met-Hb to absorb light at two wavelengths, the SpO_2 tends to drift toward 85%.[2,61] Exceptionally, the abnormal hemoglobin in sickle cell anemia may lead to spuriously high or low readings.

The use of nail polish can lead to falsely low SpO_2 readings; it has been theorized that this occurs by shunting of the light across the periphery of the finger. Although a recent study vindicates red nail polish as a cause of error, the same is probably not true for other shades which may produce a spurious fall in the hemoglobin saturations by as much as 3–6%.[40] Placing the probe sideways over the lateral aspect of the finger has been recommended to circumvent this problem.

Skin pigmentation appears to have a small but inconsistent effect on SpO_2. The pigmentation caused by hyperbilirubinemia appears to have a negligible effect on SpO_2 readings,[38] but racial pigmentation has been shown to cause as much as 4% difference in the measured oxygen saturation.[44]

In general, anemia has no impact on the SpO_2 until the hemoglobin falls to a very low level (<5 g/dL)[43]; the effect of severe anemia on oxyhemoglobin saturation appears to occur only at an SpO_2 below 80%.

When venous congestion is present, the engorged veins can lead to venous pulsations in the peripheries. These venous pulsations may be misread by the probe as arterial.

7.3 Transcutaneous Blood Gas Monitoring

Cellular animals respire exclusively through their membranes and humans have inherited to some extent the ability to breathe through their skins. In 1851, Gierlach described the property of transdermal gas exchange. In the 1960s, it was noticed that the transcutaneous partial pressures of CO_2 and O_2 reliably reflected the partial pressures of these gases in the arterial blood.[15, 46]

Transcutaneous (TCO_2) blood gas measurement involves the placement of heated electrodes directly in contact with an appropriate skin site. The application of heat at about 42°C to the skin surface in contact with the electrode causes the dermal capillaries to dilate and suffuse the dermis with arterialized blood. This increases the oxygen supply to the epidermis. The heat also causes partial dissolution of the lipid content of the epidermal stratum corneum, enhancing the epidermal permeability to blood gases.

The O_2 and the CO_2 electrodes differ in composition. Both the electrodes are covered by relatively impermeable membranes (polyethylene or polypropylene in the case of the O_2 electrode and teflon or silastic in the case of the CO_2 electrode). The membranes are necessary to maintain the required electrolyte levels in the local milieu. The electrodes are placed over a flat part of the skin (which should be devoid of hair) and secured to the chosen site by a double-sided adhesive ring over a small drop of contact solution, the purpose of which is to increase conductivity. Attention is paid to the optimization of contact between the skin and the electrode, since even a small amount of trapped air can interfere with the accuracy of readings.

Data can be analyzed after allowing the electrodes to equilibrate with the blood, a process which requires approximately 15 min. Recalibration and rotation of the site is required every 3–4 h, and failure to rotate the electrode site as frequently as this can produce burns on the part of the skin in contact with the electrode (Fig. 7.19).

Owing to the better permeability of CO_2 as compared to O_2, the CO_2 electrode has been shown to be reliable at all ages. The accuracy of the O_2 electrode is hampered in adults, since the adult dermal layer is much thicker than that of the neonate. The

Advantages of transcutaneous O_2 monitoring	**Advantages of pulse oximetry**
• Decreased susceptibility to artefactual errors during motion	• Uncomplicated caliberation
• Ability to detect fluctuation in oxygenation over higher ranges of oxygenation	• Rapid availability of data
• Accurate estimation of PaO_2 in neonates	• Lack of need to replace membranes
	• No risk of thermal injury

FIGURE 7.19. Relative advantages of transcutaneous O_2 and pulse oximetry. (Adapted from Hasan[23])

measured transcutaneous O_2 values may be lower than the arterial PaO_2 values.[20] Even in neonates, the usefulness of transcutaneous oxygen measurement may be confined to a small subgroup with arterial oxygen tensions below 80 mmHg. Although the heated electrodes facilitate gas diffusion across the skin by inducing capillary dilation as described earlier, they also increase the metabolic activity of the dermal cells, leading to an increase in O_2 consumption as well as CO_2 production, and this can lead to inaccuracies in the measurement of these gases. For these reasons, the pulse oximeter has become the preferred noninvasive monitoring device in all age-groups (Fig. 7.19).

7.4 Monitoring Tissue Oxygenation

The respiratory, and the cardiovascular system, have one common objective – to transport oxygen from the ambient air to the tissues, where the latter is used by mitochondria for the manufacture of adenosine triphosphate (ATP). ATP serves as an energy storage depot for the diverse functions of the body. Since the utilization of the O_2 occurs within the tissues, it is relevant to assess the adequacy of oxygenation at the tissue level rather than in the blood. Unfortunately, this is not easy – for several reasons. The first and the foremost reason is the lack of knowledge as to what constitutes the normal tissue PaO_2. Due to this, the level of O_2 that defines tissue hypoxia cannot be determined. It is well known, however, that the oxygen-deprived tissues change their metabolic pathways from aerobic to anaerobic. There being no reliable bedside test to measure tissue hypoxia, the markers of anaerobic metabolism serve as surrogates for tissue hypoxia.

Although the direct measurement of intracellular oxygen by special polarographic electrodes, and measurements of regional blood flow yield information about the state of the tissue oxygenation, these methods cannot be practically applied at the bedside[56] Sophisticated techniques such as nuclear magnetic resonance spectroscopy and position emission tomography (PET) for the assessment of cellular metabolism are as yet imperfectly developed.[8,27] Infrared spectrometry which quantifies the redox state of hemoglobin, myoglobin, or cytochrome-aa, is as yet a research tool,[30] and luminescent oxygen probes, which measure the redox state of the mitochondrion, are still in a nascent stage.

Tissue hypoxia often manifests with signs of organ dysfunction. When signs of organ dysfunction such as an altered sensorium or decreasing urine output are present, the presence of tissue hypoxia should be suspected. When hypoxic tissues shift from aerobic to anaerobic metabolism, they produce lactate. The consequence of this is a fall in pH, resulting in a high anion gap metabolic acidosis. The blood lactate itself can be measured directly, providing objective data about the presence and severity of the lactic acidosis. Whether an elevated lactate level in the setting of sepsis reflects tissue hypoxia or is a consequence of alternative metabolic pathways, is as yet uncertain.[11, 58]

Much attention has been focused on the effects of hypoxia on the gastrointestinal mucosa, which seems to be especially susceptible to the effects of decreased perfusion. Deprivation of O_2 causes the gastric mucosal milieu to become acidic with a rise in intracellular CO_2. Hypoperfusion of the gastric mucosa is thought to be, but one manifestation of generalized tissue hypoperfusion. Although practical difficulties exist in the implementation of gastric tonometry, it is anticipated that future developments may lead to easier ways of its measurement.

7.4.1 Oxygen Extraction Ratio and $DO_{2\,crit}$

As mentioned earlier, the amount of oxygen carried by the arterial blood depends upon the oxygen saturation of hemoglobin and the amount of hemoglobin in the blood itself (since most of the oxygen is carried in the form of oxyhemoglobin). A much smaller quantity of oxygen is carried dissolved in the plasma. Delivery of oxygen to the tissues depends on the oxygen content of the blood (CaO_2) along with an intact transport mechanism, specifically the cardiac output (Fig. 7.20).

Arteriovenous oxygen difference: The difference between the arterial and venous content of oxygen is a measure of the

These relationships can be summarized by the formula,

$$DO_2 = [(1.34 \times Hb \times SpO_2) + (0.0031 \times PaO_2)] \times CO,$$

where

DO_2	= Oxygen delivery to the tissues
Hb	= Hemoglobin concentration in the blood
SpO_2	= Percentage of hemoglobin saturation with oxygen
PaO_2	= Partial pressure of oxygen in the arterial blood (arterial blood oxygen tension)
CO	= Cardiac output

FIGURE 7.20. Oxygen delivery (DO_2).

oxygen extracted by the tissues. The oxygen content of the arterial blood (CaO_2), is approximately 20 mL of O_2/dL of arterial blood, whereas the oxygen content of the venous blood, CvO_2, is approximately 15 mL of O_2/dL of venous blood. VO_2, or oxygen consumption, can be directly measured in mechanically ventilated patients.[18] The accuracy of this method is questionable at FIO_2 in excess of 0.8.[13,50,59]

The tissue oxygen consumption can also be calculated from the Fick equation, a discussion on which is beyond the scope of this book.

Oxygen extraction ratio: Another way of looking at the O_2 consumed by tissues is the oxygen extraction ratio:

$$O_2ER = (CaO_2 - CvO_2)/CaO_2.$$

Any increase in the metabolic activity results in an increase in O_2 consumption (VO_2) by the tissues. Increased tissue oxygen consumption in metabolic stress is paralleled by an increase in the cardiac output, resulting in increased O_2 delivery to the tissues (DO_2). Since the increase in O_2 delivery is of a smaller magnitude than the increase in O_2 consumption (VO_2) by the tissues, the demand exceeds the supply. As a result, the difference in the arteriovenous O_2 content increases and the O_2 extraction ratio is consequently higher.

When DO_2 decreases for some reason such as a decreased cardiac output, for a given VO_2, the OER increases.[5] In other words, there is an increase in the tissue extraction of oxygen relative to the O_2 delivery. This relationship does not seem to hold at all levels of O_2 delivery. Below a certain limit called the critical delivery of oxygen ($DO_{2\,crit}$), the oxygen consumption by the tissues actually decreases even as the O_2 delivery falls. The $DO_{2\,crit}$ is seen to occur at relatively high levels of oxygen delivery in patients with sepsis or ARDS. Several theories have been proposed to explain this pathological dependence of VO_2 on DO_2,[53] not the least of which is a proposed decrease in the oxygen extraction or utilization process.[53] The methodology of many of the studies establishing the pathological dependence of VO_2 on DO_2 has been called into question[12] and it has been proposed that the link between VO_2 and DO_2 may be artifactual.[41] If there is indeed a pathological dependence of VO_2 on DO_2, the implication of this pathological dependency, translated into clinical terms, raises the question as to whether supernormal levels of O_2 delivery would have a favorable impact, for which at least at the present time, there seems to be no supporting evidence.

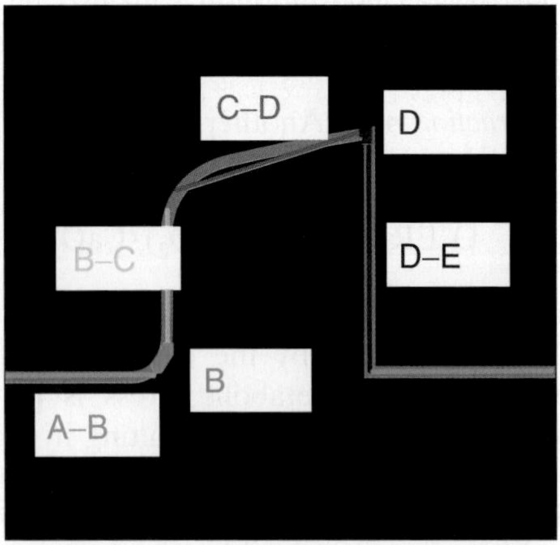
C–D
D
B–C
D–E
B
A–B

FIGURE 7.21. Parts of the capnographic waveform. (Adapted from Hasan[23])

The capnographic wave form can be divided into six distinct parts. The tracing begins with the analysis of the expired air.

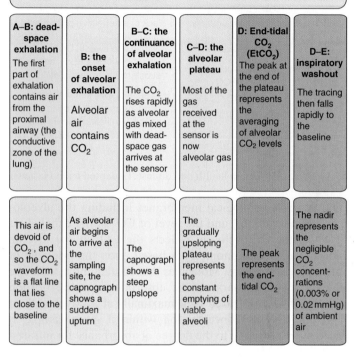

A–B: dead-space exhalation The first part of exhalation contains air from the proximal airway (the conductive zone of the lung)	**B: the onset of alveolar exhalation** Alveolar air contains CO_2	**B–C: the continuance of alveolar exhalation** The CO_2 rises rapidly as alveolar gas mixed with dead-space gas arrives at the sensor	**C–D: the alveolar plateau** Most of the gas received at the sensor is now alveolar gas	**D: End-tidal CO_2 ($EtCO_2$)** The peak at the end of the plateau represents the averaging of alveolar CO_2 levels	**D–E: inspiratory washout** The tracing then falls rapidly to the baseline
This air is devoid of CO_2, and so the CO_2 waveform is a flat line that lies close to the baseline	As alveolar air begins to arrive at the sampling site, the capnograph shows a sudden upturn	The capnograph shows a steep upslope	The gradually upsloping plateau represents the constant emptying of viable alveoli	The peak represents the end-tidal CO_2	The nadir represents the negligible CO_2 concent-rations (0.003% or 0.02 mmHg) of ambient air

FIGURE 7.21. (continued)

7.5 Capnography

As discussed in some detail in Chap. 3, section 3.6, the adequacy of alveolar ventilation can be judged by the analysis of arterial CO_2 tension ($PaCO_2$). ABG analysis involves arterial puncture which is painful, inconvenient, and capable of causing complications. Alveolar ventilation can also be monitored by analyzing the exhaled air for CO_2. Carbon dioxide, being more easily diffusible through tissues than oxygen, passes

PetCO$_2$ in health:	PetCO$_2$ in disease:
• The value of PetCO$_2$ is close to the value of PACO$_2$; and therefore to that of PaCO$_2$. PaCO$_2$ and PACO$_2$ differ by such a small amount (generally < 5mm) such as usually makes no clinical difference. • The trends in PetCO$_2$ closely match the trends in PaCO$_2$	• In disease, physiological dead-space is often increased because of patent but under-perfused alveoli. Due to the lack of an effective pulmonary circulation CO$_2$ cannot effectively diffuse into alveoli. Under such circumstances, PaCO$_2$ can substantially exceed PetCO$_2$ • In spite of this, in the absence of major *changes* in dead-space ventilation, the PetCO$_2$ trends still match those of PaCO$_2$

FIGURE 7.22. PetCO$_2$ in health and disease. (Adapted from Hasan[23])

quickly across biological membranes including the alveolo-capillary membrane, and the level of CO_2 in the exhaled air (P_ECO_2) therefore closely reflects the CO_2 in the arterial blood ($PaCO_2$). Capnometry is based upon the principle of infrared spectroscopy. Molecules that contain more than one element possess characteristic absorption spectra. Carbon dioxide absorbs infrared light maximally at a wavelength of 4.26 μm, and its concentration within a given sample is directly proportional to the degree of absorbance for infrared light that the sample possesses.

The terms capnography and capnometry are often used interchangeably, but semantically speaking, the term capnometry should be applied to the process of displaying the value of the CO_2 in the breath as a partial pressure or percentage while capnography is the analysis of the rise and fall of CO_2 over time, with continuously displayed data or waveforms. Capnography provides information about specific clinical conditions (Fig. 7.23), determines the adequacy of gas sampling, and is capable of detecting leaks in machine tubings.

Analysis of CO_2 from the end-tidal breath is accomplished by systems that sample the exhaled air either at the airway (mainstream analyzers) or draw the gas away to a sampler situated at some distance from the airway itself (sidestream analyzers). The

Factors increasing $PetCO_2$	Factors decreasing $PetCO_2$
Increase in CO_2 production: Fever and hyperpyrexia Sodium bicarbonate infusion Release of a tourniquet CO_2 embolism	**Decreased CO_2 production:** Hypothermia
Increase in pulmonary perfusion: Increase in cardiac output Increase in blood pressure	**Decrease in pulmonary perfusion:** Decreased cardiac output Fall in blood pressure Hypovolemia Pulmonary embolism
Decrease in alveolar ventilation: Hypoventilation of any cause	**Increase in alveolar ventilation:** Hyperventilation
Airway related problems Bronchial intubation Partial airway obstruction	**Airway related problems** Accidental extubation Partial or complete airway obstruction Apnea
Machine-related factors: CO_2 scrubber used up Insufficient inflow of fresh gas Leaks in circuit Malfunctioning ventilator valves	**Machine-related factors:** Circuit disconnection Leak in sampling tube Malfunction of ventilator

FIGURE 7.23. Changes in $PetCO_2$. (Adapted from Shankar[47])

end-tidal CO_2 ($P_{et}CO_2$) is measured and displayed on a breath-to-breath basis and the capnogram shows the changing CO_2 tension in the respired air throughout the respiratory cycle.

Since CO_2 is an easily diffusible gas with respect to biological membranes, the drop in the end-tidal CO_2 tension relative to arterial CO_2 is only about 2–5 mmHg.[24,36] However, this is at best a rough approximation, and in disease, the end-tidal CO_2 may be prone to substantial variation. Discrepancy between the $PaCO_2$ and the $P_{et}CO_2$ can occur when there is an increase in the dead space, or if a significant *V*/*Q* mismatch occurs.[25,40] The impact of pulmonary disease on $P_{et}CO_2$ is unpredictable and widening of the gradient often occurs. On rare occasions, when large tidal volumes are used to inflate the lungs with low-*V*/*Q* ratios, the $P_{et}CO_2$ may actually exceed the $PaCO_2$[26,35] (Fig. 7.23).

When the difference between the $PetCO_2$ and $PaCO_2$ increases, this usually means an expansion in dead space. On rare occasions, a sharp increase in CO_2 production can widen the $PetCO_2$–$PaCO_2$ difference (A–aCO_2) (see Fig. 7.24).

High concentrations of either oxygen or nitrous oxide may cause variations in the capnogram as both these gases have similar infrared spectra to CO_2[27] and correction factors should be applied when mixtures of these gases are breathed.[45] Sidestream analyzers have a significant time lag before the sampled gas values are reported. High respiratory rates can be problematic, since the response time of the instrument can be rather slow. When metered dose inhalers are used, the introduction of aerosols into the respired air can falsely elevate the $P_{et}CO_2$ (when end-tidal CO_2 analyzers that use mass spectrometry are employed). This is not the case with end-tidal CO_2 analyzers that operate on the principle of infrared spectrometry[14] (Fig. 7.25).

Sidestream analyzers are prone to blockages in the tubing system and contamination of the sampling chambers by secretions or condensate. In addition, poor gas sampling by an overly long sampling tube or an extremely high sampling rate may decrease the accuracy of the $P_{et}CO_2$. These problems can be surmounted by the use of shorter tubing, in-circuit traps, and periodic purging of the sample tubing. Sidestream analyzers can be used in the absence of an artificial airway, whereas mainstream analyzers cannot (Fig. 7.26).

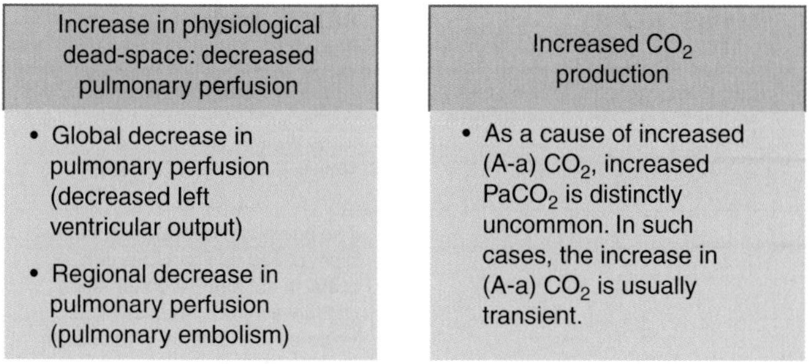
Increase in physiological dead-space: decreased pulmonary perfusion
• Global decrease in pulmonary perfusion (decreased left ventricular output)
• Regional decrease in pulmonary perfusion (pulmonary embolism)
Increased CO_2 production
• As a cause of increased (A-a) CO_2, increased $PaCO_2$ is distinctly uncommon. In such cases, the increase in (A-a) CO_2 is usually transient.

FIGURE 7.24. Increased $PetCO_2$–$PaCO_2$ gradient. (Adapted from Hasan[23])

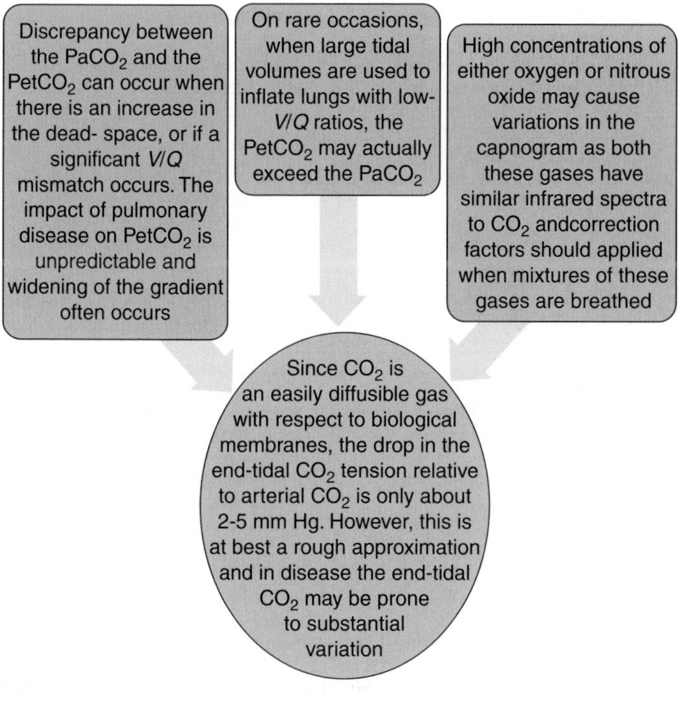
Discrepancy between the $PaCO_2$ and the $PetCO_2$ can occur when there is an increase in the dead- space, or if a significant *V/Q* mismatch occurs. The impact of pulmonary disease on $PetCO_2$ is unpredictable and widening of the gradient often occurs
On rare occasions, when large tidal volumes are used to inflate lungs with low-*V/Q* ratios, the $PetCO_2$ may actually exceed the $PaCO_2$
High concentrations of either oxygen or nitrous oxide may cause variations in the capnogram as both these gases have similar infrared spectra to CO_2 andcorrection factors should applied when mixtures of these gases are breathed
Since CO_2 is an easily diffusible gas with respect to biological membranes, the drop in the end-tidal CO_2 tension relative to arterial CO_2 is only about 2-5 mm Hg. However, this is at best a rough approximation and in disease the end-tidal CO_2 may be prone to substantial variation

FIGURE 7.25. Discrepancy between $PetCO_2$ and $PaCO_2$. (Adapted from Hasan[23])

MAINSTREAM	SIDE STREAM
The main unit incorporating a CO2 sensor is itself directly attached to a T- adapter interposed between the ET and the patient-circuit.	A relatively long sampling tube connected to the piece draws away the gas sample to a CO2 sensor located in a central unit.
	The sampling flow rate can be as high as 150 ml / min.This can result in substantial deformation of the waveform when low tidal volumes are used as in neonates and infants.
There is no sampling tube. Sensor windows are prone to clogging by secretions, aerosols or water droplets.	Sampling tube prone to becoming obstructed: secretion can be sucked in by the rapid aspiration rate.
Difficult to use in patients undergoing prone ventilation.	Relatively easy to connect in prone position
Unaffected by changes in water vapour pressure.The temperature within the mainstream sensors is maintained at around 39°C to prevent condensation.	Affected by changes in water vapour pressure.
No time lag.	Time lag in display, owing to the relatively long distance that the sensor is placed from the patient's airway.
Cannot be used in the absence of an artificial airway.	Can be used even in the absence of an artificial airway.
Sterilization is difficult	Easy to sterilize
Bulky – newer models less so. Can increase circuit dead-space & so elevate PaCO2	Side stream capnometers using micro-stream technology have been developed.These use sampling flow rates of as low as 50 ml/min. The emitted wavelength is within a narrower IR band (4.2 – 4.35 hm) and this more closely matches the absorption spectrum for CO2.

FIGURE 7.26. Mainstream and sidestream sensors.

Being closer to the airway, mainstream analyzers have a quicker response time, but the proximity also makes them prone to contamination by airway secretions. Also, a large sampling window can lead to the introduction of a substantial dead space into the ventilator circuit, itself producing a rise in the arterial CO_2 tension. The earlier models of mainstream analyzers were bulky and tended to drag on the artificial airway. The newer mainstream analyzers are smaller and lighter.

As is apparent in the discussion above, trends in arterial O_2 can be matched by the $P_{et}CO_2$ when the lungs are healthy. But in cases of pulmonary disease, especially in a situation where there is unstable or evolving lung pathology, the end-tidal CO_2 will neither reflect nor parallel changes in $PaCO_2$, and this must be kept in mind.

Capnographic tracings in various conditions are shown in Fig. 7.27.

Capnography can also help differentiate between asphyxic from primary cardiac arrest: in asphyxic cardiac arrest, $PetCO_2$ is extremely high, whereas in primary cardiac arrest the rise tends to be more moderate.[22] can prove a valuable guide to the effectiveness and outcome of cardiopulmonary resuscitation (CPR).[6, 16, 21, 42] A rise in $PetCO_2$ is often the earliest indicator of the revival of the hemodynamics during CPR. Baseline $PetCO_2$ is transiently raised with the return of spontaneous circulation following successful resuscitation. This reflects the elimination of the CO_2-buildup in tissues. Conversely, a drop in $PetCO_2$ in a patient who has just been successfully resuscitated may indicate the need for resumption of CPR A drop in $PetCO_2$ in such a patient should prompt a recheck of the pulse. In a patient with pulseless electrical activity, the $PetCO_2$ measured at 20 min after the commencement of CPR can prove a valuable guide to outcome. A $PetCO_2$ of <10 mmHg after 20 min CPR usually means that further continuation of CPR is unlikely to be fruitful, whereas $PetCO_2$ >18 mmHg usually heralds a successful outcome to the CPR. As such, no specific number can be used as a cut off value in distinguishing survivors from nonsurvivors. It is believed that the chances for survival increase by 16% for every 1 mmHg the $etCO_2$ rises.[21]

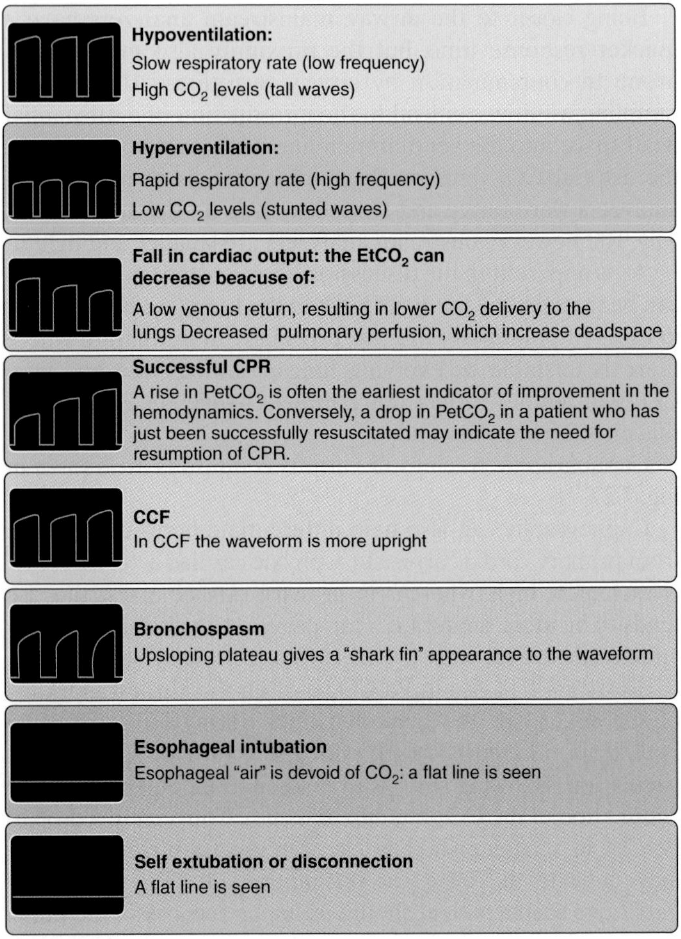
Hypoventilation:
Slow respiratory rate (low frequency)
High CO_2 levels (tall waves)
Hyperventilation:
Rapid respiratory rate (high frequency)
Low CO_2 levels (stunted waves)
Fall in cardiac output: the $EtCO_2$ can decrease beacuse of:
A low venous return, resulting in lower CO_2 delivery to the lungs Decreased pulmonary perfusion, which increase deadspace
Successful CPR
A rise in $PetCO_2$ is often the earliest indicator of improvement in the hemodynamics. Conversely, a drop in $PetCO_2$ in a patient who has just been successfully resuscitated may indicate the need for resumption of CPR.
CCF
In CCF the waveform is more upright
Bronchospasm
Upsloping plateau gives a "shark fin" appearance to the waveform
Esophageal intubation
Esophageal "air" is devoid of CO_2: a flat line is seen
Self extubation or disconnection
A flat line is seen

FIGURE 7.27. Capnographs in different medical conditions. (Adapted from Hasan[23])

It is possible to distinguish congestive cardiac failure from bronchospasm on the basis of capnography (Fig. 7.27). The capnographic tracing in bronchospasm shows a slow rise, often likened to a shark's fin. Because of bronchospasm, the CO_2 from the peripheral airspaces arrives late at the CO_2 sensor.

The capnograpic tracing can be valuable in verifying the position of the endotracheal tube after a difficult intubation. Since the source of CO_2 is the lung, any detectable CO_2 on the tracing can only mean that the endotracheal tube resides within the tracheobronchial tree (Fig. 7.27). In contrast, CO_2 will be undetectable if the endotracheal tube has been inadvertently placed within the esophagus.

References

1. Annat G, Viale JP, Percival C, et al Oxygen delivery and uptake in the adult respiratory distress syndrome. Lack of relationship when measured independently in patients with normal blood lactate concentrations. *Am Rev Respir Dis*. 1986;133:999
2. Barker SJ, Tremper KK, Hyatt J. Effects of methemoglobinemia on pulse oximetry and mixed venous oximetry. *Anesthesiology*. 1989;70:112
3. Bhavani SK, Moseley H, Kumar AY, Delph Y. Capnometry and anaesthesia. Review article. *Can J Anaesth*. 1992;39(6):617–32
4. Bhavani SK (2007) Factors influencing PetCO_2. Welcome to capnography.com. Accessed March 2007
5. Cain SM. Oxygen delivery and uptake in dogs during anemic and hypoxic hypoxia. *J Appl Physiol*. 1977;42:228
6. Callaham M, Barton C. Prediction of outcome of cardiopulmonary resuscitation from end-tidal carbon dioxide concentration. *Crit Care Med*. 1990;18:358
7. Carter BG, Carlin JB, Tibballs J, et al Accuracy of two pulse oximeters at low arterial hemoglobin-oxygen saturation. *Crit Care Med*. 1998;26:1128
8. Clark BJ, Smith D, Chance B. Metabolic consequences of oxygen transport studied with phosphorus nuclear magnetic resonance spectroscopy. In: Bryan-Brown C, Ayres SM, eds. *Oxygen Transport and Utilization*. Fullerton: Society of Critical Care Medicine; 1987:145–170
9. Criner JC, D'Alonzo GE. *Pulmonary Pathophysiology*. Madison: Fence Creek; 1999
10. Curtis SE, Cain SM. Regional and systemic oxygen delivery/uptake relations and lactate flux in hyperdynamic, endotoxin-treated dogs. *Am Rev Respir Dis*. 1992;145:348

11. Danek SJ, Lynch JP, Weg JG, Dantzker DR. The dependence of oxygen uptake on oxygen delivery on the adult respiratory distress syndrome. *Am Rev Respir Dis*. 1980;122:387
12. Dantzker D. Oxygen delivery and utilisation in sepsis. *Crit Care Clin*. 1989;5:81
13. Dantzker DR, Foresman B, Gutierrez G. Oxygen supply and utilisation relationships. *Am Rev Respir Dis*. 1991;143:675
14. Elliot WR, Raemer DB, Goldman DB, Phillip JH. The effects of bronchodilator aerosol propellants on respiratory gas monitors. *J Clin Monit*. 1991;7:175–180
15. Evans NTS, Naylor PRD. The systemic oxygen supply to the surface of human skin. *Respir Physiol*. 1967;3:21
16. Falk JL, Rackow ED, Weil MH. End-tidal carbon dioxide concentration during cardiopulmonary resuscitation. *N Engl J Med*. 1988;318(10):607–611
17. Fanconi S. Pulse oximetry for hypoxemia – a warning to users and manufacturers. *Intensive Care Med*. 1989;15:540
18. Feenstra B, et al Design and validation of an automatic metabolic monitor. *Intensive Care Med*. 1985;11:95
19. Grace RF. Pulse oximetry: gold standard or false sense of security? *Med J Aust*. 1994;160:638
20. Green GE, Hassel KT, Mahutte CK. Comparison of arterial blood gas with continuous intraarterial and transcutaneous PO_2 sensor in adult critically ill patients. *Crit Care Med*. 1987;15:491
21. Grmec S, Klemen P. Does the end-tidal carbon dioxide ($ETCO_2$) concentration have prognostic value during out-of-hospital cardiac arrest? *J Emerg Med*. 2001;8:263–269
22. Grmec S, Lah K, Tusek-Bunc K. Difference in end-tidal CO_2 between asphyxia cardiac arrest and ventricular fibrillation/pulseless ventricular tachycardia cardiac arrest in the prehospital setting. *Crit Care*. 2003;7:R139–R144
23. Hasan A. *Handbook of Blood Gas/Acid-Base Interpretation*. London: Springer; 2009
24. Hattle L, Rokseth R. The arterial to end-expiratory carbon dioxide tension gradient in acute pulmonary embolism and other cardiopulmonary diseases. *Chest*. 1974;66:352
25. Hess D. Capnometry and capnography: technical aspects, physiologic aspects, and clinical applications. *Respir Care*. 1990;35:557
26. Hess DR, Branson RD. Non invasive respiratory monitoring equipment. In: Branson RD, Hess DR, Chatburn RL, eds. *Respiratory Care Equipment*. Philadelphia: Lippincott Williams & Wilkins; 1994:184–216

27. Hotchkiss RS, Rust RS, Dence CS, et al Evaluation of the role of cellular hypoxia in sepsis by the hypoxic marker (18F) fluoromisonidazole. *Am J Physiol.* 1991;261:R965
28. Isserles S, Breen PH. Can changes in end-tidal PCO_2 measure changes in cardiac output? *Anesth Anagl.* 1991;73:808
29. Mancini DM, Bolinger L, Li K, et al Validation of near-infrared spectroscopy in humans. *J Appl Physiol.* 1994;77:2740
30. Martin L. Abbreviating the alveolar gas equation. An argument for simplicity. *Respir Care.* 1986;31:40
31. Mendelson Y. Pulse oximetry: theory and applications for noninvasive monitoring. *Clin Chem.* 1992;38:1601
32. Mengelkoch LJ, Martin D, Lawler J. A review of the principles of pulse oximetry and accuracy of pulse oximeter estimates during exercise. *Phys Ther.* 1994;74:40
33. Mira JP, Fabre JE, Baigorri F, et al Lack of oxygen supply dependency in patients with severe sepsis: A study of oxygen delivery increased by military antishock trouser and dobutamine. *Chest.* 1994;106:1524
34. Moorthy SS, Losasso AM, Wilcox J. End-tidal PCO_2 greater than $PaCO_2$. *Crit Care Med.* 1984;12:534
35. Neff TA. Routine oximetry: a fifth vital sign? *Chest.* 1988;94:22
36. Nunn JF, Hill DW. Respiratory dead space and arterial to end-tidal CO_2 tension in anesthetised man. *J Appl Physiol.* 1960;15:383
37. Palmisano BW, Severinghaus JW. Transcutaneous PCO_2 and PO_2: a multicenter study of accuracy. *J Clin Monit.* 1990;6:189
38. Poets CF, Southall DP. Noninvasive monitoring and oxygenation in infants and children: practical considerations and areas of concern. *Pediatrics.* 1994;93:737
39. Raemer DB, Frances D, Philip JH, et al Variation in PCO_2 between arterial blood and peak expired gas during anesthesia. *Anesth Analg.* 1983;62:1065
40. Ralston AC, Webb RK, Runciman WB. Potential errors in pulse oximetry. *Anesthesia.* 1991;46(3):202–206
41. Russell JA, Phang PT. The oxygen delivery/consumption controversy: approaches to management of the critically ill. *Am J Respir Crit Care Med.* 1994;149:533
42. Sanders AB, Kern KB, Otto CW, et al End-tidal carbon dioxide monitoring during cardiopulmonary resuscitation: a prognostic indicator for survival. *JAMA.* 1989;262:1347
43. Schnapp LM, Cohen NH. Pulse oximetry: uses and abuses. *Chest.* 1990;98:1244
44. Severinghaus JW. Methods of measurement of blood and gas carbon dioxide during anesthesia. *Anesthesiology.* 1960;21:717

45. Severinghaus JW, Larson CP, Eger EI. Correction factor for infrared carbondioxide pressure broadening by nitrogen, nitrous oxide and cyclopropane. *Anesthesiology*. 1961;22:429–432
46. Severinghaus JW, Kelleher JF. Recent developments in pulse oximetry. *Anesthesiology*. 1992;76:1018
47. Shankar B. Factors influencing $PetCO_2$; March 2007: Welcome to capnography.com
48. Shankar KB, Moseley H, Kumar Y. Arterial to end-tidal carbon dioxide tension differences during caesarean section anesthesia. *Anesth*. 1986;41:678
49. Shepard AP. Local control of tissue DO_2 and its contribution to the regulation of cardiac output. *Am J Physiol*. 1973;225:747
50. Shibutani K, Shirasaki S, Braaz T, et al Changes in cardiac output affect $PetCO_2$, CO_2 transport, and O_2 uptake during unsteady state in humans. *J Clin Monit*. 1992;8:175–176
51. Shoemaker WC, Appel PL, Kram HB. Role of oxygen debt in the development of organ failure sepsis and death in high-risk surgical patients. *Chest*. 1992;102:208
52. Silverman HJ. Lack of relationship between induced changes in oxygen consumption and changes in lactate levels. *Chest*. 1991; 100:1012
53. Sorbini CA, Grassi V, Solinas E, et al Arterial oxygen tension in relation to age in healthy subjects. *Respiration*. 1968;25:3–13
54. Stamlo JS, Jia L, Eu JP, et al Blood flow regulation by S-notrosohemoglobin in the physiological oxygen gradient. *Science*. 1997;276:2034–2037
55. Vallet B, Lund N, Curtis SE, et al Gut and muscle tissue PO_2 in endotoxemic dogs during shock and resuscitation. *J Appl Physiol*. 1994;76:793
56. Vary TC, Siegel JH, Nakatani T, et al Effect of sepsis on activity of pyruvate dehydrogenase complex in skeletal muscle and liver. *Am J Physiol*. 1986;250:634
57. Vermeij CG, Feenstra B, Adrichen WJ, Bruining HA. Independent oxygen uptake and oxygen delivery in septic and postoperative patients. *Chest*. 1991;99:1438
58. Weinger MB, Brimm JE. End-tidal carbon dioxide as a measure of arterial carbon dioxide during intermittent mandatory ventilation. *J Clin Monit*. 1987;3:73
59. Whitsel R, Asiddao C, Golman D, et al Relationship between arterial and peak expired carbon dioxide pressure during anesthesia and factors influencing the difference. *Anesth Analg*. 1981;60:508

60. Wood LDH, Engel LA, Griffin P, et al Effect of gas physical properties and flow on lower pulmonary resistance. *J Appl Physiol.* 1975;41:234–244
61. Wright RO, Lewander WJ, Woolf AD. Methemoglobinemia: etiology, pharmacology, and clinical management. *Ann Emerg Med.* 1999;34:646

Chapter 8
Monitoring Lung Mechanics in the Mechanically Ventilated Patient

A discussion on lung compliance and airway resistance can be found in Chap. 3.

8.1 Ventilator Waveforms

Ventilator waveforms are the graphical depictions of patient-ventilator interactions.

Ventilators are technologically limited as generators of volume, pressure, or flow. No ventilator can deliver an ideal breath: the precise waveform desired by the clinician cannot be fashioned by the machine. Because of the multiplicity of ways that the patient can interact with the ventilator, the shapes of these waveforms can be subject to considerable variation.

The graphs to follow are presented as idealized waveforms; in "real life," recordings are invariably altered by the noise that the vibration and turbulence of air flow inevitably produce. The diagrams are illustrative, and not drawn to scale.

Waveforms are classified as scalars and loops. *Scalars* are real-time displays of volume, pressure, and flow (they are the measurements of volume, pressure, and flow that are graphed against time). *Loops* are the tracings of volume plotted against pressure or of flow against volume.

A. Hasan, *Understanding Mechanical Ventilation*,
DOI: 10.1007/978-1-84882-869-8_8,

8.2 Scalars

8.2.1 The Pressure–Time scalar

8.2.1.1 Airway Pressures

Before examining the pressure–time scalar, the pressure changes that occur within the airway during a respiratory cycle will be briefly introduced here (see also sections 3.3 & 3.4).

Peak Airway Pressures

During a ventilator-driven tidal breath, the airway pressure rises rapidly to a peak. This is the peak airway pressure (peak inflation pressure, P_pk, PIP) – the maximum pressure recorded within the airway during a ventilator-delivered breath. The peak airway pressure is influenced both by airway resistance and compliance; therefore, the peak airway pressure can be high either on account of narrowed airways or stiff lung (Fig. 8.1).

Plateau Pressures

At the end of inspiration, the airway pressure falls to a plateau as the air diffuses out to the periphery of the

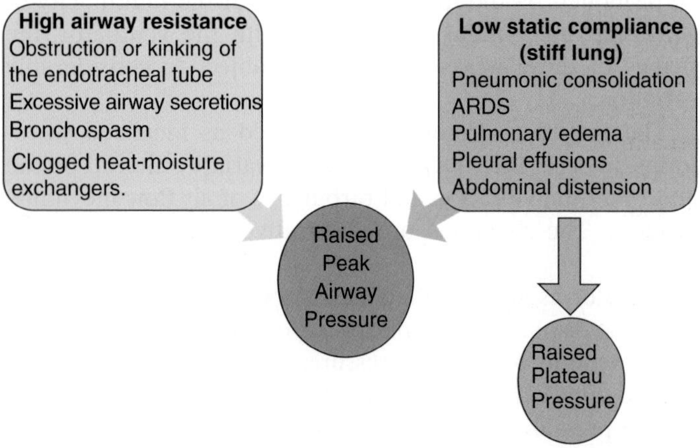
High airway resistance
Obstruction or kinking of the endotracheal tube
Excessive airway secretions
Bronchospasm
Clogged heat-moisture exchangers.
Low static compliance (stiff lung)
Pneumonic consolidation
ARDS
Pulmonary edema
Pleural effusions
Abdominal distension
Raised Peak Airway Pressure
Raised Plateau Pressure

FIGURE 8.1. Causes of raised peak airway pressure.

tracheobronchial tree. The pressure within the airway during this period of no airflow is called the pause pressure or the plateau pressure, p_{pl}. The pause pressure is a reflection of the static compliance (Section 3.1), and so, any condition that stiffens the lung will increase the pause pressure.

Mean Airway Pressure

From the hemodynamic angle, both the magnitude of the airway pressure and the time for which it is sustained are important. The level of airway pressure and the duration for which it is raised above the baseline are both factored into the mean airway pressure, which is in essence the area under the pressure–time curve. When the inspiratory flow rate is reduced, the peak airway pressure is lower; but since inspiration is now prolonged, the airway pressure is likely to remain positive for a longer duration of time. As a result, the area under the curve is not greatly reduced: manipulation of the inspiratory flow will not serve to alter the mean airway pressure to any great extent. For the same reason, when an inspiratory-hold is used at the end of inflation – with the intent of improving the oxygenation – the airway pressure will remain positive for a longer period of time, and this will elevate the mean airway pressure (Fig. 8.2).

When hemodynamic compromise occurs on account of raised airway pressures, it is the mean airway pressure that shows the closest relationship with the effect of positive pressure breathing upon the circulation.

The progress of airway pressures during a volume-targeted breath is set out in Fig. 8.3

At any given point (P) on the pressure–time curve, the pressure it takes to expand the lung (P_{ao}) is the sum of the alveolar pressure (P_{alv}) and the flow-resistive pressure (P_{ta}). The P_{ao} is measured as the peak airway pressure (*syn* peak inspiratory pressure, PIP) at the end of the breath; the P_{alv} can be measured during an applied pause (the pause pressure).

Lung Compliance

The pause pressure tends to be raised in conditions that stiffen the lung (i.e., in conditions where static compliance is

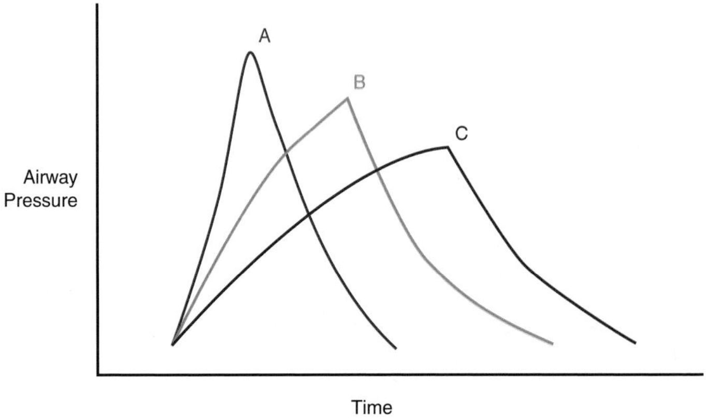
A
B
C
Airway Pressure
Time

FIGURE 8.2. Effect of flow rate on airway pressures. Three separate respiratory cycles are shown, represented by curves A, B, and C. The mean airway pressure for each breath is the area under its curve. Compared to the breath A, inspiratory flow has been deliberately lowered in breath B, and further reduced in breath C. As a consequence, a lower peak airway pressure is obtained; but it now takes longer for the breath to be completed, and the airway pressures remain elevated above the baseline for a longer time. Compared to A, although the peak airway pressure is lower, the area under curve B remains undiminished. In other words, a reduced flow rate results in a lower peak airway pressure but not necessarily a lower mean airway pressure.

reduced); conditions that increase airway resistance do not produce an appreciable rise in pause pressure. Therefore, if the peak and pause pressures are both high, the lung is likely to be stiff (noncompliant); whereas if the peak pressure is raised and the pause pressure is not, airway obstruction is likely to be present (Fig. 8.4).

The calculation of dynamic compliance is based upon peak airway pressure: a fall in *dynamic* compliance will parallel any rise in *peak* airway pressure. Similarly, calculations for static compliance take pause pressure into account: any rise in *pause* pressure will be accompanied by a fall in the *static*

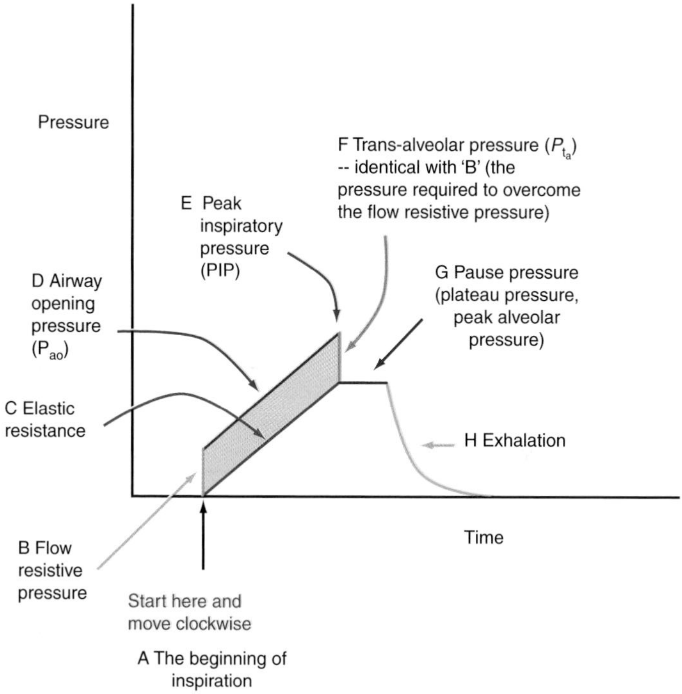
Pressure
F Trans-alveolar pressure (P_{ta}) -- identical with 'B' (the pressure required to overcome the flow resistive pressure)
E Peak inspiratory pressure (PIP)
G Pause pressure (plateau pressure, peak alveolar pressure)
D Airway opening pressure (P_{ao})
C Elastic resistance
H Exhalation
Time
B Flow resistive pressure
Start here and move clockwise
A The beginning of inspiration

A. The beginning of inspiration. The presence of a negative deflection here would mean that the breath is patient-triggered. Its absence means that the ventilator is responsible for triggering the breath.

B. The initial rise in airway pressure is on account of the resistance offered by the ETT and ventilator circuit. This pressure is called the flow resistive pressure or the trans-airway pressure (Pta) represented by the vertical print line.

C. As the lung begins to distend, pressure is required to overcome its resistive and elastic components. The pressure it takes to overcome elastic forces is the peak alveolar pressure (Palv); it is represented on the figure by the blue line that lies below and parallel to the Pao tracing red line.

D. When a constant flow is applied—the square waveform—there is a gradual but uniform rate of rise in the airway opening pressure until the entire tidal volume has been delivered.

E. The peak inspiratory pressure is reached at the end of inspiration.

F. The difference between the airway opening pressure (PAO) and the alveolar pressure (PA) is the flow-resistive pressure (also called the trans-airway pressure), that is, the pressure due to the airflow through the ventilator circuit. The flow resistive pressure rises in parallel to the alveolar pressure. The alveolar pressure is the pressure due to the elastic recoil of the airways and alveoli.

G. End inspiratory pause. This is represents the plateau pressure.

H. Exhalation

FIGURE 8.3. Pressure–time scalar of a volume-targeted breath.

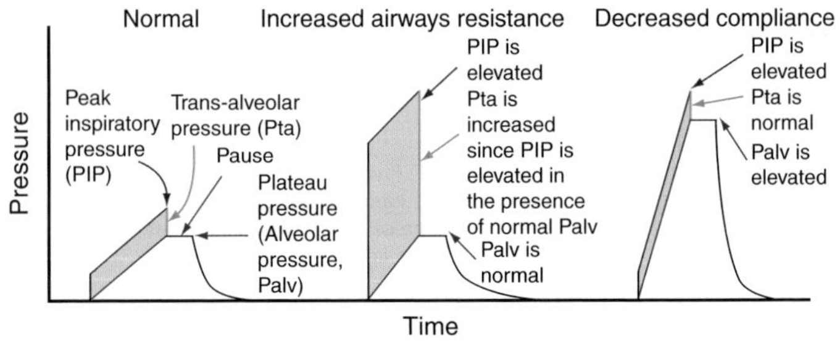
Normal
Increased airways resistance
Decreased compliance
Pressure
Time
Peak inspiratory pressure (PIP)
Trans-alveolar pressure (Pta)
Pause
Plateau pressure (Alveolar pressure, Palv)
PIP is elevated
Pta is increased since PIP is elevated in the presence of normal Palv
Palv is normal
PIP is elevated
Pta is normal
Palv is elevated

FIGURE 8.4. Pressure–time scalar: increased airway resistance and decreased compliance.

TABLE 8.1. Static and dynamic compliances in various lung conditions

Lung condition	Dynamic compliance	Static compliance
Cardiogenic pulmonary edema	Decreased	Decreased
ARDS	Decreased	Decreased
Bronchospasm without dynamic hyperinflation	Decreased	Unchanged
Bronchospasm with dynamic hyperinflation	Decreased	Decreased
Atelectasis	Decreased	Decreased
Pneumonia	Decreased	Decreased
Pneumothorax	Decreased	Decreased
Tube obstruction	Decreased	Unchanged
Pulmonary embolism	Unchanged	Unchanged

compliance. Conditions that stiffen the lung, therefore, will decrease both dynamic and static compliance, whereas, conditions that produce airway narrowing will produce a fall in dynamic compliance without affecting the static compliance much (Table 8.4). These concepts have been further developed in (Chap. 3).

Ventilator graphics can be very useful in determining whether a rise in peak pressure is due to a stiff lung or an obstructed airway.

TABLE 8.2. Information derived from the pressure–time scalar

Information obtained from the pressure–time scalar	Waveform characteristic
Volume-targeted breath	Has a peaked configuration (fig. 4.8)
Pressure-targeted breath	Has a squared configuration (fig. 4.20)
Triggering	Indicated by the presence of a negative deflection immediately preceding inspiration
I:E ratio	Calculated from the relative lengths of inspiration and expiration on the *x*-axis (the *x*-axis represents time)
Peak airway pressure	The highest point in the pressure tracing. Measured off the *y*-axis (fig. 8.3)
Plateau pressure	The "shoulder" in the pressure tracing that lies just beyond and below the peak airway pressure. Measured off the *y*-axis (fig. 8.3)
Mean airway pressure	The area under the entire inspiratory curve; includes the area under PEEP line
Set PEEP	Estimated from the distance above the baseline from where the inspiratory tracing begins
AutoPEEP/air trapping	The expiratory tracing ends well above the set PEEP level (that is, above the baseline)
Airway obstruction	A disproportionate rise in peak airway pressure relative to the pause pressure
Bronchodilator response	Decrease in peak airway pressure following administration of bronchodilators

The information that can be obtained from the pressure–time scalar is summarized in Table 8.2

This insight may not be afforded by some modes. For instance, the intent of the pressure control mode is to maintain a constant pressure throughout inspiration, and obvious as it sounds, a pause cannot be set within this mode (Fig. 8.5).

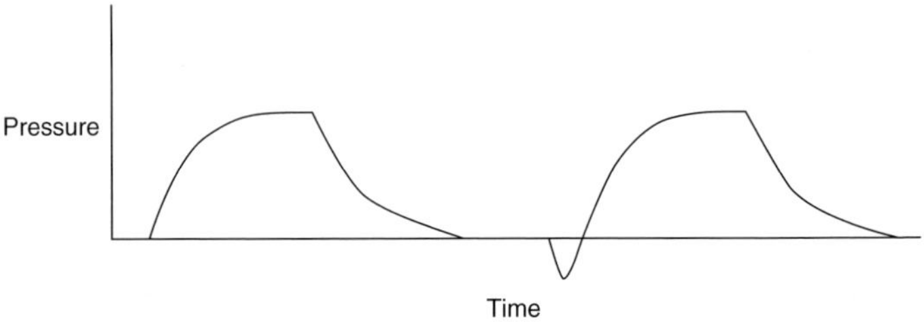
Pressure
Time

FIGURE 8.5. Pressure–time scalar during a pressure-targeted breath. Note that the second of the two breaths shown is patient-triggered.

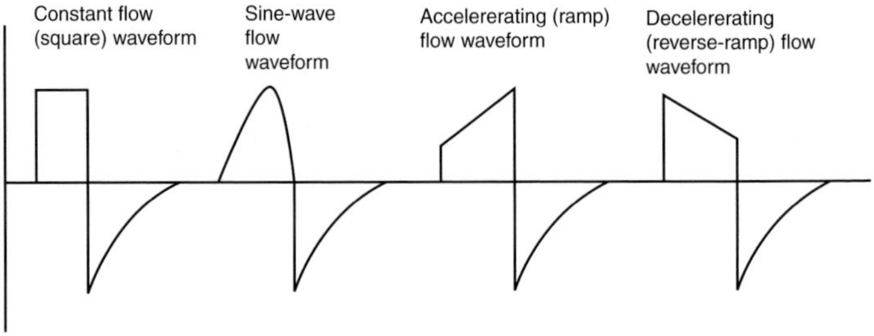
Constant flow (square) waveform
Sine-wave flow waveform
Accelererating (ramp) flow waveform
Decelererating (reverse-ramp) flow waveform

FIGURE 8.6. Flow waveforms.

8.2.2 Flow-Time Scalar

Four types of flow waveforms were introduced in Chap. 5; they are summarized in Fig. 8.6. In pressure-targeted ventilation, because the constancy of pressure within the inflating lungs has to be maintained, the flow waveform is necessarily decelerating (descending ramp flow waveform).

During volume-targeted ventilation, the most commonly used flow waveform is the square flow waveform (constant flow waveform). The events during a constant flow breath are illustrated in Fig. 8.7.

In theory, a relatively slow rise to the peak inspiratory flow – as is provided within the ascending-ramp and the sinusoidal waveforms – provides more time for gas distribution within the lungs, and thereby improves oxygenation. Slow

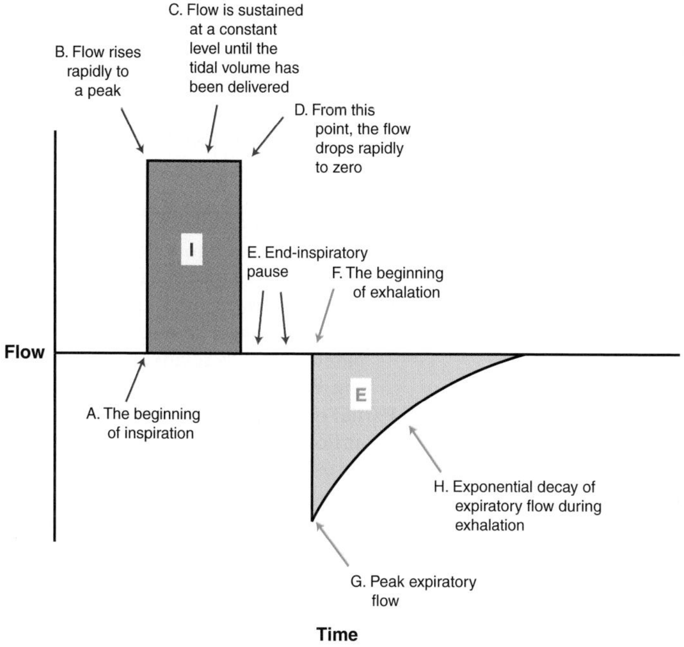
C. Flow is sustained at a constant level until the tidal volume has been delivered
B. Flow rises rapidly to a peak
D. From this point, the flow drops rapidly to zero
I
E. End-inspiratory pause
F. The beginning of exhalation
Flow
A. The beginning of inspiration
E
H. Exponential decay of expiratory flow during exhalation
G. Peak expiratory flow
Time

A. The beginning of inspiration
B. Inspiratory flow rapidly rises to a peak. In practice, inertial forces cause the ascent to be less steep than shown.
C. Thereafter, flow is sustained at a constant level (the square waveform has been applied) until the entire preset tidal volume has been delivered.
D. From this point, the flow declines sharply to zero. Again, in practice, the descent is never as steep as this.
E. During the end-inspiratory pause, the breath is briefly held within the lungs for the duration of the applied pause.
F. Commencement of exhalation
G. The peak expiratory flow is rapidly reached.
H. Exhalation is passive, and so there is an exponential decay in the inspiratory flow down to the baseline as the lung progressively empties.

FIGURE 8.7. Events during a constant flow breath.

flows can be uncomfortable for the patient. The constant flow waveform and the descending ramp flow waveform (the latter delivers high initial flows) are superior at preventing "flow starvation."

The information that can be obtained from the flow-time tracing is summarized in Table 8.3.

TABLE 8.3. Information derived from the flow-time scalar

Information obtained from the flow-time scalar	
Volume-targeted breath	Identified by a square-wave flow pattern
Pressure-targeted breath	Identified by a decelerating flow pattern
Magnitude of the inspiratory flow	Measured off the *y*-axis (fig. 8.7)
Rise time	Can be visually estimated
Auto-PEEP	Failure of the expiratory flow tracing to return to the baseline (fig. 8.9)
Airway obstruction	Expiratory flow tracing is deeply curved and takes longer to return to the baseline. PEF is relatively low (fig. 8.9)
Bronchodilator response	Partial or complete reversal of the airflow obstruction pattern after aerosolized bronchodilator
Active exhalation	Terminal part of tracing shows an upward deflection (fig… p. 56 on incoord)
Air leak	Decreased peak expiratory flow
Patient-ventilator asynchrony	Irregularities in the inspiratory or expiratory pressure tracing (fig. 8.56)

Mathematically, flow is volume divided by time; inspiratory flow is tidal volume divided by the inspiratory time.

$$\text{Flow} = \text{Tidal volume} / \text{Inspiratory time}.$$

Rearranging:

$$\text{Tidal volume} = \text{Flow} \times \text{Inspiratory time}.$$

Therefore, when flow is graphed against inspiratory time, the area under the curve will represent tidal volume. Barring some exceptions (such as air leaks), exhaled tidal volumes will be identical to inhaled tidal volumes, and so the area under the inspiratory (*I*) and expiratory (*E*) flow tracings should be the same.

The relationship holds good, provided the flow is constant, such as during constant flow waveform in volume-targeted ventilation. A normal looking flow-time scalar is set out below (Fig. 8.8). Note the absence of a pause.

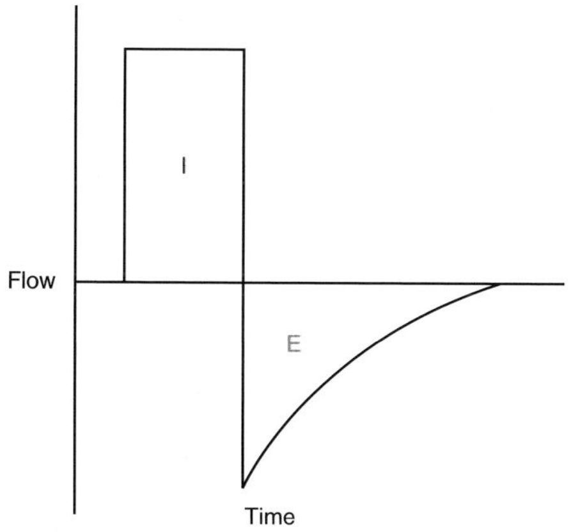
I
Flow
E
Time

FIGURE 8.8. Flow-time scalar.

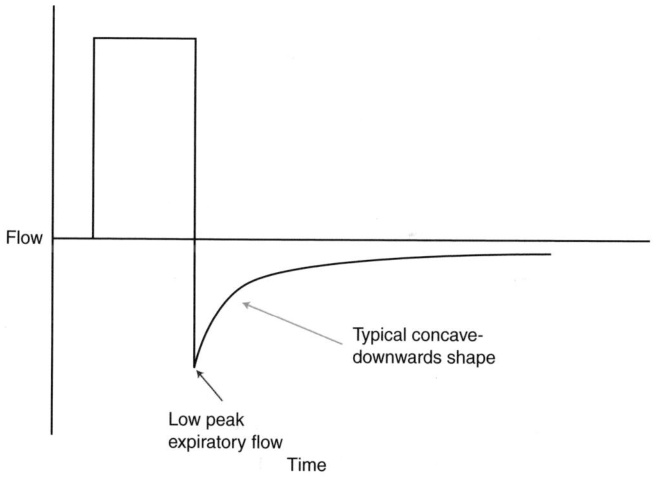
Flow
Typical concave-
downwards shape
Low peak
expiratory flow
Time

FIGURE 8.9. Flow-time scalar in obstructive airways disease.

In airflow obstruction (Fig. 8.9), a part of the tidal volume is "lost" and never delivered to the lungs owing to high ventilating pressures. The lower PEF (arrowed) illustrates the loss of volume. The expiratory flow tracing adopts a deeply curved contour (concavity downward), and takes much

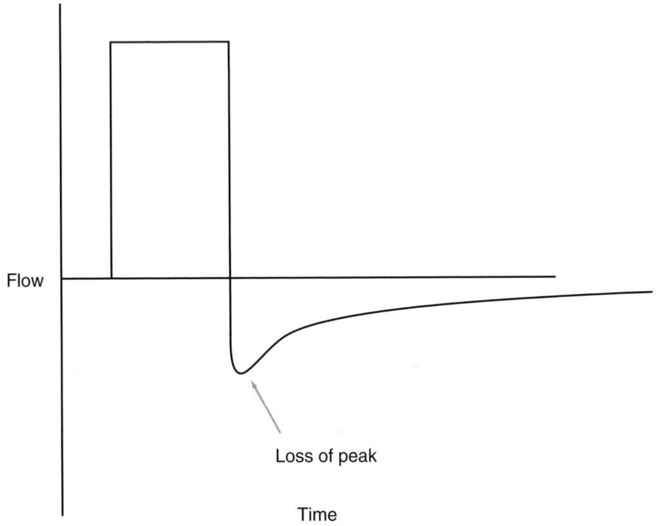
Flow
Loss of peak
Time

FIGURE 8.10. Flow-time scalar in emphysema.

longer to return to the baseline. In the presence of auto-PEEP, the expiratory tracing may still be well below the baseline by the time the next breath is triggered (Fig. 8.9).

Emphysema is a common cause of airflow limitation, but here, the waveform is slightly different. Because of the extensive loss of lung parenchyma and the resultant loss of elastic recoil, the usual peaked configuration of the PEF is replaced by a more relaxed, rounded contour (Fig. 8.10).

On the other hand, when lung compliance is low, the greater elastic recoil leads to a higher PEF; expiratory time is shortened, and the lung empties more quickly (Fig. 8.11).

8.2.3 Volume–Time Scalar

The volume–time scalar in constant flow, volume-targeted ventilation is shown below (Fig. 8.12). Flow being constant, the volume rise is linear. Because expiration is passive, the expiratory flow falls exponentially.

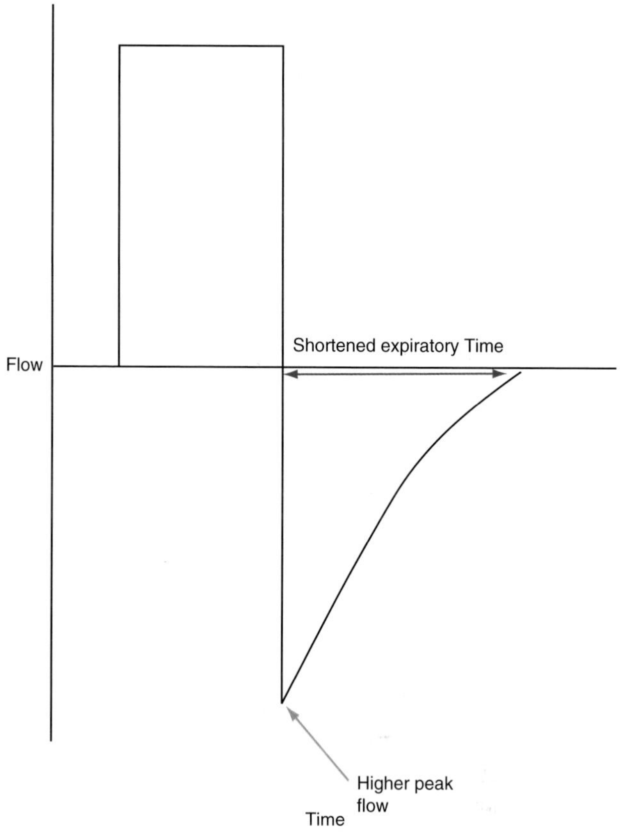
Shortened expiratory Time
Flow
Higher peak
flow
Time

FIGURE 8.11. Flow-time scalar: low compliance.

Information derived from the volume-time scalar	
Tidal volume	Indicated on the *y*-axis
AutoPEEP	Expiratory part of the tracing fails to return to the baseline before the commencement of the next breath
Active exhalation	Tracing continues beyond the baseline
Air leak	Tracing fails to return to baseline (fig. 8.13)
Patient-ventilator asynchrony	(*See text*)

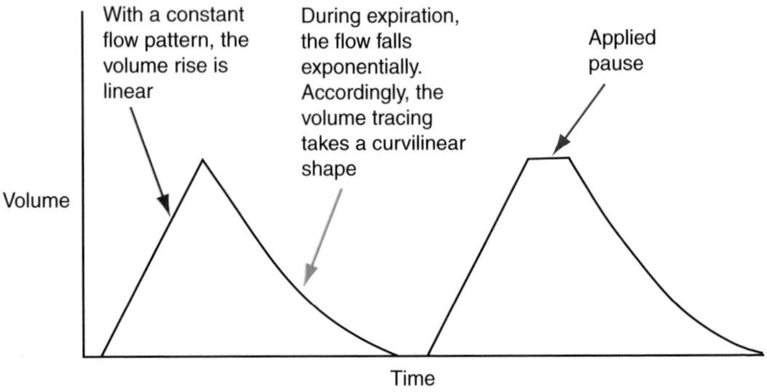
With a constant flow pattern, the volume rise is linear
During expiration, the flow falls exponentially. Accordingly, the volume tracing takes a curvilinear shape
Applied pause
Volume
Time

FIGURE 8.12. Volume–time scalar in constant flow, volume-targeted ventilation.

The length of the inspiratory limb of the tracing should normally be roughly the same as that of the expiratory limb. When the latter fails to reach the baseline, some of the gas provided by the ventilator to the patient has not returned to the machine – a part of the inspired tidal volume has been lost. A leak in the ventilator circuit or a bronchopleural fistula can produce such a tracing. A similar graphic can be produced during dynamic hyperinflation when air trapping permits only the partial exhalation of the tidal volumes that have been inhaled (Fig. 8.13).

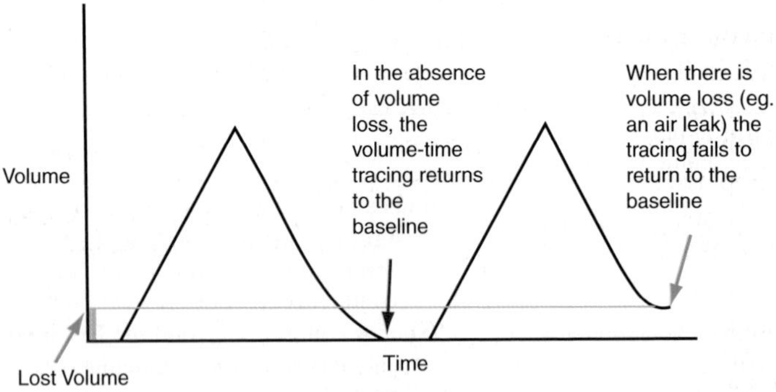
In the absence of volume loss, the volume-time tracing returns to the baseline
When there is volume loss (eg. an air leak) the tracing fails to return to the baseline
Volume
Lost Volume
Time

FIGURE 8.13. Volume–time scalar: incomplete exhalation.

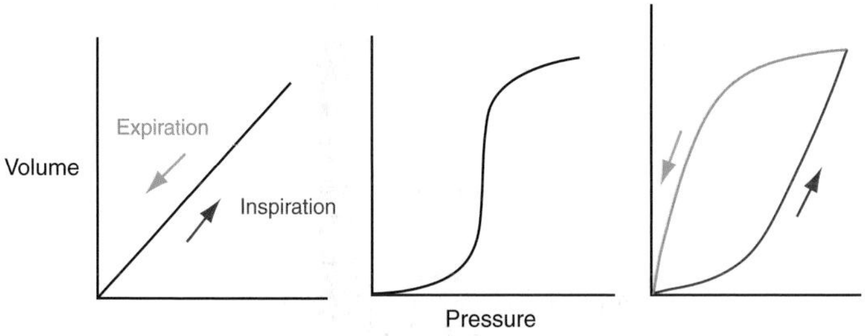
Volume
Expiration
Inspiration
Pressure

FIGURE 8.14. The pressure–volume loop.

8.3 The Loops

8.3.1 Pressure–Volume Loop

Volume graphed against pressure yields the compliance curve. If the forces of surface tension could be eliminated – as they can in a saline-filled experimental lung preparation – this "curve" would actually be a straight line (see Fig. 8.14). The PV tracing moves up this diagonal line with inspiration (red arrow) and down the same line with expiration (green arrow). In intact animals, air–fluid interfaces within the lung generate forces of surface tension, and the inspiratory and expiratory tracings follow different paths – tracing out not a curve, but a loop. The pressure–volume loop normally tends to be slightly warped: it does not appear symmetrical (as a biconvex lens would when viewed side on), but bulges to the left in its upper half, and to the right in its lower.

Spontaneous breath: During spontaneous breathing – without any form of support such as CPAP or PSV – the PV loop assumes the characteristic shape just described. The spontaneous breath is traced clockwise (in contrast to the assisted breath – see later – which is traced anticlockwise). With inspiration, as the intrapleural pressure becomes negative, the tracing moves to the left of the *y*-axis, and air is drawn into the lungs. With increasing tidal volume, the lungs fill up with air and the negativity of the intrapleural pressure decreases: the tracing returns to the zero pressure line (the *y*-axis) (Fig. 8.15).

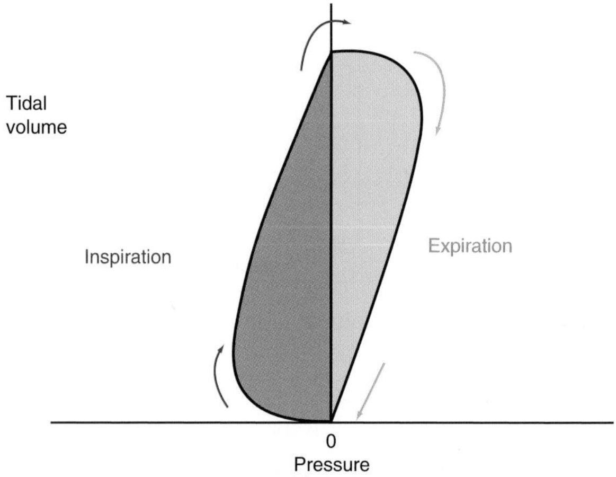
Tidal
volume
Inspiration
Expiration
0
Pressure

FIGURE 8.15. The pressure–volume loop during spontaneous breathing.

Machine breath: With a ventilator-delivered breath, the tracing begins in the lower left hand corner of the graph and moves counterclockwise (in opposite direction to that during a spontaneous breath); at end expiration, it has returnes to the point where it originally began. The highest point of the PV loop read off on the y-axis represents the tidal volume. The same point read against the x-axis represents the PIP.

With exhalation, the tracing follows the expiratory curve downward, culminating at the point representing zero tidal volume and zero PEEP (note the absence of set PEEP).

Volume change in relation to pressure change naturally defines compliance, and so, the PV loop is a useful way of monitoring the compliance of the respiratory system. Since the loops are plotted during airflow, the PV loop also provides useful information about airway resistance (Fig. 8.27).

Airway pressures: With the movement of the tidal breath into the lungs, the airway pressure tracing follows the inspiratory curve (red) upward to the point at the extreme right: the peak airway pressure (Fig. 8.17), also known as the PIP (PIP and P_{pk}).

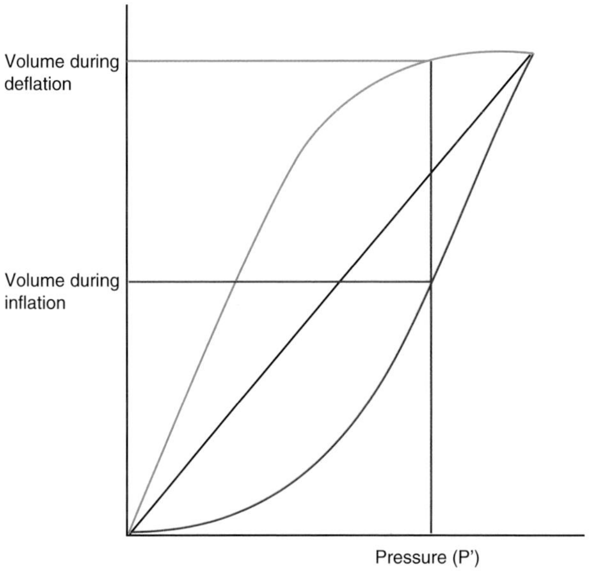
Volume during
deflation
Volume during
inflation
Pressure (P')

FIGURE 8.16. The pressure–volume loop: lung volume during inflation and deflation.

Note: That at a given pressure (P'), the volume is greater during deflation than during inflation.

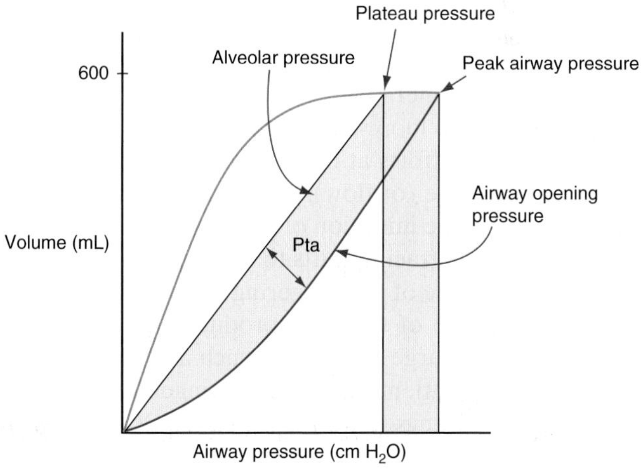
Plateau pressure
Alveolar pressure
Peak airway pressure
600
Airway opening
pressure
Volume (mL)
Pta
Airway pressure (cm H_2O)

FIGURE 8.17. The pressure–volume loop: airway pressures.

When a pause is set, the tidal volume is briefly held within the lungs. With the dissemination of gas into the periphery of the lungs, the tracing shifts a little to the left – to say that the PIP drops slightly – to its new level, the plateau pressure or the pause pressure (P_{ps}). Up to this point, there is as yet no discernible fall in the tidal volume: the tracing has not yet begun to lose height.

The transalveolar pressure gradient: The gradient between alveolar pressure (P_{alv}) and intrapleural pressure (P_{pl}) is the transpulmonary pressure (P_{ta}), also known as the flow-resistive pressure. P_{ta} is the difference between the peak alveolar pressure (P_{alv}) and the airway opening pressure (P_{ao}) – represented at end-inspiration as the difference between the peak airway pressure (P_{pk}) and the pause pressure (P_{ps}). In the upright individual, P_{ta} is greater at the lung apices than at the lung bases.

At a given transpulmonary pressure, lung volume is higher during deflation than during inflation (Fig. 8.16). Most diagrams show only the deflation limb of the pressure – volume loop. The P_{ta} gradient is smaller in the saline-filled lung (it takes a smaller pressure to inflate the saline-filled lung) because now only the elastic resistance needs to be overcome.

With the square wave (constant flow) pattern, once the peak *flow* is reached, the P_{ao} (red) and the P_{alv} (blue) parallel each other (Fig. 8.18). In other words, once the peak inspiratory flow has been attained, the transairway pressure (P_{ta} – the difference between the P_{ao} and the P_{alv}) will remain constant for the rest of the inspiration.

Triggering: In panel b of Fig. 8.19, a patient-triggered breath is shown. The loop seen to the left of the *y*-axis represents the patient's efforts at triggering. The ventilator senses the negative pressure (or flow), and is triggered into delivering a breath. With the initiation of a machine-driven positive-pressure breath, the tracing shifts to the right hand side of the *y*-axis. The magnitude of the triggering effort by the patient is reflected in the size of the loop produced by the patient's effort. A relatively large sized "tail" such as this indicates an inordinately high patient-effort due to inadequate machine settings (trigger settings not sensitive enough).

PEEP: Fig. 8.20 shows the effect of applied PEEP on the pressure–volume loop. In the panel on the left, the tracing starts adjacent to the *y*-axis, at a pressure of zero, which

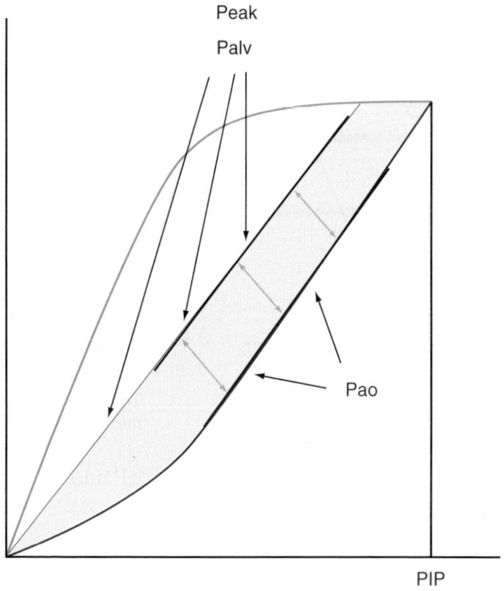
Peak
Palv
Pao
PIP

FIGURE 8.18. The pressure–volume loop: transairway pressure. Machine-triggered and patient-triggered breaths.

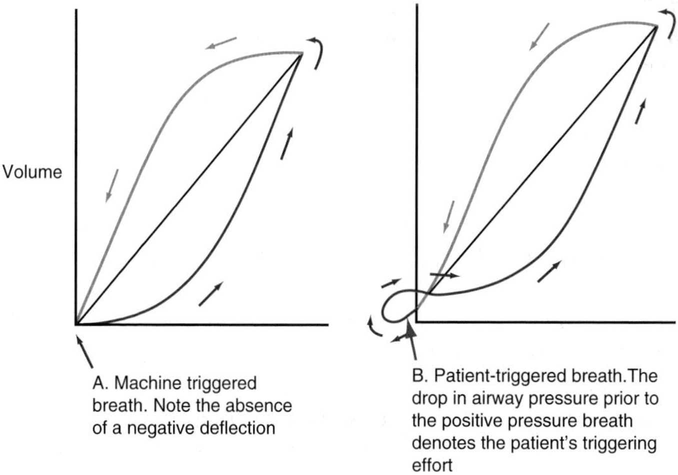
Volume
A. Machine triggered breath. Note the absence of a negative deflection
B. Patient-triggered breath.The drop in airway pressure prior to the positive pressure breath denotes the patient's triggering effort

FIGURE 8.19. The pressure–volume loop: triggering.

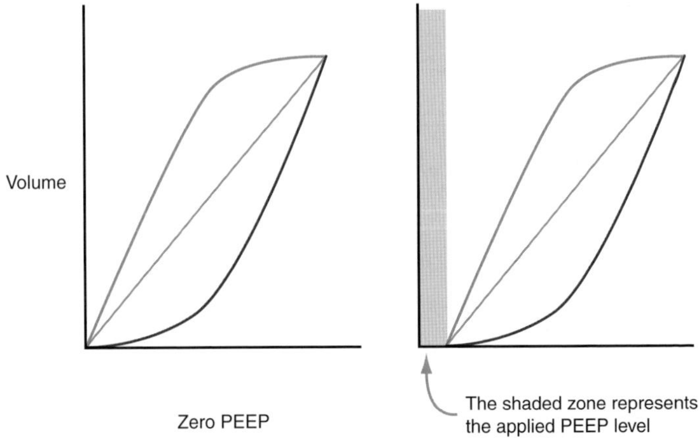
Volume
Zero PEEP
The shaded zone represents the applied PEEP level

FIGURE 8.20. The pressure–volume loop: ZEEP and PEEP.

means that there is no set PEEP. On the panel to the right, the loop begins further to the right of the *y*-axis, and the shaded zone represents the magnitude of the set PEEP.

Compliance: In Fig. 8.21, B represents the pressure–volume axis of a lung with normal compliance. Conventionally, the PV loop representing a lung with normal compliance is represented at an angle of approximately 45° to the horizontal (B). The more upright line (A) represents a lung with increased compliance (as in emphysema), whereas the relatively rightward-tilted line (C) represents a stiffened lung. Note that the pressure required to move a given volume of air into the lung (V_t) would be the least for A and the most for C. In other words, lung (A) has the best compliance and C the worst.

Shown in Fig. 8.22 are two pressure–volume loops generated during volume-controlled ventilation. The tidal volume is the same for both the breaths (horizontal red line), since every breath is volume limited. The green loop to the left is representative of a lung with relatively good compliance: note its upright position and the relatively low pressure change (P_1) it takes to produce the given change in volume (V_t). The blue loop on the right represents a relatively noncompliant

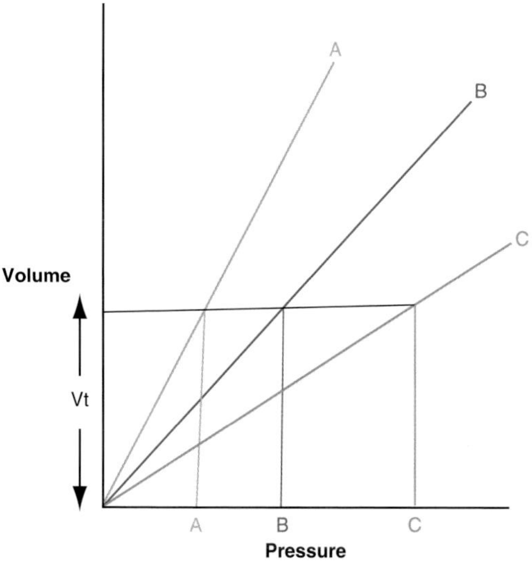
A
B
C
Volume
Vt
A
B
C
Pressure

FIGURE 8.21. Effect of decreased compliance on the pressure–volume loop.

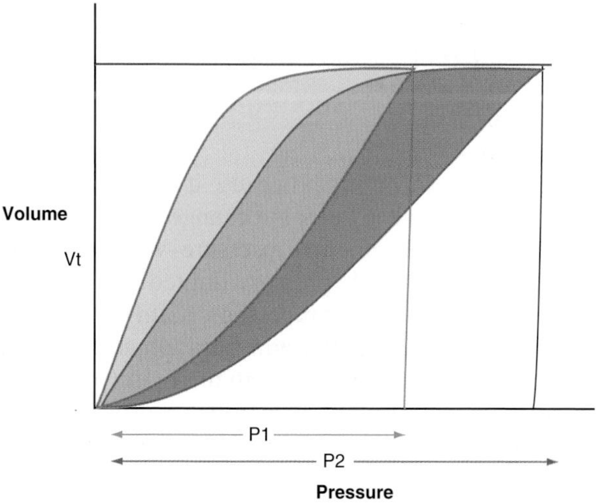
Volume
Vt
P1
P2
Pressure

FIGURE 8.22. Effect of decreased compliance on the PV loop during volume-targeted ventilation.

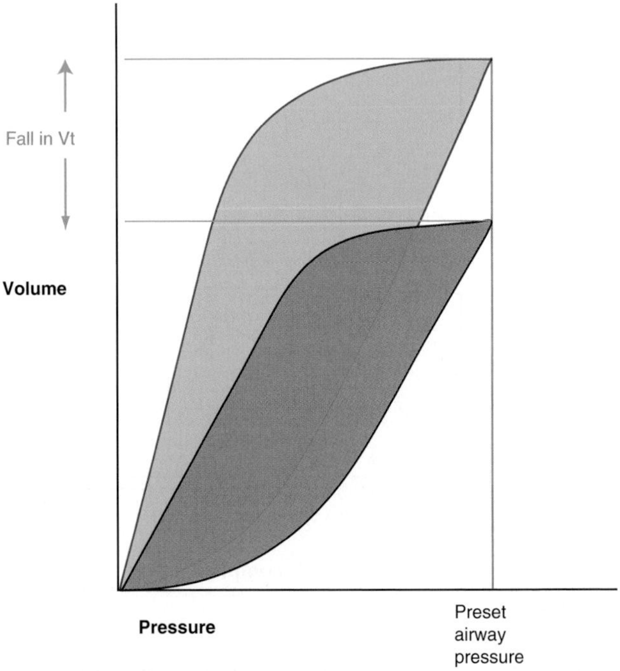
Fall in Vt
Volume
Pressure
Preset
airway
pressure

FIGURE 8.23. Effect of decreased compliance on the PV loop with pressure-targeted ventilation.

lung. The loop sits less upright because it takes a much higher pressure (P_2) to produce the same change in volume (V_t).

Shown in Fig. 8.23 are two pressure–volume loops that have been obtained with pressure-limited ventilation. The upright blue loop at the left represents a lung with relatively normal compliance. With the deterioration in lung compliance, the loop tilts downward and to the right (pink loop). In the pressure control mode, as compliance worsens, it is the tidal volume that falls. The pressure is controlled at the preset value (vertical gray line).

If the pressure limit in the pressure control mode is deliberately lowered, the point that represents the PIP retreats leftward. Smaller tidal volumes can now be administered

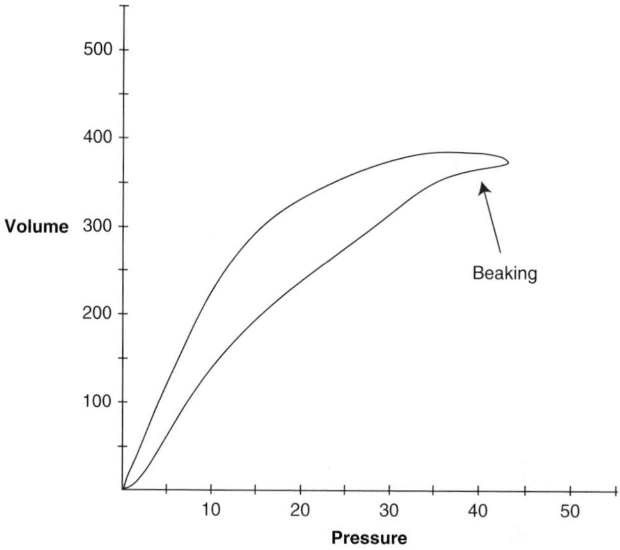
500
400
Volume 300
200
100
Beaking
10
20
30
40
50
Pressure

FIGURE 8.24. Pressure–volume loop: overdistension of the lung.

within the lowered pressure limit, and so the height of the loop becomes reduced as well.

When overdistended, the lung is noncompliant and less accommodative of tidal volumes. As it fills up, it increasingly stiffens, and so there is less volume change for a given applied pressure toward the end of the breath, than there is at the beginning of the breath. The flattening of the terminal part of the inspiratory curve gives a characteristic beaked shape to the pressure–volume loop (Fig. 8.24).

In contrast to the rightward-tilted PV loop of the noncompliant lung, the loop of the highly compliant – for instance, emphysematous – lung is more vertical (Fig. 8.25).

Elastic work and resistive work: The area shaded in green (Fig. 8.26) represents the elastic work of breathing. As can be envisaged, a rightward shift of the pressure–volume loop (when the static compliance is decreased) will cause its area to expand (in other words, the elastic work of breathing will increase).

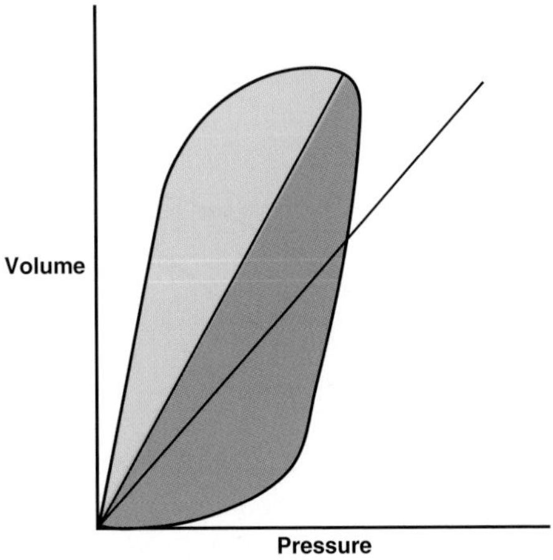
Volume
Pressure

FIGURE 8.25. Pressure–volume loop of a highly compliant lung.

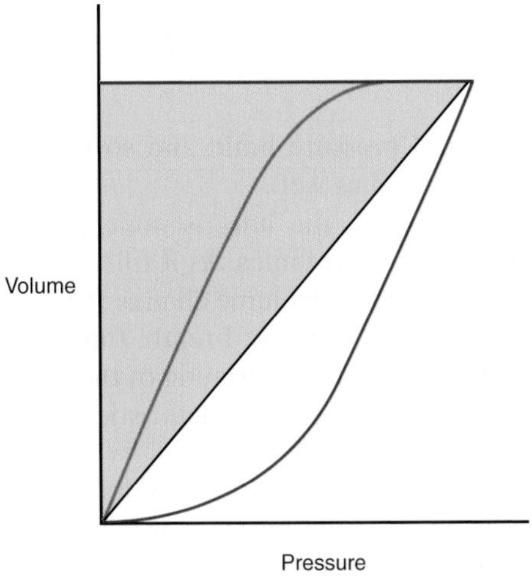
Volume
Pressure

FIGURE 8.26. The elastic work of breathing.

In Fig. 8.27, the panel on the left shows a relatively normal pressure–volume loop. The area shaded yellow represents the flow-resistive pressure of the system (flow-resistive pressures

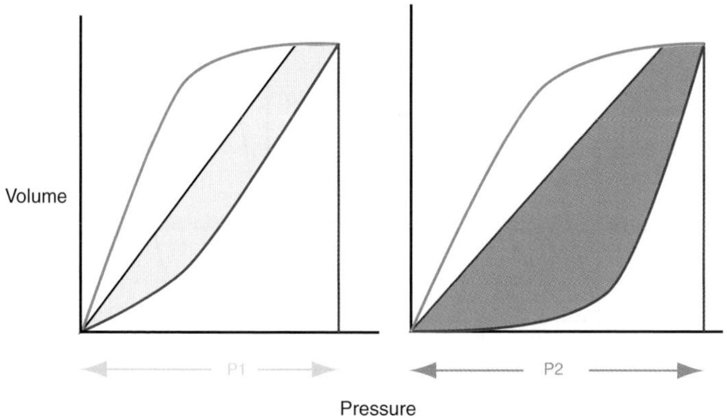
Volume
P1
P2
Pressure

FIGURE 8.27. Pressure–volume loop: increased flow-resistive work during volume-targeted ventilation.

have been dealt with earlier in this chapter). In panel B, increased flow-resistive work has resulted in the change in inspiratory volume lagging behind the change in pressure. The noticeable sag in the inspiratory curve has resulted in expansion of the area that represents the flow-resistive work (shaded pink).

In the volume-targeted mode, an increase in airflow resistance will cause the PIPs to increase. The tidal volumes being preset, are naturally unchanged. As a matter of fact, the tidal volume can also get limited if the airway pressure exceeds the set upper airway pressure limit (see chap. 6).

Note that the peak pressure in the second loop (P2) is slightly higher than that in the first (P1), reflecting a decrease in the dynamic compliance. Sometimes, the loop is tilted downward, indicating a decrease in static compliance as well.

In the pressure-control ventilation (PCV) mode, increased airway resistance will cause tidal volumes to drop slightly (Fig. 8.28, right-sided panel). Since in PCV the PIP is preset, it can be seen to be unchanged in both panels; but note the altered shape of the loop with increasing resistance.

Volume loss: The height of the inspiratory curve (red line) above the baseline represents the inspiratory volume – the

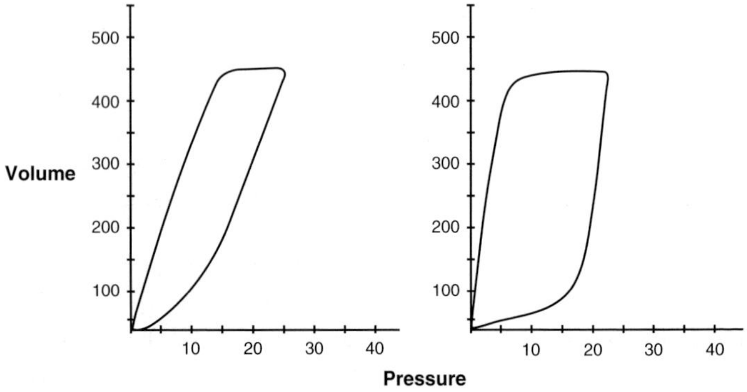

500
400
300
200
100
Volume
10
20
30
40
Pressure

FIGURE 8.28. Pressure–volume loop: increased flow-resistive work during pressure-targeted ventilation.

volume of the machine-delivered tidal inspiration (Fig. 8.29). The height of the expiratory curve (green line) above the baseline represents the exhaled volume, i.e., the volume returning to the machine. The difference between the inhaled and the exhaled tidal volume (arrowed) is the volume that has been lost (see earlier in this chapter for causes of incomplete exhalation).

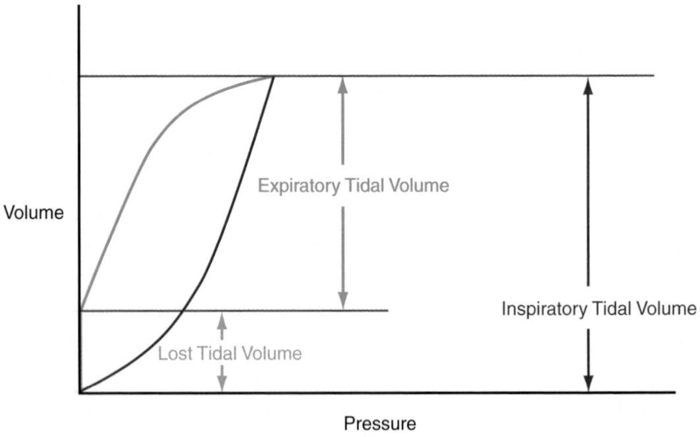

Volume
Expiratory Tidal Volume
Inspiratory Tidal Volume
Lost Tidal Volume
Pressure

FIGURE 8.29. Pressure–volume loop: incomplete exhalation (volume loss).

8.3.2 The Flow–Volume Loop

The flow–volume loop is another useful way of looking at data. Flow (*y*-axis) is graphed against volume (*x*-axis). The loop differs in some respects from the flow–volume loop obtained on the office spirometer. Most ventilators display the inspiratory curve above, and the expiratory curve below the *x*-axis: this orientation is the reverse of that which is familiar to physicians from office spirometry reports.The usual loop obtained in the PFT lab is generated from a maximal expiratory effort that follows a deep inspiration; on the ventilator, the inspiratory flow rate is set by the clinician/therapist, and expiration is passive. The nadir of the expiratory loop represents the peak expiratory flow (PEF).

On the ventilator, a spontaneous breath is recognizable by the slightly irregular contour of its inspiratory portion (Fig. 8.30), especially if the peak flow is relatively low. *Volume-targeted ventilation:* With the sine-wave flow pattern

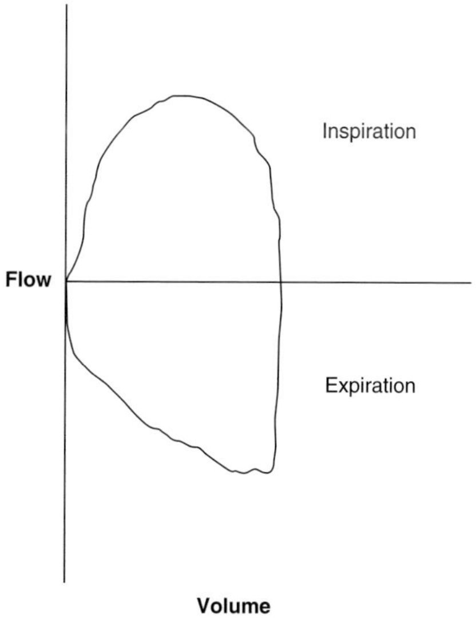
Inspiration
Flow
Expiration
Volume

FIGURE 8.30. Flow–volume loop: spontaneous breath.

of volume-targeted (volume control) ventilation (Fig. 8.31, panel A), the inspiratory flow rises gradually to a crescendo and then decreases. The inspiratory tracing describes a curve. With a constant flow pattern, the flow waveform is predictably square (panel B).

In (Fig. 8.32), the effect of varying the set inspiratory flow rate during square-wave ventilation is shown.

Pressure-control ventilation: During PCV, the peak flow is attained early during inspiration, and the waveform shows a decelerating flow that is a defining characteristic of any pressure-targeted mode (e.g., pressure control mode, pressure support mode, etc.). The waveform retains its typical morphology at all the three levels of the pressure level represented. As the pressure level is increased from A–C, the peak flow is seen to increase (Fig. 8.33).

Pressure support ventilation (PSV): the pressure support mode is one of the pressure-targeted modes of ventilation. One of the hallmarks of pressure supported ventilation is the rather abrupt decline in flow (arrowed) toward the end of inspiration

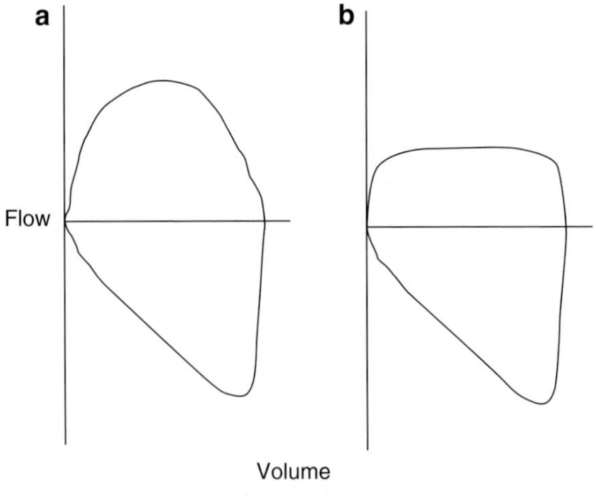
a
b
Flow
Volume

FIGURE 8.31. Flow–volume loop during volume controlled ventilation. (a) Sine-wave flow pattern. (b) Square-wave flow pattern.

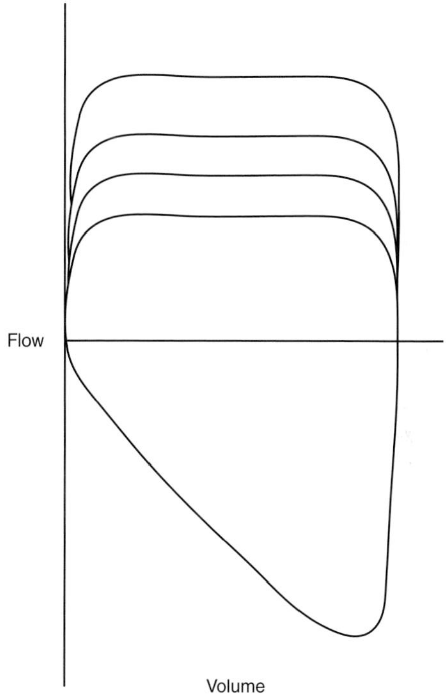
Flow
Volume

FIGURE 8.32. Flow–volume loop: the effect of varying the set inspiratory flow rate during square-wave volume-targeted ventilation.

(Fig. 8.34). This feature is produced by the cycling off of the ventilator as the flow-threshold is reached (see section 4.8).

Increased airway resistance: In Fig. 8.35, a flow–volume loop obtained with PCV is represented – note the decelerating waveform. With increased airway resistance, tidal volumes become constrained by the set airway pressures (the inspiratory time is unchanged). Since flow is volume divided by time, a decrease in flow will translate into lower tidal volumes if the inspiratory time is unchanged.

In Fig. 8.36, two flow–volume loops obtained with square-wave volume control ventilation are depicted. A normal looking flow–volume loop is represented on the left panel. The panel on the right shows a flow–volume loop under conditions

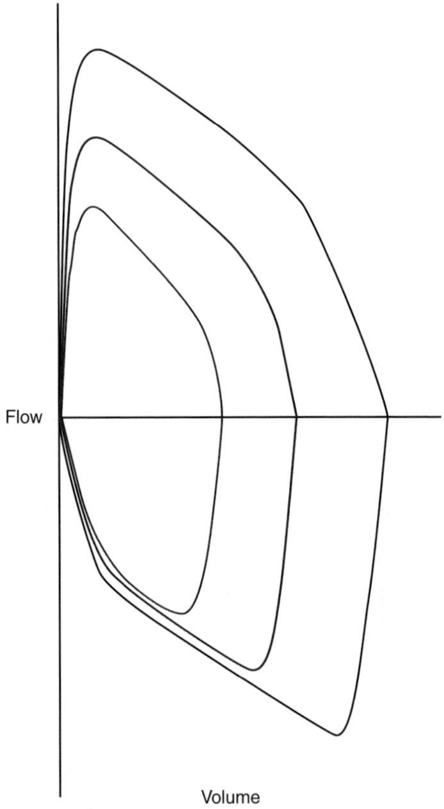
Flow
Volume

FIGURE 8.33. Flow–volume loop: the effect of varying the set airway pressure during a pressure-targeted ventilation. Shown in purple is a flow–volume loop obtained during pressure-targeted ventilation at a relatively low pressure setting. The effect of progressively increasing the airway pressure is shown in the tracings in *blue* and *black*, respectively.

Note: The decelerating flow that is characteristic of pressure targeted ventilation.

of increased inspiratory *and* expiratory resistance. With a mild to moderate increase in airways resistance, there should be no great difference in the morphology of the inspiratory limbs, since most ventilators are capable of driving airflows that overcome the additional resistive load. A subtle clue, however,

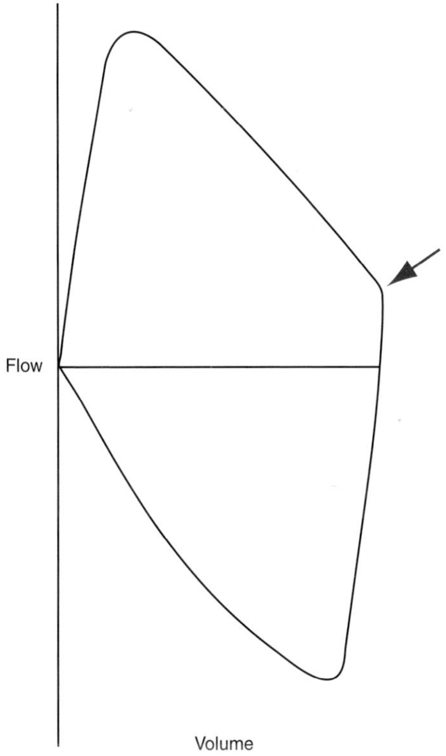
Flow
Volume

FIGURE 8.34. Flow–volume loop in pressure support ventilation. Note the abrupt decline in flow toward the end of ventilation as the ventilator cycles from inspiration to expiration (*red arrow*).

is a slight blunting of the initial part of the inspiratory waveform as the machine begins coping with the increased resistance. The PEF is decreased, indicating a large airways component to the airflow obstruction. The slightly scalloped expiratory limb of the loop suggests that there is a small airway component to the expiratory obstruction as well.

Auto PEEP: Fig. 8.37 shows a constant flow–volume-targeted breath in dynamic hyperinflation. The expiratory flow tracing fails to return to the baseline at the end of exhalation (green line). The normal terminal part of the expiratory tracing is shown in blue.

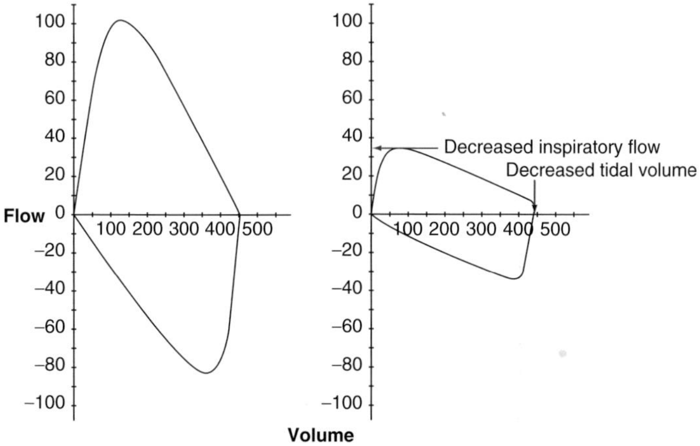

Flow
Volume
100
80
60
40
20
0
–20
–40
–60
–80
–100
100 200 300 400 500
Decreased inspiratory flow
Decreased tidal volume

FIGURE 8.35. Flow–volume loop: effect of increased airway resistance on flow and volume. Shown in the panel on the left is a normal looking flow–volume loop obtained during pressure-targeted ventilation. The effect of increased airway resistance is shown in the panel on the right. Both flow and volume have decreased.

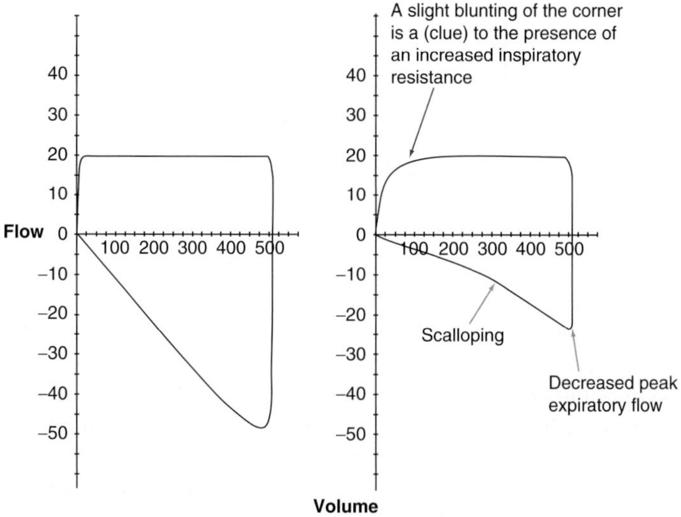

Flow
Volume
40
30
20
10
0
–10
–20
–30
–40
–50
100 200 300 400 500
A slight blunting of the corner is a (clue) to the presence of an increased inspiratory resistance
Scalloping
Decreased peak expiratory flow

FIGURE 8.36. Flow–volume loop: effect of increased inspiratory and expiratory resistance.

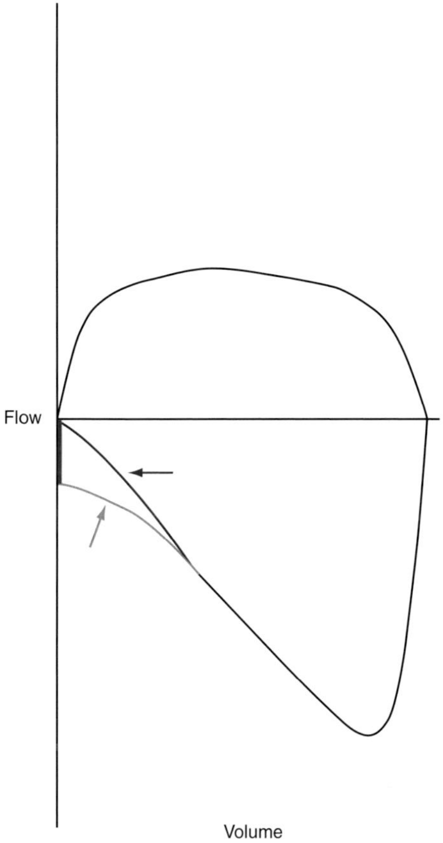
Flow
Volume

FIGURE 8.37. Flow–volume loop: dynamic hyperinflation (*see text*).

Decreased compliance: The effects of reduced compliance on a flow–volume loop are relatively subtle compared to those on a pressure–volume loop. Because of the increased elastic recoil in a stiff lung, the lung deflates rapidly; this becomes noticeable as a PEFR which is high relative to the tidal volume (Fig. 8.38).

Volume loss: The expiratory tracing stops well short of the *y*-axis – this can happen when there is air leakage (circuit or

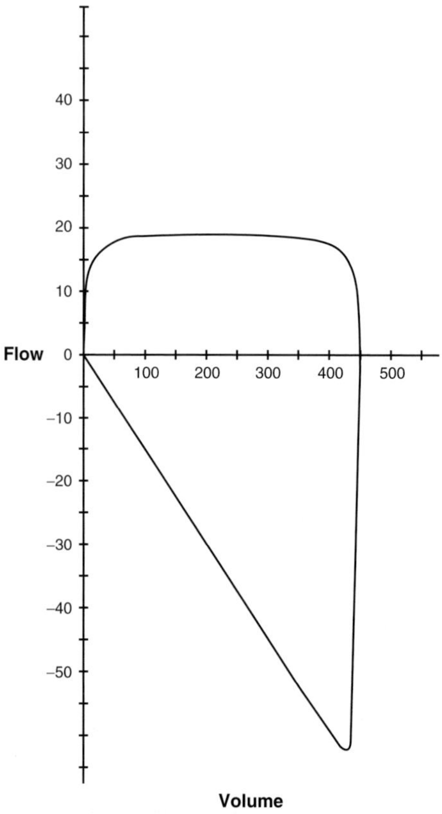
40
30
20
10
Flow 0
–10
–20
–30
–40
–50
100
200
300
400
500
Volume

FIGURE 8.38. Flow–volume loop: effect of a decrease in compliance.

ET cuff leak; or a bronchopleural fistula), and a part of the inhaled volume fails to return to the expiratory sensor. The difference between the inhaled and the exhaled tidal volume can be quantified.

Tubing compressibility: The expiratory limb of the flow–volume loop (Fig. 8.40) is similar in appearance to the flow–volume loop of the airflow obstruction shown (compare with Fig. 8.36B). That there is no airway obstruction is indicated by the absence of scalloping on the expiratory waveform (double green arrow). The prominent spike at the commencement of expiration (red

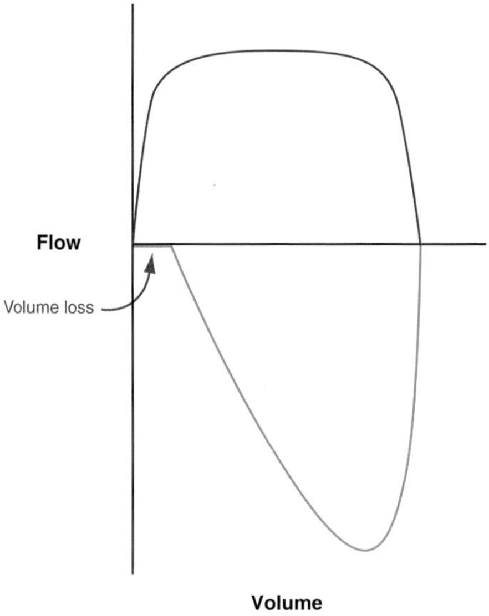
Flow
Volume loss
Volume

FIGURE 8.39. Flow–volume loop: lost tidal volume.

arrow) represents the expiratory "rebound" of air that has distended the circuit during inspiration. The ventilator tubing can often be seen to contract visibly at the onset of expiration.

Airway secretions: Secretions within the proximal airway or the endotracheal (or tracheostomy) tube can impart a saw-toothed appearance to the tracing [13] (Fig. 8.41).

8.4 Patient-Ventilator Asynchrony

8.4.1 Level of Ventilator Support and Work of Breathing

One of the goals of mechanical ventilation is to fully unload the respiratory muscles when they are fatigued and to allow them to participate in the work of breathing when they have recovered, such that disuse atrophy is prevented.

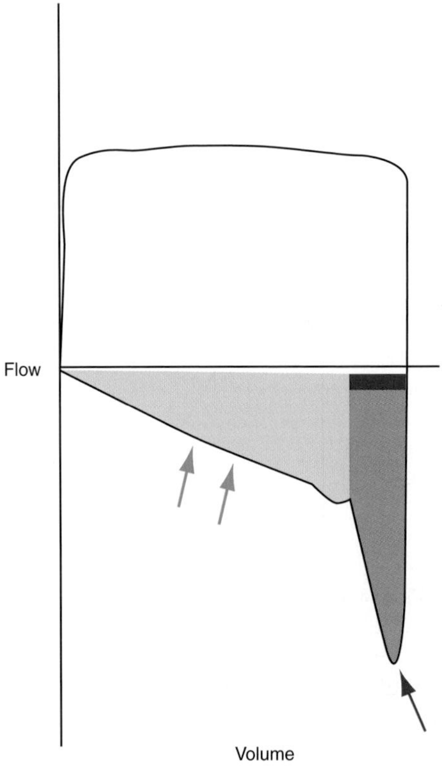
Flow
Volume

FIGURE 8.40. Flow–volume loop: effect of tubing compressibility.

8.4.2 Complete Support

The completely supported patient theoretically spends energy only during triggering the ventilator. The work of breathing during the reminder of inspiration is performed by the machine.

8.4.3 Partial Support

During partial support, the work of breathing is shared between the patient and the ventilator.

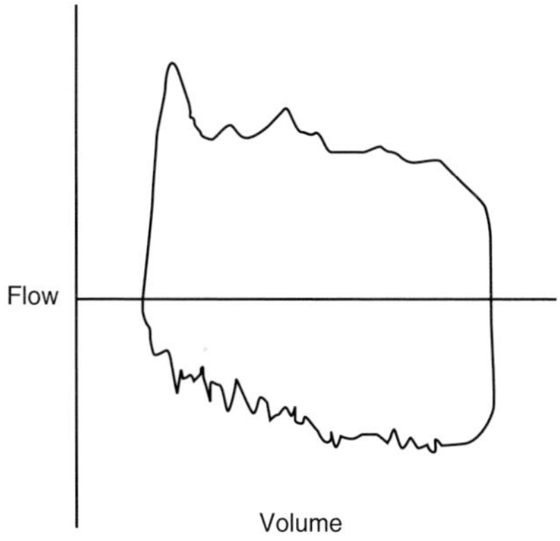
Flow
Volume

FIGURE 8.41. Flow–volume loop: effect of airway secretions.

8.4.4 Patient-Ventilator Asynchrony

Patient-ventilator asynchrony can have widespread ramifications. The work of breathing can increase oxygen consumption, impair myocardial performance, cause considerable discomfort to the patient and even impact upon the weaning process. Graphics provide vital insight into the cause of asynchrony, and thereby enable optimization of ventilator settings.

Box 8.1 Causes of Patient-Ventilator Asynchrony

Tidal volumes too low
Inspiratory flow too slow
Inspiratory time too long
Trigger sensitivity too negative
Increased resistance of patient-tube or respiratory circuit (e.g., blocked endotracheal tube, clogged HME, "water" in circuit)
Auto-PEEP
Change in patient's lung mechanics
Pain, discomfort, and agitation

8.4.5 Triggering Asynchrony

8.4.5.1 Response Time

During spontaneous breathing, because of the distance the neural signal needs to travel – from the respiratory center in the medulla oblongata to the diaphragm – there is necessarily a time delay between the onset of neural inspiration and the respiratory muscle response. To this, the mechanical ventilator adds another dimension. The time taken by the machine to respond to the patient's effort once the trigger sensitivity level has been reached is termed as the response time. Response time is a function of the intensity of the patient's respiratory effort, the trigger sensitivity, the set peak flow level, and the response time of the inspiratory valve itself. A degree of insensitivity is deliberately incorporated into the sensors that detect a patient's inspiratory effort, in order to prevent autotriggering (see section 5.6). However, asynchrony can occur because of the delays in signal processing and the inherent mechanical inertia of the demand valves – which may take up to 100 ms to open.

Respiratory muscles have been shown to contract isometrically before flow is actually initiated and this can substantially increase the work of breathing (Fig. 8.42).

When the respiratory drive is high, it helps if the trigger is reset to a higher sensitivity – for instance, to –0.5 cm H_20 rather than the usual –2.0 cm H_2O – especially if a higher peak flow has been set. On the other hand, lowering the

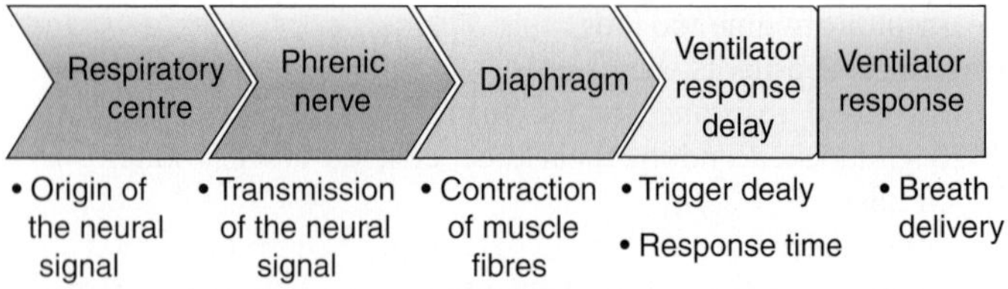
Respiratory centre
Phrenic nerve
Diaphragm
Ventilator response delay
Ventilator response
• Origin of the neural signal
• Transmission of the neural signal
• Contraction of muscle fibres
• Trigger dealy
• Response time
• Breath delivery

FIGURE 8.42. Time delay between the commencement of neural inspiration and breath delivery.

trigger sensitivity even slightly (say, to 4 or 5 cm H_2O) can substantially increase the work of breathing.[15]

8.4.5.2 Type of Trigger

There may also be some advantages of flow triggering over pressure-triggering. With an applied pressure, the trigger gas does not flow into the lungs until the end of the response time. If the ventilator manometer underestimates the negative pressures generated by the inhaling patient, the work done during triggering can be considerable. With flow triggering, on the other hand – this can be shown mathematically – the energy expended in triggering the ventilator is zero; so at least in theory , the flow trigger should be superior to the pressure trigger.[21] With the newer generation of ventilators, however, such an obvious difference in benefit has not been demonstrated.[10]

8.4.5.3 Ineffective Triggering

Trigger asynchrony is common with the pressure support mode, but no more so with other conventional modes such as the assist control.[23] Trigger delays, as discussed above, may be inherent to the system: although some modern ventilators provide a breath within 40 ms of the patient-effort, older versions took as long as 400 ms,[22] and could cause considerable asynchrony. Ineffective triggering ("wasted efforts") appears to be, by far, the most common type of asynchrony during pressure support ventilation, and commonly occur in the setting of dynamic hyperinflation (see section 9.5 COPD). Inadvertent oversupport is another common but less appreciated reason for ineffective triggering during pressure support ventilation.[23]

8.4.6 Flow Asynchrony

When the patient's flow demands are not matched by suitably high set tidal volumes or flows, asynchrony occurs. The flow-starved patient's attempts to breathe deeply leads to a drop in airway pressures, and this can show up as an inward buckling on the initial part of the ascending limb of the pressure waveform (Fig. 8.43).

On the other hand, with volume starvation, the initial part of the ascending limb of the pressure–time graph is fairly normal looking: the flow demands of the patient are met, at least during the initial phase. Rather, there is sagging of its terminal portion (Fig. 8.44).

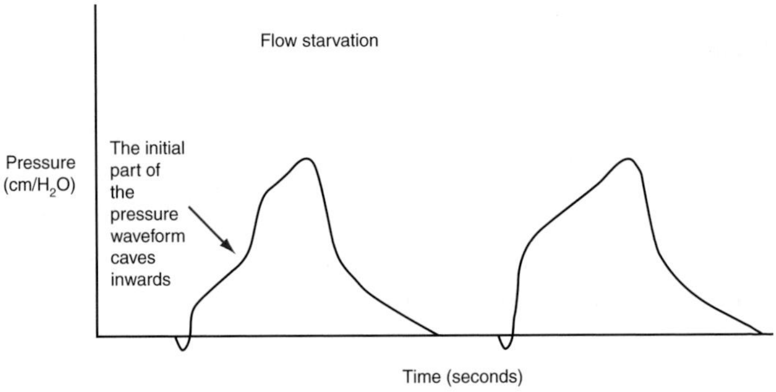
Flow starvation
Pressure
(cm/H_2O)
The initial part of the pressure waveform caves inwards
Time (seconds)

FIGURE 8.43. Constant flow–volume-targeted ventilation: flow starvation.

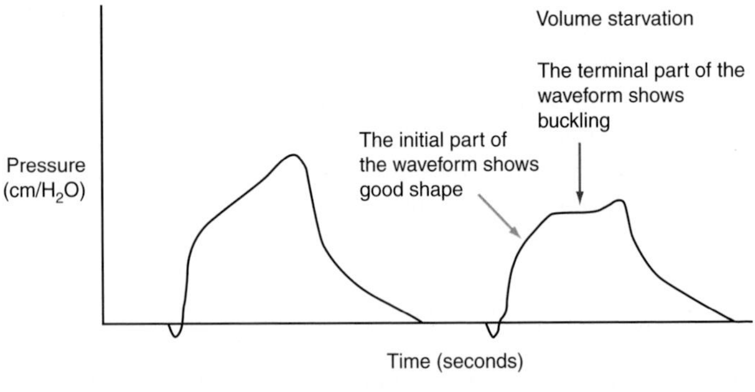
Volume starvation
The terminal part of the waveform shows buckling
The initial part of the waveform shows good shape
Pressure
(cm/H_2O)
Time (seconds)

FIGURE 8.44. Constant flow–volume-targeted ventilation: volume starvation.

The appropriate action will be to titrate the tidal volume upward. Increasing the peak flow may also help to sate the patient's air hunger by delivering tidal volumes more quickly.

Flow starvation during PSV results in a loss of the usual peak on the *flow*-time waveform. During PSV, the normal flow-time scalar shows an early peak followed by a ramping decline – the descending ramp pattern of course is one of the defining features of any pressure-limited mode – followed by a steeper fall. With flow starvation, the steep descent at the end of the breath occurs much earlier, to enable the successive breath to be quickly drawn in. On the *pressure*–time scalar, such increased efforts are also evident during the triggering phase, as deep negative deflections that precede the machine assisted breaths.

Figure 8.45 depicts flow starvation during PSV. When the patient attempts to inhale during the machine's expiratory cycle, there is a transient increase in the rate of decay of the expiratory flow. Incidentally, the patient's attempts at exhalation during a machine-delivered inspiration can also be

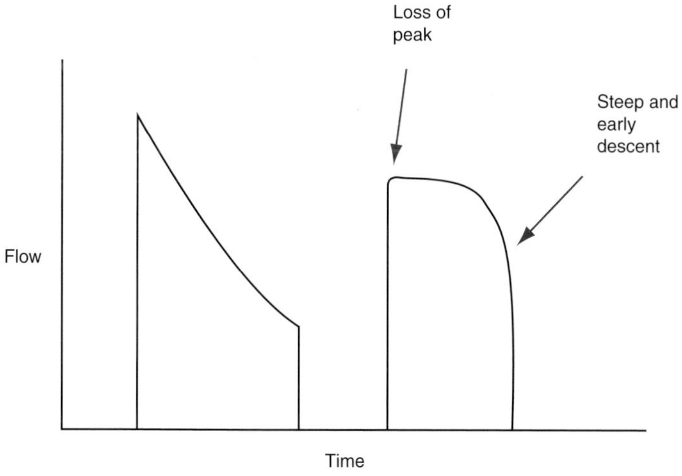
Loss of peak
Steep and early descent
Flow
Time

FIGURE 8.45. Flow-time scalar in pressure support ventilation: flow starvation.

seen – as a temporary cessation of flow; the inspiratory tracing is seen to drop briefly to the baseline.

Flow starvation on the pressure–volume loop manifests as an indentation on the inspiratory segment of the loop (Figs. 8.46 and 8.47).

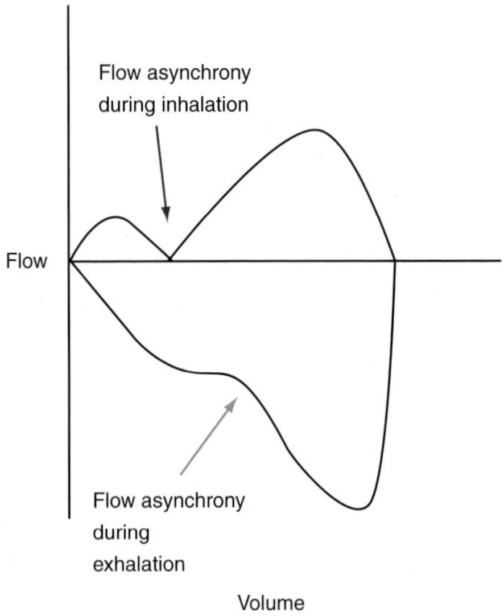
Flow asynchrony
during inhalation
Flow
Flow asynchrony
during
exhalation
Volume

FIGURE 8.46. Flow–volume loop in pressure support ventilation: flow starvation.

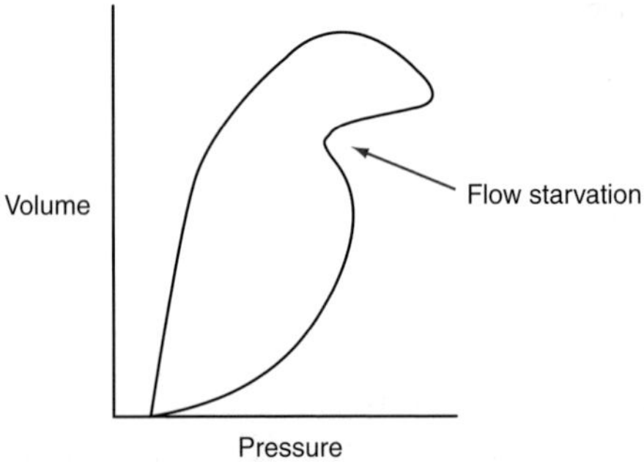
Volume
Flow starvation
Pressure

FIGURE 8.47. Pressure–volume loop: flow starvation.

8.4.6.1 Expiratory Asynchrony

Expiratory asynchrony can present in two forms: delayed termination of the ventilator flow, and premature termination of the ventilator flow.[3]

Delayed Termination of Ventilator Flow

In the PSV mode, once it is triggered, the machine rapidly boosts the flow rate until the preset level of pressure support has been attained. To hold the pressure constant for the rest of inspiration, flow must necessarily be decelerating. The rate of decay of the flow is a factor of the patient's respiratory time-constant, which is the product of the resistance and compliance (see p…). With a short time-constant (as in a stiff lung), decay is fast, and vice versa. In COPD, not only is the airway resistance high, but also the lung compliance low (due to emphysema). As a result of this the time-constant is inordinately prolonged, and the patients will have a delayed termination of their inspiration (Fig. 8.48).

Expiration in PSV is flow cycled (p…). Expiration begins when the flow falls to a predetermined fraction of the peak flow rate. This preselected flow (expiratory trigger sensitivity

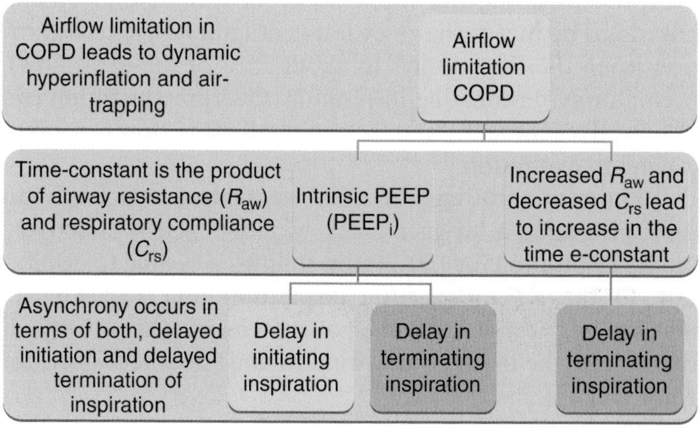
Airflow limitation in COPD leads to dynamic hyperinflation and air-trapping
Airflow limitation COPD
Time-constant is the product of airway resistance (R_{aw}) and respiratory compliance (C_{rs})
Intrinsic PEEP ($PEEP_i$)
Increased R_{aw} and decreased C_{rs} lead to increase in the time e-constant
Asynchrony occurs in terms of both, delayed initiation and delayed termination of inspiration
Delay in initiating inspiration
Delay in terminating inspiration
Delay in terminating inspiration

FIGURE 8.48. Patient-ventilator asynchrony in COPD.

or ETS) varies considerably between different ventilator brands (Drager Evita 4, Macquet Servo 900, and Bird 8400: ETS is 25% of the peak flow; Macquet 300:5% of the peak flow). It is no surprise therefore, that a given machine may not match the special requirements of different individuals with diverse time-constants. Other ventilators have user-selectable ETS criteria (Puritan Bennet 840: 1–45% of the peak flow; Hamilton-Galileo 10–40% of the peak flow). This innovation, however, introduces perhaps, an undesirable complexity into ventilator management[3] (see also Proportional Assist Ventilation, see section 4.8.1).

Premature Termination of Ventilator Flow

Autotriggering: Autotriggering is a form of expiratory asynchrony due to the premature termination of ventilator flow. Autotriggering (see section 8.4.6.1) can occur due to system leaks (e.g., a ruptured endotracheal tube cuff or a connection leak in the circuitry) or the vibration of fluid in waterlogged tubing. Autotriggering is the likely cause of new-onset tachypnea, if an obvious triggering deflection at the onset of the breath is absent.

Multiple triggering: Multiple triggering (e.g., "double breaths") can be the result of autotriggering or overpressurization. With overpressurization, the rapid decay in flow allows cycling criteria to be met earlier (several ventilators cycle to expiration when the flow decays to about 25% of the peak flow), prematurely terminating inspiration. Overpressurization can also produce air leaks, and the rapid fall off in flow can cause cycling to expiration.

To prevent autotriggering, most ventilators have built into their programs, a "trigger block window" which effectively blocks inspiration for 150–300 ms following cycling to inspiration. If the patient's neural inspiration time exceeds the machine inspiration time, the patient's inspiratory effort will span across the trigger block window and "double triggering" will occur.

Early cycling off can also result in multiple triggering. If the ventilator inspiratory cycle is too short in relation to the patient's inspiration time – that is, if the patient is yet to complete his inspiration while the ventilator has already cycled to expiration – the patient's inspiratory demands can result in multiple triggering; more usually, a negative pressure deflection is apparent in early expiration.

On the other hand, if the ventilator's inspiratory cycle outlasts the patient's inspiration time – that is, if the patient has already begun to exhale while the ventilator is still in the process of delivering its breath – the pressure scalar at end expiration remains positive (Figs. 8.49 and 8.50).

Asynchrony Due to Auto-PEEP

In Fig. 8.51, the patient is clearly having difficulty in exhaling. The expiratory flow falls smoothly to a point indicated by the green arrow at which point there is a perceptible fall off in the rate of decay (green arrow). This is followed by a complete cessation in the airflow (blue arrows): the patient has been trying to inhale before the machine's exhalation time has been completed. Following this futile/abortive attempt at inhalation the patient exhales some more of the trapped gas (purple arrow), until the ventilator time-cycles into inspiration.

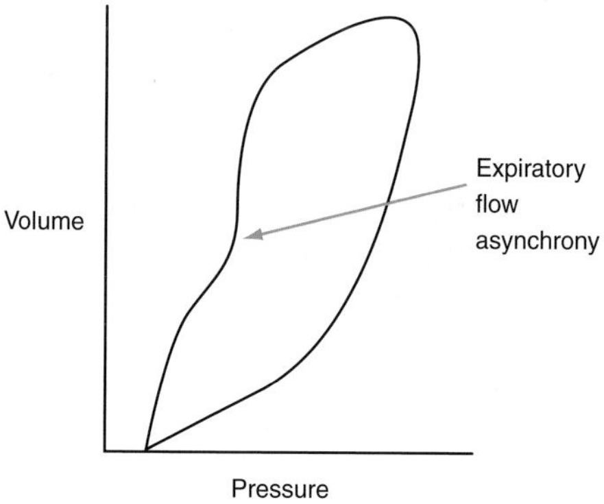
Expiratory
flow
asynchrony
Volume
Pressure

FIGURE 8.49. Pressure–volume loop: expiratory flow asynchrony.

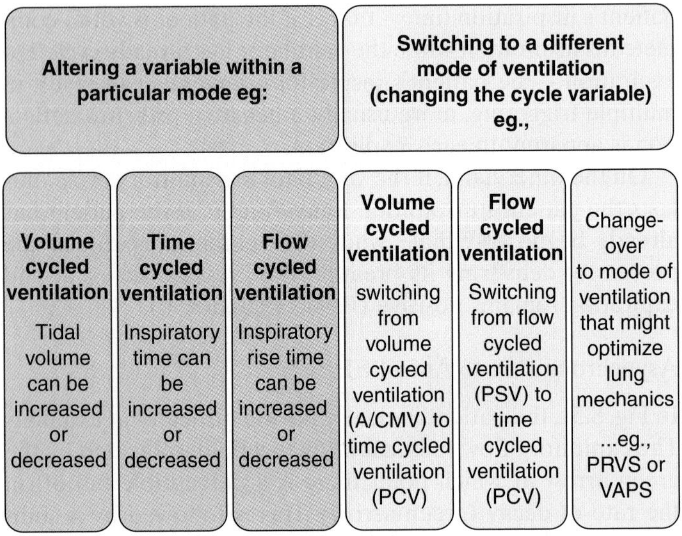
Altering a variable within a particular mode eg:
Switching to a different mode of ventilation (changing the cycle variable) eg.,
Volume cycled ventilation
Tidal volume can be increased or decreased
Time cycled ventilation
Inspiratory time can be increased or decreased
Flow cycled ventilation
Inspiratory rise time can be increased or decreased
Volume cycled ventilation
switching from volume cycled ventilation (A/CMV) to time cycled ventilation (PCV)
Flow cycled ventilation
Switching from flow cycled ventilation (PSV) to time cycled ventilation (PCV)
Change-over to mode of ventilation that might optimize lung mechanics
...eg., PRVS or VAPS

FIGURE 8.50. Treatment approach to cycle asynchrony.

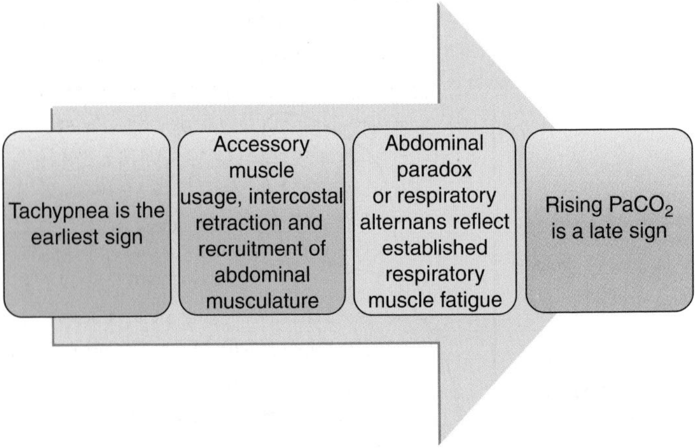
Tachypnea is the earliest sign
Accessory muscle usage, intercostal retraction and recruitment of abdominal musculature
Abdominal paradox or respiratory alternans reflect established respiratory muscle fatigue
Rising $PaCO_2$ is a late sign

FIGURE 8.51. Clinical signs of asynchrony.

Active exhalation on the part of the patient usually indicates air trapping (though such a pattern can also be produced artifactually by a defective expiratory flow transducer). Every time the patient makes an attempt to exhale the excess of gas, the expiratory tidal volume will substantially exceed the inspiratory tidal volume (Fig. 8.52). Shown on the pressure–volume loop (Fig. 8.53, below) is an active expiratory effort. At end-exhalation, when all the inspiratory tidal volume has returned, to the expiratory transducer the machine displays zero tidal volume at the baseline. With active exhalation, the intrathoracic pressure continues to remain positive, and so

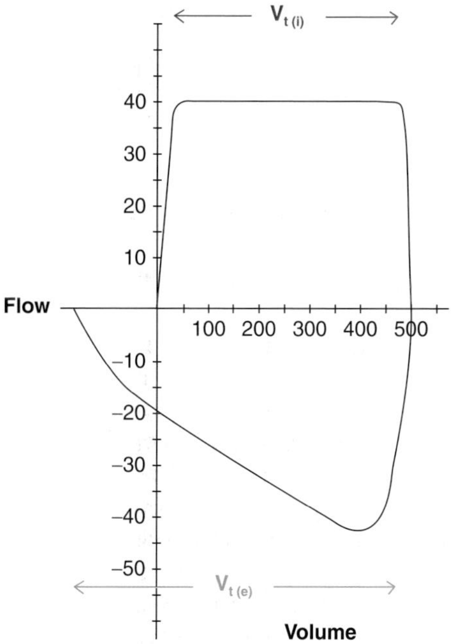
$V_{t(i)}$
40
30
20
10
Flow
100 200 300 400 500
−10
−20
−30
−40
−50
$V_{t(e)}$
Volume

FIGURE 8.52. Flow–volume loop: active exhalation. Inspiratory tidal volume ($V_{t(i)}$) is shown by the red arrow, and expiratory tidal volume $V_{t(e)}$ by the *green arrow*.

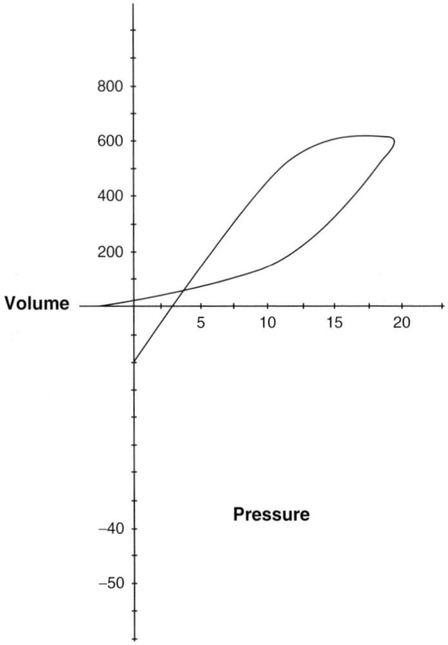
800
600
400
200
Volume
5
10
15
20
Pressure
–40
–50

FIGURE 8.53. Pressure–volume loop: active exhalation.

even though the volume has returned to zero, the pressure has not: the tracing stays on the positive side of *y*-axis until the exhalation has been completed.

In Fig. 8.54 active exhalation is demonstrated on the volume–time scalar.

Measuring Auto-PEEP

Auto-PEEP as a cause of expiratory cycle asynchrony can be unmasked by using the expiratory pause option. The breath is held briefly at end expiration, and the pressure between the proximal and distal airways then gradually

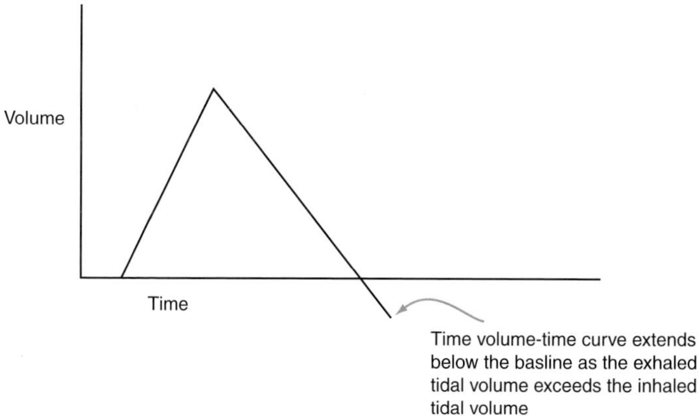
Volume
Time
Time volume-time curve extends below the basline as the exhaled tidal volume exceeds the inhaled tidal volume

FIGURE 8.54. Volume–time scalar: active exhalation.

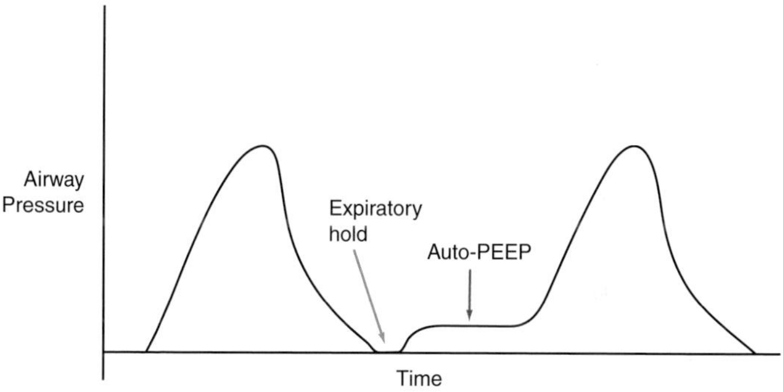
Airway Pressure
Expiratory hold
Auto-PEEP
Time

FIGURE 8.55 Auto-PEEP.

equalizes. As the ventilator transducers begin to sense the increased end-expiratory pressure within the distal airways, the airway pressure tracing gradually rises to reflect the auto-PEEP.

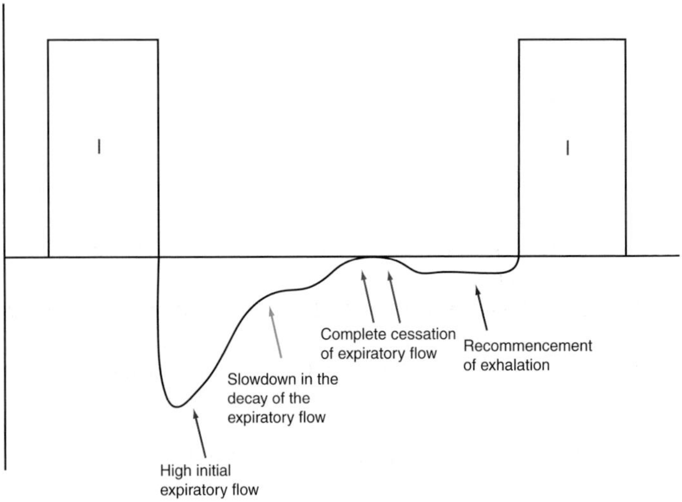
I
I
Complete cessation of expiratory flow
Recommencement of exhalation
Slowdown in the decay of the expiratory flow
High initial expiratory flow

FIGURE 8.56 Patient-ventilator asynchrony.

References

1. Aslanian P, El Atrous S, Isabey D, et al Effects of flow triggering on breathing effort during partial ventilatory support. *Am J Respir Crit Care Med*. 1998;157:135–143
2. Beck J, Tucci M, Emeriaud G, et al Prolonged neural expiratory time induced by mechanical ventilation in infants. *Pediatr Res*. 2004;55:747–754
3. Boneto C, Calo MN, Delgado MO, Mancebo J. Modes of pressure delivery and patient-ventilator interaction. *Respir Care Clin N Am*. 2005;11:247–263
4. Chang DW. *Clinical Applications of Mechanical Ventilation*. 3rd ed. New York: Delmar Learning; 2006
5. Cinnella G, Conti G, Lofaso F, et al Effects of assisted ventilation on the work of breathing: volume-controlled versus pressure-controlled ventilation. *Am J Respir Crit Care Med*. 1996;153: 1025–1033
6. Dubois AB. Resistance to breathing. In: Fenn WO, Rahn H, eds. *Handbook of Physiology and Respiration*, vol. 1. Washington, DC: American Physiology Society; 1964:451–462

7. Forster RE, DuBois AB, Briscoe WA, Fisher AB. *The Lung: Physiological Basis of Pulmonary Function Tests*. Chicago: Yearbook Medical Publishers; 1986
8. Gattinoni L, Brazzi L, Pelosi P, et al A trial of goal-oriented hemodynamic therapy in critically ill patients. *N Engl J Med*. 1995; 33:1025
9. Gay CG, Rodarte JR, Hubmayer RD. The effects of positive expiratory pressures on isovolume flow and dynamic hyperinflation in patients receiving mechanical ventilation. *Am Rev Respir Dis*. 1989;139:621–626
10. Goulet R, Hess D, Kacmarek RM. Pressure vs flow triggering during pressure support ventilation. *Chest*. 1997;111(6):1649–1653.
11. Imanaka H, Nishimura M, Takeuchi M, et al Autotriggering caused by cardiogenic oscillation during flow-triggered mechanical ventilation. *Crit Care Med*. 2000;28:402–407
12. Jubran A, Tobin MJ. The effect of hyperinflation on rib cage-abdominal motion. *Am Rev Respir Dis*. 1992;146:1378–1382
13. Jubran A, Tobin MJ. Use of flow-volume curves in detecting secretions in ventilator-dependent patients. *Am J Respir Crit Care Med*. 1994;150:766
14. Lofaso F, Brochard L, Hang T, et al Home vs intensive-care pressure support devices: experimental and clinical comparison. *Am J Respir Crit Care Med*. 1996;153:1591–1599
15. Marini JJ, Capps JS, Culver BH. The inspiratory work of breathing during assisted mechanical ventilation. *Chest*. 1985;87:612.
16. Marini JJ, Ravenscraft SA. Mean airway pressure: physiologic determinants and clinical importance: 2. Clinical implications. *Crit Care Med*. 1992;20:1604–1616
17. Oakes DF, Shortall SP. *Ventilator Management: A Bedside Reference Guide*. 2nd ed. Orono: Health Educator Publications; 2005
18. Prinianakis G, Kondili E, Georgopoulos D. Effects of the flow waveform method of triggering and cycling on patient ventilator interaction during pressure support. *Intensive Care Med*. 2003;29: 1950–1959
19. Richard JC, Carlucci A, Breton L, et al Bench testing of pressure support ventilation with three different generations of ventilators. *Intensive Care Med*. 2002;28:1049–1057
20. Sassoon CSH, Girion AE, Ely EA, Light RW. Inspiratory work of breathing on flow-by and demand flow continuous positive airway pressure. *Crit Care Med*. 1989;17:1108–1114
21. Slutsky AS. Mechanical ventilation. American College of Chest Physicians' Consensus Conference. *Chest*. 1993;104:1833

22. Stell I, Paul G, Lee K, Ponte J, Moxham J. Noninvasive ventilator triggering in chronic obstructive pulmonary disease: A test lung comparison. *Am J Respir Crit Car Med.* 2001;164:2092–2097
23. Thille A, Lellouche F, Brochard L. Patient-ventilator asynchrony during mechanical ventilation: prevalence and risk factors. *Intensive Care Med.* 2004;30:S71
24. Tobin MJ. Advances in mechanical ventilation. *N Engl J Med.* 2001;344:1986–1996
25. Tobin MJ, Jubran A, Laghi F. Patient–ventilator interaction. *Am J Respir Crit Care Med.* 2001;163:1059–1063
26. Tokioka H, Tanaka T, et al The effect of breath termination criterion on breathing patterns and the work of breathing during pressure support ventilation. *Anesth Analg.* 2001;92:161–165
27. Uchiyama A, Imanaka H, Taenaka N. Relationship between work of breathing provided by a ventilator and patients inspiratory drive during pressure support ventilation: effects of inspiratory rise time. *Anaesth Intensive Care.* 2001;29:349–358
28. Waugh JB, Deshpande VM, Harwood RJ. *Rapid Interpretation of Ventilator Waveforms.* Upper Saddle River, NJ: Prentice Hall; 1999.
29. Yamada Y, Du HL. Analysis of the mechanisms of expiratory asynchrony in pressure support ventilation: a mathematical approach. *J Appl Physiol.* 2000;88:2143–2150
30. Yang SC, Yang SP. Effects of inspiratory flow waveforms on lung mechanics, gas exchange, and respiratory metabolism in COPD patients during mechanical ventilation. *Chest.* 2002;125:2096–2104
31. Younes M. Control of breathing during mechanical ventilation. In: Slutsky AS, Brochard L, eds. *Mechanical Ventilation: Update in Intensive Care and Emergency Medicine*, vol. 40. Berlin: Springer; 2004:63–82
32. Younes M, Kun J, Webster K, Roberts D. Response of ventilator dependent patients to delayed opening of exhalation valve. *Am J Respir Crit Care Med.* 2002;166:21–30

Chapter 9
Mechanical Ventilation in Specific Disorders

9.1 Myocardial Ischemia

In myocardial ischemia, the goal of mechanical ventilation is to decrease the work of breathing and thereby the oxygen demands of the respiratory muscles. When the work of breathing is high, as much as 40% of the cardiac output can be diverted to the respiratory muscles[69]: myocardial ischemia will worsen, and a positive feedback cycle is established (Fig. 9.1). Ventilating patients with strategies that unload the respiratory muscles can be expected to improve myocardial perfusion and break the vicious cycle.

The normal heart is preload dependent and relies on adequate filling to generate a sufficient stroke volume. Positive pressure ventilatory support will reduce venous return and frequently aggravate the problem in a hypovolemic patient. On the other hand, the initiation of positive pressure ventilatory support in heart failure (where an increased preload is a problem) can improve cardiac function by decreasing the preload. Positive pressure breathing can also lower the afterload by reducing the transmural aortic pressure and thereby result in a better stroke volume (see Fig. 9.2).

As the myocardial function improves, so does the perfusion of other organs. Moreover, by opening up the lung, positive pressure ventilation can improve systemic oxygenation.

Inappropriate ventilator settings, such as an unduly high PEEP, can increase the work of breathing. Myocardial

A. Hasan, *Understanding Mechanical Ventilation*,
DOI: 10.1007/978-1-84882-869-8_9,

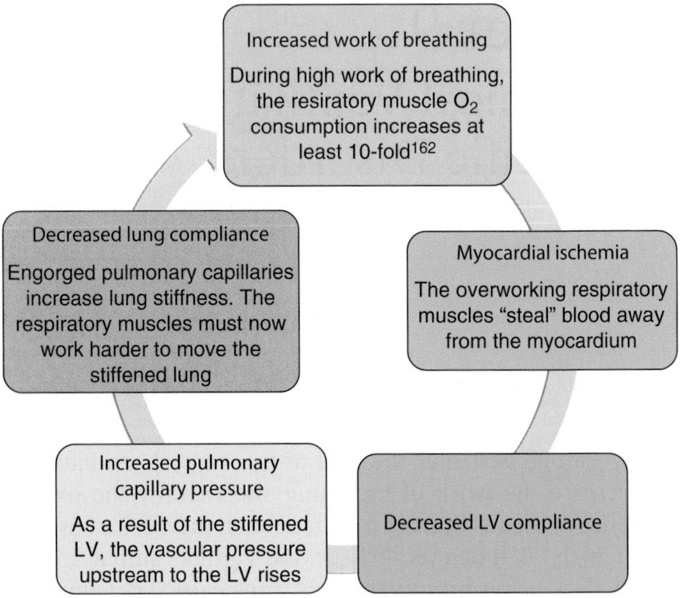
Increased work of breathing
During high work of breathing, the resiratory muscle O2 consumption increases at least 10-fold162
Myocardial ischemia
The overworking respiratory muscles "steal" blood away from the myocardium
Decreased LV compliance
Increased pulmonary capillary pressure
As a result of the stiffened LV, the vascular pressure upstream to the LV rises
Decreased lung compliance
Engorged pulmonary capillaries increase lung stiffness. The respiratory muscles must now work harder to move the stiffened lung

FIGURE 9.1. The effect of increased work of breathing and myocardial perfusion.

ischemia might then occur and reduce the LV compliance. Since the complex interplay of events never guarantees the effect of mechanical ventilation on the heart one way or another, the patient should be carefully monitored to ensure that positive pressure breathing does not increase oxygenation at the cost of the cardiac output, poor tissue perfusion due to a falling cardiac output will negate the benefit of an increased oxygen content of the blood.

Arrythmias are common in the ventilated patient on account of primary illness, cardiac injury, dyselectrolytemias, hypoxemia, and beta-adrenergic drugs – and also directly due to the effects of positive pressure breathing.[135] The size of tidal volumes can influence the autonomic control of the heart[27] (see Fig. 9.3).

Both hypocapnia and hypercapnia have a bearing on autonomic control. Acute hypocapnia can increase both myocardial contractility and systemic vascular resistance, and thereby

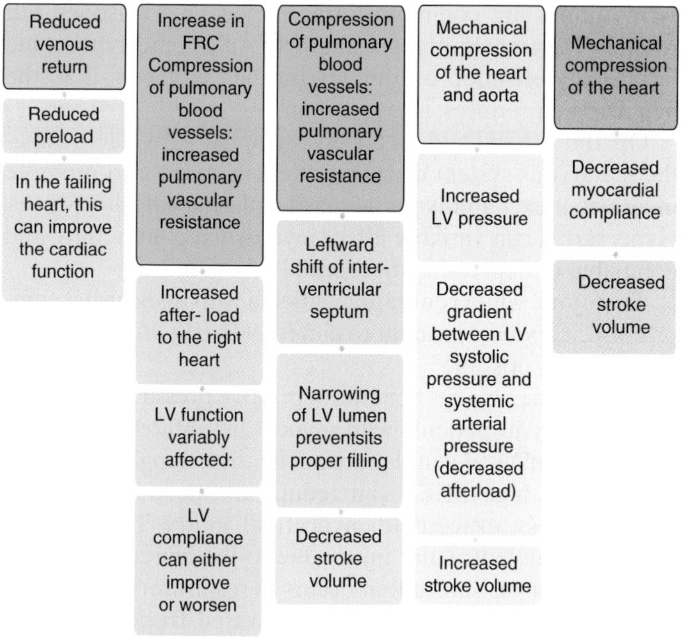
Reduced venous return
Reduced preload
In the failing heart, this can improve the cardiac function
Increase in FRC Compression of pulmonary blood vessels: increased pulmonary vascular resistance
Increased after- load to the right heart
LV function variably affected:
LV compliance can either improve or worsen
Compression of pulmonary blood vessels: increased pulmonary vascular resistance
Leftward shift of inter-ventricular septum
Narrowing of LV lumen preventsits proper filling
Decreased stroke volume
Mechanical compression of the heart and aorta
Increased LV pressure
Decreased gradient between LV systolic pressure and systemic arterial pressure (decreased afterload)
Increased stroke volume
Mechanical compression of the heart
Decreased myocardial compliance
Decreased stroke volume

FIGURE 9.2. Potential effects of PEEP on cardiac function.

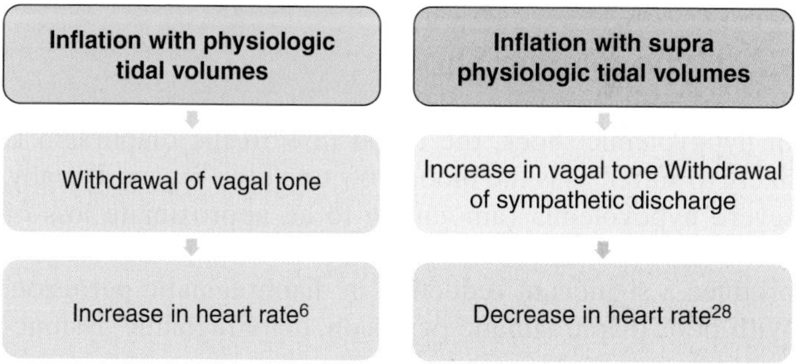
Inflation with physiologic tidal volumes
Withdrawal of vagal tone
Increase in heart rate[6]
Inflation with supra physiologic tidal volumes
Increase in vagal tone Withdrawal of sympathetic discharge
Decrease in heart rate[28]

FIGURE 9.3. Effect of tidal volume on heart rate.

increase the myocardial oxygen demand. This is the reason for episodes of variant angina being more common in the setting of hypocapnia. It also appears that hypocapnia, by promoting platelet aggregation, might be thrombogenic.

Arrhythmias are common during hypocapnic episodes, but whether the arrhythmias are a direct result of the hypocapnia or are an offshoot of the myocardial ischemia that the hypocapnia produces, is less certain.

On the other hand, acute hypercapnia – by the sympathetic nervous system discharge it elicits – can also promote myocardial excitability by increasing plasma catecholamines. Hypercarbia can variably affect myocardial contractility and is capable of depressing myocardial function.

Therefore, while ventilating patients with myocardial compromise, it appears prudent to aim for a $PaCO_2$ that is as close to normal as possible.

Despite the obvious benefits of positive pressure breathing, the mortality in patients with myocardial infarction who do require mechanical ventilation can be disturbingly high.[94] An inordinately high PEEP can reduce coronary blood flow[15] and doubtless, exacerbate myocardial injury. To confound matters, right ventricular injury due to the increased pulmonary vascular resistance that occurs in respiratory failure can falsely elevate Troponin-I levels.[73] Elevated Troponin-I levels nevertheless appear to be a marker for increased mortality in such patients.[12]

9.2 Hypovolemic Shock

In hypovolemic shock, the blood flow to the diaphragm is likely to suffer, as is the blood flow to all the organs. Usually, severe hypovolemia (amounting to an approximate loss of more than 40% of circulating blood volume) is necessary to produce a significant reduction in diaphragmatic perfusion. With poor diaphragmatic perfusion, diaphragmatic dysfunction can occur. Also, the decrease in cardiac output will decrease the pulmonary blood flow, thereby decreasing the perfusion of patent alveoli. With supranormal tidal volumes, an inflation-vasodilation response can occur and LV contractility can decline on account of this as well.[165]

In well ventilated but ill-perfused alveoli, the dead space will expand, and this can increase the minute ventilation requirement. With an already compromised diaphragm, any increase in the work of breathing can unfavorably impact the failing heart. In this setting, positive pressure breathing can, by increasing the intrathoracic pressure, further diminish preload, unless the body fluids are adequately replenished.

If large amounts of crystalloid are required for the replenishment of circulatory volume, fluid sometimes spills out into the lung tissues. Pulmonary edema will not only impair gas exchange, but also increase the work of breathing by reducing lung compliance. Nevertheless, rapid volume resuscitation – and not mechanical ventilation – should be the priority in such situations. Intubation and ventilation should be carried out when cardiopulmonary arrest is impending, or when specific issues such as pulmonary edema or contusion, cervical cord injury, head, or maxillofacial injuries require better control of the situation.

Spontaneous modes of ventilation produce relatively modest elevations in mean airway pressure, and so do not depress the circulation as much as the other modes. In view of its propensity to depress the circulation in hypovolemia, PEEP is better kept at a minimum until the circulatory dynamics are improved.

9.3 Neurological Injury

The lungs of patients with head injury can be compromised for a variety of reasons. A vulnerable airway predisposes patients to aspiration, acid pneumonitis and aspiration pneumonia. Neurogenic pulmonary edema, which is thought to be mediated by sympathetic reflexes, can cause alveolar filling and further worsen gas exchange.[113,178]

Cerebral autoregulation normally protects the cerebral circulation from major swings in systemic arterial pressure. A preserved gradient between arterial pressure and cerebral venous pressure are critical to cerebral blood flow. The cerebral perfusion pressure (CPP) is the difference between the mean arterial pressure (MAP) and the ICP. It is generally agreed that CPP needs to exceed 60 mmHg to sustain cerebral perfusion.[40,171]

When cerebral autoregulation fails, any rise in intracranial pressure narrows the difference between the MAP and mean intracranial pressure. Consequently, there is a decrease in the CPP and cerebral blood flow.[76] By reducing the venous return from the head, positive pressure ventilation is capable of increasing the intracranial pressure and decreasing the CPP further. Positive pressure breathing – and PEEP in particular – will often reduce the cardiac output by several mechanisms (see sections 3.8 and 9.1), and the MAP and CPP can decrease on account of this.[25]

Patients in whom intracranial pressure is already raised – such as those with closed head injuries and cerebral tumors, as well as postneurosurgical patients – seem to be more vulnerable to develop cerebral hypoperfusion as a result of positive pressure breathing. By contrast, patients with normal intracranial dynamics do not seem to develop raised intracranial pressure with the application of positive pressure ventilation.

The brain, its blood vessels, and the interstitium are contained within the rigid confines of the cranium: strategies directed at shrinking the vascular compartment will often help reduce ICP.[65] Since the relationship between the cerebral blood flow and the $PaCO_2$ is roughly linear, lowering the $PaCO_2$ will produce cerebral vasoconstriction and bring about a parallel reduction in the cerebral blood flow.[76]

Unless the degree of injury is extremely severe, brainstem reflexes are generally intact, and the respiratory drive is therefore preserved. In spite of this, the degree of hyperventilation that occurs as a physiological response to the raised intracranial pressure may not be enough to lower the $PaCO_2$ to a level that is required for cerebral vasoconstriction.

ICP, normally around 10 mmHg, will require intervention for its control if it rises above 20 mmHg. Occasionally, ICP can be much higher, and pressures above 40 mmHg can lead to herniation of the brain.[195]

A brief spell of hypocapnic ventilation a– deliberate hyperventilation – can prove to be lifesaving by the dramatic physiological changes it evokes. Lowering the $PaCO_2$ to the mid or low 20 s often brings about a rapid fall in intracranial pressure. A decrease of cerebral blood flow by about 4% can be anticipated for every 1 mmHg of acute reduction in $PaCO_2$. It is rather less certain that hypocapnic ventilation will be beneficial when used for prolonged periods in critically ill patients.

The cerebral vasoconstriction that hypocapnia induces can worsen cerebral ischemia and produce cerebral lactic acidosis.[101] Hypocapnia results in alkalosis, and the leftward shift of the oxyhemoglobin dissociation curve that occurs as a consequence of this impairs oxygen release from the hemoglobin to the cerebral tissues. Compensatory mechanisms then gradually restore the pH in the local milieu toward normal over the next few hours; cerebral blood flow also slowly normalizes. If at a subsequent point of time an attempt is made to normalize the systemic $PaCO_2$ by reducing the level of hyperventilation, a rebound increase in intracranial pressure can occur; cerebral hyperemia can result in reperfusion injury or cerebral hemorrhage in previously ischemic regions of the brain. Most authors therefore do not recommend the use of hypocapnic ventilation within the first 24 h, when the cerebral blood flow is generally low,[74,107,188] and then only where monitoring of ICP is available.[25]

Since the compensation for hypocapnic cerebral vasoconstriction occurs fairly quickly, deliberate hyperventilation can at best be considered a temporizing measure for the urgent control of intracranial hyperventilation until more definitive measures for the control of the latter are taken.

In cases of neurological injury with normal intracranial pressure, prophylactic hyperventilation is certainly not desirable.[166] Hyperventilating the patient whose intracranial pressures are normal might reduce the option of hyperventilation at a later stage, should the intracranial pressure subsequently rise. Furthermore, the large minute volumes required – for the degree of hyperventilation that would be required to drop the CO_2 to a new low – could by themselves increase the intrathoracic pressure.

In the setting of high ICP, the role of PEEP has predictably come under scrutiny. A PEEP level of up to 12 cm H_2O does not seem to dangerously increase ICP.[74] Higher levels of PEEP – around 15 cm H_2O – are tolerated when the lung is noncompliant,[25,54] since a stiff lung will not transmit airway pressures to the vasculature as well as a compliant lung (see section 9.4 below).

9.4 Acute Respiratory Distress Syndrome (ARDS)

The first descriptions of ARDS appear in Rene Laennec's account of idiopathic anasarca of the lungs, published in 1821. Since then, ARDS has been described in medical literature under various appellations – principally due to a general failure to realize that this syndrome could be encountered under widely disparate circumstances. During World War I and in the years that followed, descriptions of ARDS surfaced under different names. Thus, posttraumatic massive pulmonary collapse, white lung, shock lung, and Da Nang lung were frequently witnessed on battlefields. The occurrence of ARDS in diverse scenarios led to the coinage of terms representative of those situations, such as adult hyaline membrane disease, respirator lung, pump lung, hemorrhagic lung syndrome, and congestive atelectasis.

It took Ashbaug and colleagues to recognize in 1967 that the above descriptions were all of a single entity. In 1994, the American–European Consensus Conference defined ARDS in tangible and unambiguous terms, proposing four criteria for its characterization:

1. Acute onset
2. Diffuse, bilateral radiological involvement
3. Severe hypoxemia
4. The absence of a raised pulmonary artery occlusion pressure (PAOP)

Fulfillment of all four criteria in a compatible clinical setting defines ARDS.

Hypoxemia has been quantified by the PaO_2/FIO_2 ratio (the ratio of the pulmonary arterial oxygen tension to the fraction of inspired oxygen concentration). A value of less than 200 (regardless of the level of applied PEEP) in the presence of the other criteria defines ARDS; a value between 200 and 300 (regardless of the applied PEEP level) defines acute lung injury (ALI). The difference between ARDS and ALI lies in the severity of the pathological process. The SpO_2/FIO_2 ratio – the calculation of which does not require arterial puncture – has been proposed as a surrogate for the $PaO_2/$

FIO_2 ratio. A PaO_2/FIO_2 ratio of 235 has been shown to equate with a PaO_2/FIO_2 ratio of 200, and a PaO_2/FIO_2 ratio of 315 with a PaO_2/FIO_2 ratio of 200.[154]

Since cardiogenic pulmonary edema and the pulmonary edema of fluid overload closely mimic ARDS, it is necessary to exclude them by applying the fourth criterion: the absence of raised pulmonary artery occlusion pressure (PAOP > 18 mmHg). In the absence of the means to measure PAOP, lack of evidence of congestive cardiac failure or fluid overload are sometimes used as rough surrogates for a normal (or at least, not elevated) PAOP. It must be borne in mind that an elevated PAOP does not decisively rule out ARDS, since left ventricular dysfunction can complicate about 20% of all patients with ARDS.[193]

9.4.1 Primary and Secondary ARDS

More than 60 causes of ARDS are now listed. The etiological processes leading to ARDS or ALI have traditionally been classified as primary and secondary. Processes such as pneumonia, aspiration, inhalation, or near-drowning have been classified as primary because they are direct inciting causes of lung injury. Events such as major trauma, pancreatitis, burns, or multiple blood transfusions are thought to injure the lung as a consequence of the systemic inflammatory response that they produce, and have therefore been classified as secondary (extrapulmonary) causes of ARDS/ALI.

The division of ARDS into the two syndromes may have merit. The dominant pattern of injury in the primary form ("pulmonary ARDS") is airspace consolidation, with a dense exudate of neutrophils and hyaline membranes within the air spaces. There is a widespread alveolar epithelial cell injury,[133] with relative sparing of the pulmonary endothelium. In contrast, in the secondary ("extrapulmonary") form, the alveolar epithelial cells are preserved, and the distribution of pulmonary edema is mainly into the interstitium rather than into the airspaces. The two syndromes also differ slightly in their patterns of radiological involvement, respiratory mechanics, and in their response to treatment modalities such as PEEP and proning.

9.4.2 Pathophysiology

Fluid dynamics within the lung are governed by the Starling equation (see Box 9.1). The movement of fluid between the interstitium and the pulmonary capillaries is determined by the resultant of two opposing forces, that is, the hydrostatic pressure and the fluid oncotic pressure. The latter is mainly on account of small protein molecules in the fluid, principally albumin.

Since the forces that encourage transudation of fluid from the capillaries into the interstitium exceed the forces that oppose this effect, there is normally a net outflow of small quantities of fluid from the pulmonary capillaries into the interstitum. If this fluid were to leak into the alveoli, this could seriously compromise gas exchange. In health, alveolar flooding does not occur because the fluid that transudes into the interstitium is promptly removed by the interstitial lymphatics.[115] Also, the alveolar epithelium is rendered leakproof by intercellular "tight junctions," preventing oozing of fluid into the alveoli. Furthermore, the fluid oncotic pressure within the capillaries exerts a moderating influence on fluid migration out of the vasculature.

Box 9.1 The Starling Equation

According to the Starling equation, the net flow of fluid across the capillaries (Q) can be summarized by the following equation:

$$Q = K(P_c - P_i - \sigma(\pi_c - \pi_i),$$

where

Q = net flow of fluid across the pulmonary capillaries
P_c = pulmonary capillary hydrostatic pressure
P_i = interstitial fluid hydrostatic pressure
π_c = pulmonary capillary oncotic pressure
π_i = interstitial fluid oncotic pressure
K = permeability coefficient, which basically represents the endothelial leakiness for the transuding fluid
σ = reflectance, which is a property of the fluid molecules

In ARDS, due to the loss of the integrity of the alveolocapillary membrane, protein-rich fluid escapes from the vasculature. The presence of protein-rich fluid in the interstitium diminishes the oncotic pressure gradient, and one of the mechanisms that protects against excessive fluid accumulation in the interstitum is thereby lost.[24] When this occurs, the pulmonary interstitium becomes waterlogged and the lymphatics are no longer able to cope with the excess of fluid that they are presented with. Proteinaceous fluid, debris, and hyaline membranes fill up the airspaces, severely compromising gas exchange. A shift in the normal fibrinolytic state of the lung to a procoagulant one leads to the formation of hyaline membranes – mostly composed of fibrin and the detritus of Type 1 alveolar epithelial cells.[118]

Large areas of lung tissue become atelectatic and poorly ventilated. Because atelectatic lung units resist expansion, the overall lung compliance falls.[56] The shutting off of large numbers of lung units means that fewer alveoli are now available for gas exchange, in effect offering a smaller lung for ventilation (tiny tidal volumes ought to be used while ventilating these so called "baby lungs,"[56] lest airway pressures rise dangerously or alveolar overdistension occurs)[159] – see discussion later on.

Presumably, on account of the hypoxia as well as direct vascular compression by the raised intrathoracic pressure that mechanical ventilation produces, pulmonary artery hypertension (PAH) frequently occurs.[170,191] It is uncertain as to what role PAH actually plays in this complex interplay of events: because hypoxic vasoconstriction actually improves *V/Q* matching by closing down the blood supply to atelectatic air units, PAH may rather be a compensatory response directed at reducing hypoxemia.

The histologic hallmark of ARDS is diffuse alveolar damage (DAD). However, there is less than perfect correlation between the clinical syndrome – as defined by the AECC criteria – and DAD[125]; since this association appears closer for extrapulmonary ARDS than pulmonary ARDS,[44] it could be that these two pathologies represent distinct syndromes.[126]

9.4.3 Ventilatory Strategies

9.4.3.1 Modes of Ventilation

Due to the volatility and uncertainty of the clinical situation that often prevails, some form of a control mode of ventilation is required, at least initially. Both volume-and pressure-limited modes are acceptable.

Because the control of airway pressure often presents a challenge in ARDS-ventilation, pressure-limited modes are preferred by many clinicians (see Pressure-Controlled Ventilation in Chap. 4). As the lung mechanics do not usually change rapidly in ARDS patients, either volume control ventilation or pressure control ventilation may be equally appropriate. It has been proposed that the choice between these two modes should be dictated by physician-familiarity with a particular mode rather than the relative merits of the modes themselves.[166] It is, however, important to distinguish the different objectives of these two modes. While the goal of volume control mode is to tightly control the tidal volumes while monitoring airway pressures, that of the pressure control

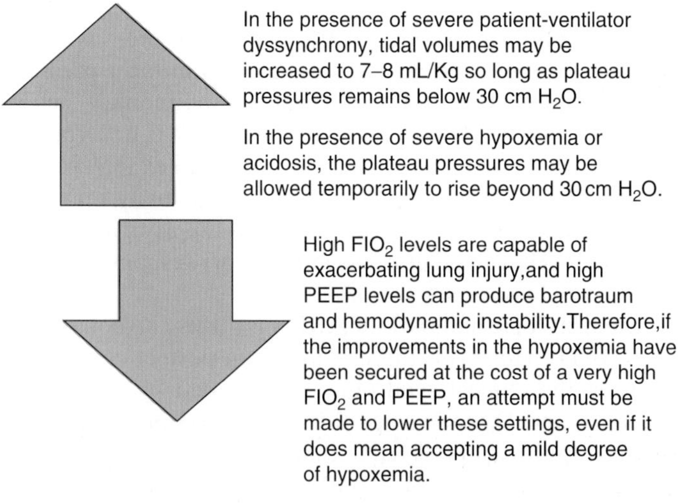
In the presence of severe patient-ventilator dyssynchrony, tidal volumes may be increased to 7–8 mL/Kg so long as plateau pressures remains below 30 cm H_2O.
In the presence of severe hypoxemia or acidosis, the plateau pressures may be allowed temporarily to rise beyond 30 cm H_2O.
High FIO_2 levels are capable of exacerbating lung injury,and high PEEP levels can produce barotraum and hemodynamic instability.Therefore,if the improvements in the hypoxemia have been secured at the cost of a very high FIO_2 and PEEP, an attempt must be made to lower these settings, even if it does mean accepting a mild degree of hypoxemia.

FIGURE 9.4. Compromises in ventilator settings in ARDS.

mode is to tightly control airway pressures while monitoring the tidal volumes.

Airway pressure release ventilation and high frequency oscillation have been discussed in Chaps. 4 & 17 respectively.

9.4.3.2 Tidal Volumes

The lungs are functionally small in ARDS, and low tidal volumes are used in order to avoid alveolar overdistension, barotrauma, and hypotension.[7]

Mechanical ventilation *per se* can be considered to be proinflammatory, and it is now well recognized that even physiologic tidal volumes are capable of causing or perpetuating lung injury in ARDS. Ventilation with relatively high tidal volumes (e.g., upward of 10 mL/kg) results in alveolar overdistension, and the lung operates above the upper deflection point on the pressure–volume curve. Above the deflection point, any increase in the distending pressures will fail to achieve a commensurate increase in lung expansion in lung volume: this is typical of a stiff and overdistended lung (see Fig. 5.7 Chap. 5).

Of all the ventilation strategies currently in vogue for ALI/ARDS the employment of a low tidal volume ventilation strategy is the one shown to have the most powerful mitigating effect on ARDS mortality.[141] Tidal volumes have been considered safest below 10 mL/kg (probably to the order of around 7–8 mL/kg), and ventilation with even smaller tidal volumes may sometimes become necessary. With these tiny tidal volumes, the minute volume requirements may not be satisfied even at relatively high respiratory frequencies, and some amount of hypercarbia may need to be accepted: the $PaCO_2$ accordingly needs to be allowed to rise in a controlled manner[83] (see Sect. 9.5.3.10 below).

9.4.3.3 Airway Pressures

Wherever possible, the plateau pressure should be kept below 30 cm H_2O, even if this entails ventilating the patient with extremely small tidal volumes. In fact, there is no plateau pressure level that can be regarded as absolutely safe: ventilation with a relatively low plateau pressure can still injure the lung, and a goal of 28 cm H_2O has been suggested.[177] In view of this fact, it appears sensible to ventilate patients with the low tidal volume strategy even if the plateau pressures are not overly raised.[70]

9.4.3.4 Respiratory Rate

The respiratory rate is frequently high in the spontaneously breathing ARDS patient; this is in response to the need to preserve the minute ventilation in the face of the restricted tidal volumes afforded by a stiffening lung. With the adoption of a low tidal volumes strategy in the ventilated patient, the respiratory rate must necessarily be set high enough to avoid a buildup in the $PaCO_2$.

9.4.3.5 Flow Waveforms

Increasing the respiratory rate decreases the respiratory cycle time. The expiratory time becomes proportionately shortened as well, resulting in insufficient time being available for expiration. This can lead to auto-PEEP.[38]

Increasing the inspiratory flow rate will allow delivery of the set tidal volumes within a shorter inspiratory time – leaving more time for expiration. Although this strategy can be expected to decrease the airway pressures to some extent, it is often seen that notwithstanding these manipulations, airway pressures still continue to be perilously high. This is because given a stiff lung rather than an obstructed lung, manipulation of inspiratory flow (which mostly affects the resistance) is less likely to be effective than manipulation of the tidal volume (which mostly affects the compliance).[109] The trade-off here is to decrease the tidal volumes or respiratory rate (or both) even further, thus bringing down the airway pressures to as safe a level as possible; but the price to pay would be the acceptance of a higher $PaCO_2$, since hypoventilation would now become inevitable.

Within volume-controlled ventilation, manipulating the waveforms can also help in decreasing airway pressures. With a decelerating waveform, the inspiratory flow decreases as inspiration progresses, and rise in airway pressures is of a lesser magnitude. This may prove to be advantageous when high airway pressures are the limiting factor for adequate ventilation. However, with the slowing of airflow that the decelerating wave pattern produces, the inspiratory time lengthens, and the available expiratory time is encroached upon. The air trapping thus produced can raise the airway pressures by itself.

9.4.3.6 PEEP

Treatment of ARDS is mainly supportive. Mechanical ventilation is the most important supportive modality in evolved ARDS, and PEEP – the maintenance of a positive pressure in the airway at the end of expiration – forms a crucial part of this support strategy.

Normally, expiration is passive, with a few exceptions (e.g., an obstructed patient who uses his expiratory muscles to exhale through narrowed airways). This is true of a patient who is spontaneously breathing, as well as a patient on intermittent positive pressure support. Expiration ends when the alveolar pressure equates with the pressure at the mouth. In a ventilated patient, by closing the expiratory valve before the exhalation is quite complete – and while the airway pressure is yet higher than the pressure at the mouth – positive end-expiratory pressure is created within the airways.

The glottis in health maintains a small amount of PEEP to prevent alveolar collapse. Emphysematous patients augment their intrinsic PEEP by pursed-lip breathing. Physiological PEEP is the small amount of PEEP (generally 3 cm H_2O) that is applied to a ventilated patient to compensate for the loss of glottic function that the endotracheal tube causes.

It is as yet unclear whether patients at risk of *developing* ARDS benefit from the application of PEEP as a prophylactic measure, and evidence so far has not been supportive of this fact.[49,139] The usage of PEEP in *established* ARDS, however, is of proven benefit. PEEP results in improvement in tissue oxygenation by several important mechanisms.[102,151] By opening up collapsed alveoli, PEEP increases FRC. Alveolar recruitment decreases the shunt fraction; PEEP also decreases the blood supply to the collapsed alveoli and thereby shuts off wasteful perfusion of unventilated alveoli, further improving V/Q matching. These effects translate into better oxygenation of the blood leaving the pulmonary capillaries. By increasing the alveolar recruitment and FRC, PEEP makes the lungs more compliant.

Several large trials have shown no significant difference in outcome between a high-PEEP (about 15 cm H_2O) and a low-PEEP (about 8 cm H_2O) strategy.[23,120,122] This, however, should not be taken to mean that a low PEEP strategy is better: it has been established that low PEEP levels (<5 cm H_2O) can exacerbate lung injury.[48] In practice, a level of at least 15 cm H_2O PEEP has been shown to optimize the lung compliance.[28]

9.4.3.7 Overdistension

Since the inspiratory force that is required to distend the alveoli that are already open is less than that required to open up collapsed alveoli, compliance is relatively normal in the recruited parts of the pulmonary parenchyma. Due to the relatively high compliance of these regions, most of the tidal volumes are directed here during inspiration.[56] When comparatively large tidal volumes are received into portions of the lung that are already well expanded, regional alveolar overdistension can occur, with compliance once again falling, as the upper deflection point on the pressure–volume curve is exceeded (see below).[37]

Even in the normal lung, ventilation is never uniform; the greater negativity of intrapleural pressures in the upper parts of the lung causes the alveolar units here to be more distended at end-expiration. The dimensions of the alveolar units in the lower portions of the lung are relatively small at end-expiration, and so these units are capable of a greater *change* in volume during inspiration. In ARDS, closed alveoli

coexist along with normal lung units, making for a heterogeneous population within the lung parenchyma. With the addition of PEEP, a proportion of closed alveoli open up – and stay open – decreasing the inhomogeneity of ventilation.

For the reasons just mentioned, the nondependent lung zones by virtue of their position are vulnerable to overdistension by inappropriately high levels of PEEP, or with high tidal volumes.[57] In the supine position, PEEP mostly recruits alveoli in the apical and parasternal regions of the lung, but can derecruit alveoli in the paraspinal and juxtadiaphragmatic areas. PEEP seems to be rather more beneficial in ARDS of nonpulmonary etiologies where the increase in lung water is by and large confined to the interstitium (at least in the initial stages), than in ARDS of pulmonary origin (such as pneumonia) where *alveolar* filling is the dominant pathology (Fig. 9.5).

High PEEP may cause difficulties at several levels.[142] An inappropriately high PEEP can elevate airway pressures, causing alveolar overdistension and barotrauma. The rise in intrathoracic pressure produced by PEEP can decrease the venous return to the heart; hypotension can occur especially

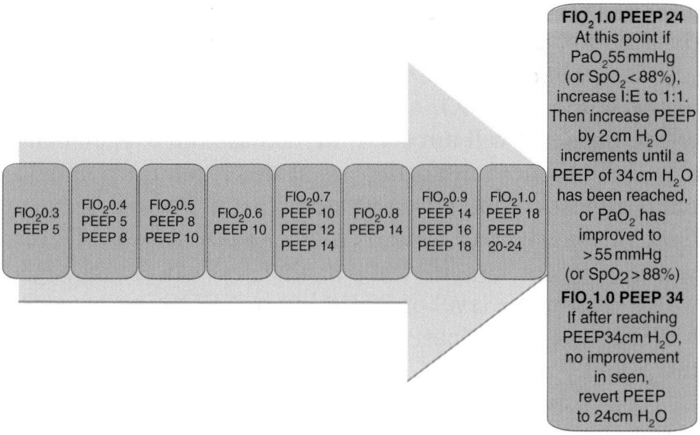
FIO2 0.3 PEEP 5
FIO2 0.4 PEEP 5 PEEP 8
FIO2 0.5 PEEP 8 PEEP 10
FIO2 0.6 PEEP 10
FIO2 0.7 PEEP 10 PEEP 12 PEEP 14
FIO2 0.8 PEEP 14
FIO2 0.9 PEEP 14 PEEP 16 PEEP 18
FIO2 1.0 PEEP 18 PEEP 20-24
FIO2 1.0 PEEP 24
At this point if PaO2 55 mmHg (or SpO2 < 88%), increase I:E to 1:1. Then increase PEEP by 2 cm H2O increments until a PEEP of 34 cm H2O has been reached, or PaO2 has improved to > 55 mmHg (or SpO2 > 88%)
FIO2 1.0 PEEP 34
If after reaching PEEP34cm H2O, no improvement in seen, revert PEEP to 24cm H2O

FIGURE 9.5. Incremental increase in PEEP and FIO2 for optimization of oxygenation.[7???]

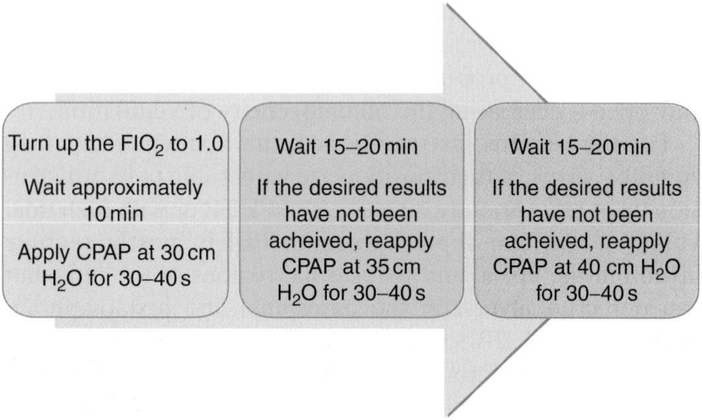
Turn up the FIO2 to 1.0
Wait approximately 10 min
Apply CPAP at 30 cm H2O for 30–40 s
Wait 15–20 min
If the desired results have not been acheived, reapply CPAP at 35 cm H2O for 30–40 s
Wait 15–20 min
If the desired results have not been acheived, reapply CPAP at 40 cm H2O for 30–40 s

FIGURE 9.6. Recruitment by sustained inflation (CPAP) technique.

if the patient is hypovolemic.[100,158] PEEP can, by elevating the right atrial pressure, produce intracardiac shunting across a patent foramen ovale.[36] To ensure optimization of PEEP, and to protect against alveolar distension and depression of cardiac output, PEEP is added at a relatively low level (e.g., at 5 cm H_2O) and then gradually boosted in small increments of 3–5 cm H_2O at periodic intervals, until the desired level of oxygenation is achieved (Fig. 9.6).[142]

It is worth reemphasizing that the target for oxygenation of the blood is a PaO_2 much above 60 mmHg. PaO_2 much above this level will not serve to increase the oxygen delivery to the tissues any further, as at this level, the hemoglobin is almost completely saturated. The aim is to achieve at least this much PaO_2 with as low an FIO_2 as possible, certainly of 0.6 or less. It is hoped that this can be managed with a reasonable level of PEEP, but in ARDS, it is usual for a PEEP level of at least 15 cm H_2O to be needed to bring this about.[28]

The construction of pressure–volume curves and the relevance of ventilating the patient at a level between the lower inflection point and the upper deflection point has been discussed in 5.10.

9.4.3.8 Inspiratory Time

Increasing the inspiratory time (T_i) can also help in decreasing the hypoxemia. Because of the heterogeneity of involvement in ARDS, alveoli with varying time constants are dispersed throughout the lungs: during inspiration, diseased alveoli take longer to fill up (see 3.5). With longer inspiratory time settings, diseased units are given the extra time they need to open up, and as a result, can now participate in ventilation.

The inspiratory time can be increased by reducing the inspiratory flow rate. Inspiratory time can also be increased by using a decelerating waveform, wherein the inspiratory flow slows down progressively as inspiration advances. By adding an inspiratory pause, the lung can be held open at end-inspiration for the duration of the applied pause, achieving the same goal. Increasing the inspiratory time has been shown to improve blood oxygenation in ARDS.

9.4.3.9 Inverse Ratio Ventilation

A mode of ventilation that has emerged as a logical extension of the above strategy is the inverse ratio ventilation (IRV) mode. Normally, inspiratory time occupies about a third of the respiratory cycle; two thirds of the respiratory cycle is spent in expiration. IRV is the reversal of this ratio; the inspiratory time is actually made to equal or exceed the expiratory time to enable improvement in oxygenation by the mechanisms just discussed. Controversies still surround the use of IRV.[105,123] (see 5.4 & 5.12.3). It is also unclear whether the better oxygenation translates into improved survival.[8]

Owing to the prolongation of T_i (with the consequent decrease in expiration time) air trapping is possible, with its potential to cause barotrauma and hypotension in an already fragile situation. This problem usually occurs when the I:E ratio exceeds 2:1.[106] Since the pattern of breathing in IRV is so different from the physiological pattern, patients generally tend to tolerate it poorly, and frequently require heavy sedation if not actual pharmacological paralysis.

9.4.3.10 Recruitment Maneuvers

When alveoli are atelectatic, the need for high pressures to achieve a given change in volume translates into poor lung compliance. Also, by repeatedly opening and closing during the respiratory cycle, unstable alveoli generate shear forces at their interface with relatively normal alveoli, increasing the probability of injury in these regions (atelectrauma).[128,173]

Lungs ventilated with low tidal volumes are likely to develop regional atelectasis. Since the dependent regions bear the weight of the lung above them, it is reasonable to suppose that some of the airspaces in these regions may be collapsed: therefore these should theoretically be recruitable (this concept is undoubtedly oversimplistic). Although PEEP is helpful in keeping the functioning lung units open, it cannot prize open up collapsed airspaces. Lung recruitment can be performed by several methods,[80] but which of these is best, is currently uncertain. The most usually employed of these techniques is the sustained inflation (or CPAP) method.[96,132] The incremental PEEP technique – used with pressure control ventilation – is generally used when there is a lack of response to sustained inflation. Lung recruitment by intermittent sighs (approximately 150% of tidal volume) may be effective in extrapulmonary ARDS or during prone ventilation (Fig. 9.7).[136]

Compared to the secondary (extrapulmonary) form, not only is the primary ARDS less responsive to recruitment, but is also more susceptible to hemodynamic compromise during the maneuver.[97]

Lung recruitment maneuvers are potentially harmful, and can cause severe hemodynamic compromise and barotrauma. They are contraindicated when the patient is hemodynamically unstable, or in the presence of intracranial hypertension, bronchospasm, lung bullae, or an untreated pneumothorax. Finally, not all patients respond to lung recruitment[67]; any improvements in hypoxemia may be transient.

Still, despite their theoretical potential to overdistend the lung, recruitment maneuvers appear to be reasonably safe when used carefully. It should be kept in mind that the

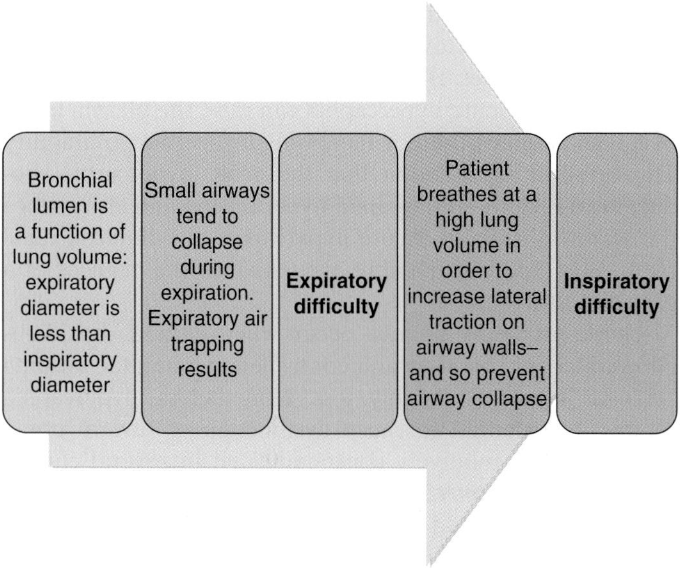
Bronchial lumen is a function of lung volume: expiratory diameter is less than inspiratory diameter
Small airways tend to collapse during expiration. Expiratory air trapping results
Expiratory difficulty
Patient breathes at a high lung volume in order to increase lateral traction on airway walls– and so prevent airway collapse
Inspiratory difficulty

FIGURE 9.7. Pattern of breathing with dynamic hyperinflation.

pressures used in "cranking" the lung open are far in excess of those considered safe during tidal ventilation. The exercise should be aborted if the MAP falls to <60 mmHg (or by 20 mmHg), or should severe tachycardia (HR >140) or bradycardia (HR <60) supervene. For the time being at least, attractive as the concept may appear, the routine use of recruitment maneuvers cannot be recommended.

9.4.3.11 Permissive Hypercapnia

The application of low tidal volumes frequently means the acceptance of a degree of hypercapnia.[83] Permissive hypercapnic ventilation is a strategy where the carbon dioxide is gradually allowed to rise by limiting minute ventilation in order to prevent an inordinate elevation in the airway pressures.

Acute elevations in the carbon dioxide tension of blood can lead to severe acidemia, cardiac arrhythmias, and severe neurologic injury. In theory, large fluxes of CO_2 across cellular membranes can overwhelm the substantial intracellular buffering resources. By increasing sympathetic nervous system discharge, acute hypercapnia can raise the plasma levels of catecholamines, thereby increasing myocardial excitability. The cerebral vasodilation that the acute hypercarbia produces can result in intracranial hypertension and also reduce the seizure threshold. Acute hypercarbia can diminish renal blood flow and can possibly also enhance the chances of a gastrointestinal bleed.

These problems do not occur when carbon dioxide is allowed to rise in a slow and controlled manner; the ensuing acidosis is understandably less. Nonetheless, hypercapnia retains its potential to cause dysfunction of several organ systems and is relatively contraindicated in several clinical circumstances (Box 9.2).

All attempts should be made to reduce all possible external deadspace, and this may include shortening the ventilator tubing[156] and replacing a HME with a heated humidifier.[147] Tracheal gas insufflation (TGI) – a technique during which fresh gas is streamed into the trachea through small channels in the walls of the endotracheal tube – has been used to flush out the CO_2

Box 9.2 Physiological Effects of Hypercapnia

Pulmonary effects
Bronchodilation
Increased pulmonary vascular resistance
Rightward shift of the oxyhemoglobin dissociation curve
Cardiovascular effects
Tachycardia
Increased stroke volume
Decreased afterload
Cerebral effects
Increased cerebral perfusion
Increased intracranial pressure

resident in the lower trachea and beyond. Auto-PEEP, mucosal injury and inspissations of airway secretions are common, and the technique awaits further refinement.Whether the acidosis that the hypercarbia produces, should be corrected by bicarbonate infusion, remains a moot point. The carbon dioxide generated from the infused bicarbonate can itself worsen the acidemia. Bicarbonate as such is relatively inefficient at controlling the acidemia, and it often takes large amounts of bicarbonate to change the pH to any significant degree. Large bicarbonate infusions can involve considerable sodium or fluid loading and this in itself may have adverse implications. With respect to the brain, the blood brain barrier is in any case poorly permeable to bicarbonate, and that bicarbonate loading has a cerebroprotective effect is by no means certain. It has been the practice to correct a pH of below 7.2 with bicarbonate.

In spite of its drawbacks, it appears that respiratory acidosis can actually have a mitigating effect on ventilator-associated lung injury,[20] but again, the clinical implications of this are uncertain.

9.4.3.12 Prone Ventilation

The ability of prone ventilation to improve oxygenation was first noticed many years ago, but the mechanisms whereby it achieves these effects are as yet obscure.[143] As many as 60–80% of all patients show an appreciable reduction in their oxygen requirements with prone positioning.[17,172] Yet, to date, there is no proof that this modality actually improves the outcome in ARDS.

Several mechanisms appear to operate together in bringing about the improvement in oxygenation. The transpulmonary pressure – the difference between airway pressure and the pleural pressure – is the net force that governs alveolar patency. A complex interplay of several factors causes the transpulmonary pressure to decrease anteroposteriorly in the supine position, along a gradient determined in part by gravity.[9] It has been seen that proning the patient decreases this gradient and ensures better V/Q matching in the erstwhile dependent zone of the lungs.

It is also conjectured that in the prone position, the now dependent heart no longer hinders lung expansion as it might possibly do, where the patient supine.[85] Upward diaphragmatic displacement seems to be less marked in the prone than in the supine position, and this may result in less pulmonary compression by the weight of the abdominal contents.[137] Indeed, it has been shown that proning significantly improves FRC, and hence oxygenation. However, that improvements in FRC do actually occur as a result of proning has not been universally appreciated.[2,137] Most of the pulmonary parenchyma is located posteriorly: proning allows gravitational drainage of water out of large areas of the lung. It has also been proposed that proning the patient results in better perfusion of the ventral lung. The latter does not necessarily seem to be the case however, and other explanations need to be sought for the improvements in oxygenation.[87,130]

Some advantage might also accrue from the clearance of airway secretions, and from the redistribution of the edema fluid occasioned by gravitational shift.

A lack of a clear perception of the mechanisms contributing to the improvement in oxygenation makes it difficult to predict who might benefit from prone ventilation. Prone ventilation appears to confer advantages when much of the fluid is thin – as in ARDS – rather than viscous, possibly because viscous fluid is more refractory to gravitational shift. Also, oxygenation tends to show greater improvement when most of the pathology affects the dependent lung units – again because in the prone position, there would presumably be a gravitational shift of fluid from the consolidated dorsal zones toward the ventral zones.

A short test of proning the patient has been suggested to select potential responders.[88] It has been suggested that if oxygenation fails to improve by the end of half an hour, subsequent improvement in oxygenation will be unlikely to occur. The reason behind this seems to be that while proning can be expected to continue improving oxygenation over several hours, a rapid response seems to be the rule in responders. Absence of a *rapid* response is usually predictive of failure of this strategy. A brief spell of desaturation immediately on turning the patient may precede the improvement in blood gases, and this drop in PaO_2 can be prevented by adequate preoxygenation before proning. It is interesting to note that a large number of patients tend to sustain the improvements that they have shown on proning even after a return to the supine position. Conceivably, this could be due to the other strategies already in place that are aimed at keeping the lung open (PEEP), and this very likely reflects the fact that "it is easier to keep an open lung open, than to open up a closed lung."[29,52]

As of now, it is unclear how long to maintain the prone position in responders, but proponents of prone ventilation believe that the prone position may need to be maintained as long as the oxygenation continues to benefit. In the supine patient, as long as there is a need to administer high fractions of inspired concentration – despite usage of other conventional strategies – "proning" should be considered.[52]

As can be anticipated, nursing prone patients is challenging to say the least, and every precaution should be taken while changing the position of the patient in order to prevent inadvertent extubation or displacement of other cannulas.

Obvious as it may sound, it is impossible to give effective CPR in the prone position, and patients who have suffered a cardiac arrest must be immediately placed in a supine position for resuscitation. For this reason, dysrrhythmias and hemodynamic instability constitute contraindications to prone ventilation.

Box 9.3 Relative Contraindications to the Use of Permissive Hypercapnia

Cerebrovascular disease
Epilepsy
Patients at risk of developing intracranial hypertension
Coronary artery disease,
Cardiac dysrythmias
Pulmonary artery hypertension
Metabolic acidosis.

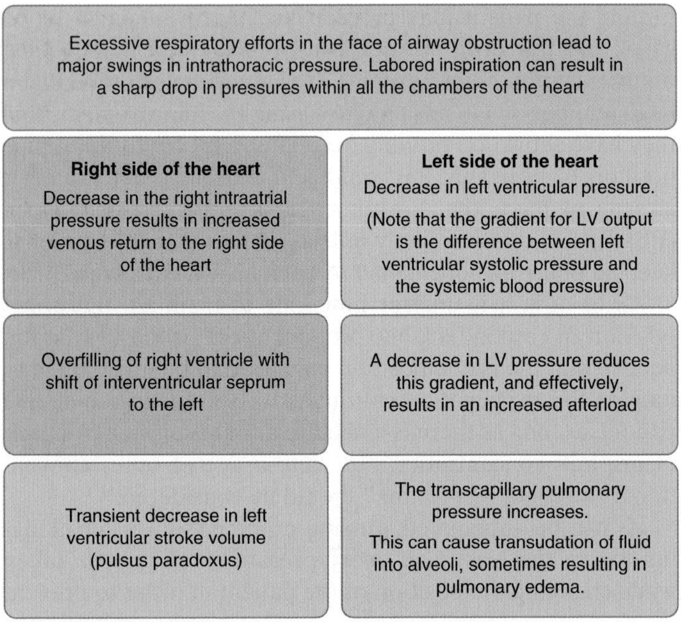
Excessive respiratory efforts in the face of airway obstruction lead to major swings in intrathoracic pressure. Labored inspiration can result in a sharp drop in pressures within all the chambers of the heart
Right side of the heart
Decrease in the right intraatrial pressure results in increased venous return to the right side of the heart
Left side of the heart
Decrease in left ventricular pressure.
(Note that the gradient for LV output is the difference between left ventricular systolic pressure and the systemic blood pressure)
Overfilling of right ventricle with shift of interventricular seprum to the left
A decrease in LV pressure reduces this gradient, and effectively, results in an increased afterload
Transient decrease in left ventricular stroke volume (pulsus paradoxus)
The transcapillary pulmonary pressure increases.
This can cause transudation of fluid into alveoli, sometimes resulting in pulmonary edema.

FIGURE 9.8. Effect of labored respirations upon the heart.

9.5 Obstructive Lung Disease

Patients with obstructed airways present a special problem in ventilatory care. In such patients airway resistance is increased, often to extremely high levels. The narrowed airways impede airflow so that the time available for expiration is insufficient for the lungs to empty. This leads to dynamic hyperinflation and air trapping within the lungs. Dynamic hyperinflation can itself lead to alveolar distension and barotrauma, and may hamper the venous return to the heart (Fig. 9.8).

The heart being an intrathoracic structure, is just as vulnerable to variations in intrathoracic pressure as are the lungs. With the fall in the intrathoracic pressure at the commencement of *spontaneous* inspiration, pressures within all the cardiac chambers (relative to the atmospheric pressure) fall. Any lowering in right atrial pressure in the face of preserved

Increased respiratory loading

- Increased resistive load (decreased diameter of airway lumen)
  - Bronchial smooth muscle hypertrophy and spasm
  - Mucosal inflammation and edema
  - Increased airway secretions
  - Increased collapsibility of degenerated bronchial cartilage
  - Loss of tethering of bronchial wall to surrounding lung parenchyma
- Increased elastic load
  - Dynamic hyperinflation results in a decrease in compliance (see 10.2.5.1)

Decreased respiratory muscle effeciency

- Decreased diaphragmatic curvature: forces of contraction directed medially rather than downwards
- Decreased zone of diaphragmatic apposition with the chest wall
- Shortened diaphragmatic fibre length: sub-optimal length-tension relationships translate into decreased force of contraction
- Inflamatory infiltration of diaphragmatic sarcomeres
- Possibly decreased blood supply to diaphragmatic muscle

FIGURE 9.9. Respiratory impairment in COPD.

systemic venous pressure will increase the gradient for blood flow from the periphery to the thorax. The increased venous return dilates the right ventricle (RV) and in accordance with Starling's law, augments the right ventricular output. Although right ventricular stroke volume increases as a consequence of this, left ventricular output does not (see Fig. 9.9).

The decrease in left ventricular stroke volume during inspiration is transient and is clinically manifest as a decreased pulse pressure. This phenomenon (pulsus paradoxus) is exaggerated in patients with obstructive lung disease who are making strenuous attempts to draw air into overfilled lungs. Pulsus paradoxus is actually a misnomer, for it is in fact an exaggeration (≤10 mmHg) of the normal inspiratory drop in arterial pressure (≤5 mmHg). The magnitude of pulsus paradoxus can be estimated either with a sphygmomanometer or deduced from the variation in amplitude of the pulse-oximetric tracing.

In obstructed patients, the stroke volume of the left ventricle can be diminished by another mechanism. The arterial circuit, into which the LV pumps blood, is surrounded and influenced by atmospheric pressure and is therefore not subject to variations in intrathoracic pressure. The gradient for LV output is the difference between the force developed during systole within the left ventricle itself and the systemic blood pressure. If large decrements in intrathoracic pressure (such as those that occur during inspiration in obstructed patients) should decrease the pressure within the LV, the gradient for LV outflow decreases, and the LV pumps against what is effectively an increased afterload. An increased afterload increases the pulmonary transcapillary pressure and this can potentiate the transudation of fluid into alveoli.

Indeed, patients with severe airways obstruction have been seen to develop acute pulmonary edema, and the increase in afterload that occurs due to the large inspiratory effort has been invoked to explain this. Overhydration in a situation such as this could further promote the spillage of fluid into the alveoli. Patients with congestive cardiac failure are fluid overloaded and have a greater circulating blood volume. It has been proposed that negative swings in intrathoracic pressure enhance venous return in volume-overloaded patients and this can worsen the hemodynamics by the mechanisms described above.

9.5.1 $PaCO_2$

Patients with acute severe asthma often have to breathe against extremely high inspiratory loads. This may render them vulnerable to respiratory muscle exhaustion, one of the earliest signs of which may be a normalization of a previously low $PaCO_2$.

In COPD patients, a high $PaCO_2$ does not by itself have the same implications as it does in a patient with status asthmaticus. The asthmatic patient most usually has a normal premorbid $PaCO_2$ and will wash CO_2 out from the blood while hyperventilating during the asthmatic attack. Consequently, a low $PaCO_2$ is the rule rather than the exception in acute asthma: a normal $PaCO_2$ in such a patient implies that the $PaCO_2$ has begun to rise with the onset of respiratory muscle fatigue. An asthmatic with a normal $PaCO_2$ level must be closely watched and intubated as soon as it is clear that respiratory muscle fatigue has set in, as is evinced by a rising $PaCO_2$ and a falling pH.

The mechanisms leading to CO_2 retention in COPD patients are complex, and have been discussed 10.4.3.

In acute exacerbations of COPD that progress to respiratory failure, the indication for mechanical ventilation is often respiratory muscle fatigue, or occasionally, depression of the respiratory center (either due to injudicious sedation, or as a result of administration of excessive oxygen). In either case, there is a rise in the $PaCO_2$ level with a fall in pH (respiratory acidosis), which if uncontrolled, can lead to convulsions, arrhythmias, or respiratory arrest (Fig. 9.9).

The hypercapnia that is manifest at presentation may respond to appropriate therapy, and does not always presage the initiation of mechanical ventilatory support. Sometimes, the COPD patient in exacerbation remains hypoxemic despite the administration of low flow oxygen. In such cases, the danger inherent in increasing the level of delivered oxygen is the potential suppression of the respiratory drive. When a high level of oxygen is mandated in such a patient and yet cannot be safely given because of the above constraints, some form of mechanical ventilation is often the only rational option. The option of noninvasive ventilation should now be considered in all COPD patients with severe acute hypercapnic respiratory failure. NIV is presently considered a first-line intervention in this setting, and will frequently obviate the need for invasive mechanical ventilation (Fig. 9.10).[5]

9.5.2 Modes of Ventilation in Obstructed Patients

The modes and settings used in obstructed patients are targeted at reducing dynamic hyperinflation.

Due to the impressive impact of bronchial narrowing on airway resistance, the work done by an obstructed patient can be considerable. This may not only predispose the patient to respiratory muscle exhaustion, but also render weaning difficult. On the other hand, if the patient is completely rested for a prolonged duration of time, the lack of stimulus to the

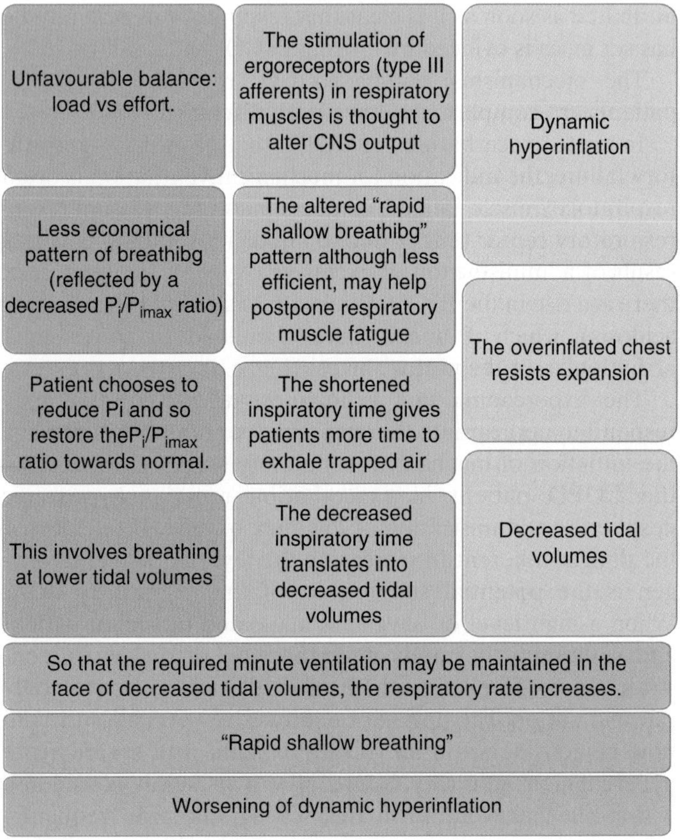
Unfavourable balance: load vs effort.
The stimulation of ergoreceptors (type III afferents) in respiratory muscles is thought to alter CNS output
Dynamic hyperinflation
Less economical pattern of breathibg (reflected by a decreased P_i/P_{imax} ratio)
The altered "rapid shallow breathibg" pattern although less efficient, may help postpone respiratory muscle fatigue
The overinflated chest resists expansion
Patient chooses to reduce Pi and so restore theP_i/P_{imax} ratio towards normal.
The shortened inspiratory time gives patients more time to exhale trapped air
This involves breathing at lower tidal volumes
The decreased inspiratory time translates into decreased tidal volumes
Decreased tidal volumes
So that the required minute ventilation may be maintained in the face of decreased tidal volumes, the respiratory rate increases.
"Rapid shallow breathing"
Worsening of dynamic hyperinflation

FIGURE 9.10. The reason why COPD patients breathe at low tidal volumes.

respiratory muscles can promote respiratory muscle atrophy. Although the ideal mode of ventilatory support to an obstructed patient should balance these two considerations, at the present time, there seems to be no single mode which fulfills these requirements.

NIV has emerged as an important mode for the initial therapy of COPD in exacerbation and is considered in some detail in chapter 13.

The mode that is optimal for the initial management of the patient with obstructive airways disease is as yet unclear, and clinicians may be justified in using modes that they have used successfully in this situation.[166] Patient triggered modes like assist-control mode, intermittent mandatory mode, and pressure support mode present a stimulus to the respiratory muscles that is important for the prevention of disuse atrophy of the respiratory muscles. The volume cycled assist-control mode in the initial management of an awake patient with active bronchospasm will sometimes produce significant air trapping and dynamic hyperinflation.[166]

Contrary to the earlier thinking, the energy expended in triggering the ventilator may be considerable and might itself impose a considerable burden on respiratory muscles.[111,112] When a significant amount of intrinsic PEEP ($PEEP_i$, auto-PEEP) exists in the lung, the patient may additionally be required to overcome the $PEEP_i$ before the ventilator is triggered into delivering the tidal volume.[138] Furthermore, if the flow delivered to the patient does not meet the requirements of his or her ventilatory drive, the work of breathing can be substantial.[61,161]

It may seem reasonable that the IMV mode should spare patient effort in direct proportion to the number of set mandatory breaths, but this has not been shown to be the case.[112] Possibly because of the fact that the respiratory muscles cannot adapt to the changing burden imposed on them by the alternation of the spontaneous and mandatory breaths, the work of breathing (resulting from an excess of input to the respiratory muscles from the respiratory center) may be quite high.[77]

Supporting the inspiratory breaths with the PSV mode generally helps in reducing the patient's inspiratory work. However, the effect of this approach is to a large extent unpredictable in the individual patient and at high levels of pressure support, patients may exhibit inordinately high levels of expiratory muscle activity.[79] Although in the PSV mode the patient has the freedom to determine his own respiratory rate and so directly influence his respiratory cycle time, he may be constrained to breathe at a higher respiratory frequency (see Fig. 9.11).

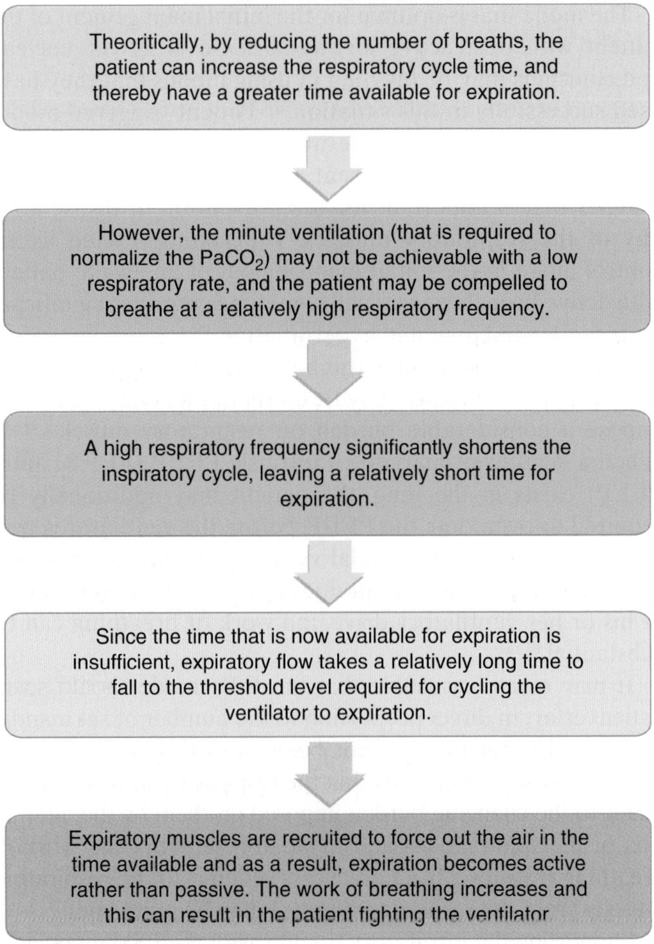
Theoritically, by reducing the number of breaths, the patient can increase the respiratory cycle time, and thereby have a greater time available for expiration.
However, the minute ventilation (that is required to normalize the $PaCO_2$) may not be achievable with a low respiratory rate, and the patient may be compelled to breathe at a relatively high respiratory frequency.
A high respiratory frequency significantly shortens the inspiratory cycle, leaving a relatively short time for expiration.
Since the time that is now available for expiration is insufficient, expiratory flow takes a relatively long time to fall to the threshold level required for cycling the ventilator to expiration.
Expiratory muscles are recruited to force out the air in the time available and as a result, expiration becomes active rather than passive. The work of breathing increases and this can result in the patient fighting the ventilator

FIGURE 9.11. Pressure support mode: asynchrony in COPD patients.

9.5.3 Ventilator Settings in Airflow Obstruction

9.5.3.1 Tidal Volume

During the past few years, it has emerged that lower tidal volumes than that employed previously, should be used while ventilating patients on volume-assisted modes. Higher tidal volumes as used in the past (for instance, 10–15 mL/kg body weight) are liable to produce alveolar distension and injury. It has now become usual to ventilate patients with smaller tidal volumes (in the range of 5–7 mL/kg body weight).

9.5.3.2 Respiratory Rate

The rate is set according to the needs of the patient. Usually, once stabilized, patients will themselves choose a respiratory rate that satisfies their demands. In such cases, it is sufficient to set the backup rate *less* than the spontaneous rate the patient chooses to breathe at, by about 4 breaths/min. This will serve as a safety measure, should the patient hypoventilate for any reason.[78]

Within the IMV or the SIMV mode, the appropriate frequency of the backup (mandatory) breaths should be determined not only by the trend in the patient's $PaCO_2$, but also by the adequacy of the spontaneous breaths (the breaths that the patient takes in between the mandatory breaths), and by patient comfort. Just as in the pressure support (PSV) mode, if the frequency of the spontaneous breaths is seen to be rising or the tidal volumes of the spontaneous breaths falling, the minute ventilation being delivered to the patient is clearly inadequate, and either the level of pressure support must be boosted or the frequency of the mandatory breaths increased.

Since on the PSV mode the patient chooses his own respiratory frequency, no rates as such can be "set." The pressure support should be adjusted to a level that enables satisfactory tidal volumes to be delivered. If the tidal volumes being delivered are adequate for the patient's needs, this will manifest in the patient comfortably breathing at relatively low respiratory rates, say 20 breaths/min or even lower.

9.5.3.3 Inspiratory Flow Rate

Setting an appropriate inspiratory flow can be vital to patient comfort and can greatly help reduce the work of breathing.

Box 9.4 The Hyperventilating Patient on Assist-Control Mode with a Low Backup Rate Runs the Risk of Over Distending His Lungs.

With some older ventilators, the inspiratory time is automatically assigned according to the backup rate chosen. For example, if an I:E ratio of 1:2 is chosen and a backup rate of 10 breaths/min is set, each respiratory cycle will last for 60 s/10 breaths per min = 6 s.

Of these 6 s (given an I:E ratio of 1:2), 2 s will be spent in inspiration and 4 s in expiration. This 2 s inspiration will now be applied to all breaths irrespective of the respiratory rate. If the patient were now to increase his respiratory rate to 20 breaths/min, each of these breaths would contain a 2 s inspiration despite the shortened respiratory cycle.

New respiratory cycle time = 60 s/20 breaths per min = 3 s.

Of these 3 s, 2*s would still be spent in inspiration* (as the inspiration duration is linked to the backup rate, which is still 10 breaths/min), leaving just 1 s for expiration.

Most patients demand relatively high flow rates. A high flow rate achieves the important objective of shortening the inspiratory time (the same tidal volume is delivered more quickly with a faster flow rate than with a slower flow) leaving ample time for expiration. The lung consequently has a better chance of emptying itself.[33]

A faster flow rate is likely to elevate the peak airway pressure; but the more complete lung emptying results in a lower *plateau pressure*. Since it is the plateau pressure which correlates more closely with barotrauma than does the peak airway pressure, there is merit (at least in theory) in ventilating obstructed patients using high flow rates.[166]

In practice, increasing the inspiratory flow rate is less effective at shortening the inspiratory time than reducing the respiratory frequency.

9.5.3.4 Trigger Sensitivity

As in the case of the flow rate, setting the right trigger sensitivity plays an important role in preventing patient-ventilator asynchrony. A trigger sensitivity that has been set too high results in unnecessary loading of the inspiratory muscles and predisposes to respiratory muscle fatigue. In the presence of auto-PEEP, greater effort is necessary to trigger the ventilator: the change in airway pressure required to trigger the machine must equal the sum of trigger sensitivity and auto-PEEP. This may prove a daunting task for the COPD patient.[181]

9.5.3.5 External PEEP

Where auto-PEEP is significant, addition of external PEEP of a level of approximately 50–75% of the auto-PEEP may succeed in narrowing the gradient, as explained by the analogy of the cascade or waterfall.[179] With the application of external PEEP, the patient requires to produce a smaller change in airway pressure to trigger the ventilator,[140,167] and this can substantially reduce the work of breathing.[34] However, external PEEP should be used with caution, for it has been shown that when the level of applied PEEP exceeds 80% of the auto-PEEP, dynamic hyperinflation can actually be worsened.[152] External PEEP does not seem to reduce the inspiratory work of breathing in acute exacerbations of asthma as it does in COPD, but on the contrary, may actually worsen dynamic hyperinflation.

9.5.3.6 NIV

Noninvasive positive pressure ventilation (NIPPV, NIV) has been shown to reduce the rate of intubation for exacerbations of COPD and to shorten ICU stays.[22] The patient on NIV, particularly the severely obstructed patient, must be closely monitored – for, as many as 26–31% of patients treated with NIV will worsen and eventually require invasive mechanical ventilation (see also chapter 13).[22]

9.5.3.7 General Principles of Treatment in Asthma and COPD

The principles of treatment of acute severe attacks of asthma parallel those of COPD, since the mechanisms of disease are very similar. Asthmatic patients have more airways inflammation than COPD patients and are therefore likely to have much more mucosal edema of the airways and mucus hypersecretion. For this reason, airway resistance in asthmatic patients is likely to be greater. COPD patients are much more tolerant of hypercapnia than asthmatics and, in fact, may have baseline $PaCO_2$ levels that are well in excess of that considered normal for other subjects.

In general, although baseline CO_2 levels are higher for COPD patients than for asthmatics, control of CO_2 levels in mechanically ventilated patients present fewer difficulties in COPD patients than they do in status asthmaticus. When control of CO_2 is problematic in intubated COPD patients, severe bronchospasm, pneumothorax, atelectasis due to mucus plugging etc., should be looked for.

COPD patients who are habitual retainers of CO_2 should have their minute ventilation titrated to the pH and not to their CO_2 level.

9.5.3.8 FIO_2

The FIO_2 should be set to achieve an arterial oxygen tension of above 60 mmHg. At this level of arterial oxygen tension, the hemoglobin is near-saturated and a higher FIO_2 does not confer any further advantage. The fraction of inspired oxygen being delivered is also important at the time of weaning, when as low a level of supplemental oxygen as safely possible should be given, in order to avoid suppression of the hypoxic drive.

9.5.3.9 ET Size

From weaning considerations, it is also necessary to use an endotracheal tube of as large a bore as possible, in order to decrease airway resistance. The benefit of even a small increase in ET tube caliber is profound, and a change of endotracheal tube to a higher luminal diameter may accomplish succcssful weaning in a difficult situation.

If despite optimal ventilatory settings, patient-ventilator asynchrony is still manifest, sedation and paralysis may become necessary. A pharmacologically aided decrease in the activity of the patient's respiratory muscles will translate into lower intrathoracic pressures during expiration, with less dynamic collapse of the airways. This is likely to result in better lung emptying – despite the absence of active expiratory effort on the part of the patient – much in the same way as the slow vital capacity is larger than the forced vital capacity during spirometry in obstructed patients.

9.5.3.10 Permissive Hypercapnia

When airway pressures are very high despite optimization of the flow rates and I:E ratio, reducing the tidal volumes and/or respiratory rate may help to decrease airway pressures. This may be easier said than done, since reduction in either of these parameters may decrease the minute volume to a point where maintenance of a near-normal $PaCO_2$ is no longer possible. Since the primary objective is to normalize the pH and not the $PaCO_2$,[59,166] it may be necessary to nevertheless reduce the minute ventilation and allow the $PaCO_2$ to rise in a controlled fashion (permissive hypercapnia). In certain centers, it has been the practice to control the resulting respiratory acidosis by infusion of bicarbonate, such that the pH does not drop below 7.2.[122] These issues have been discussed section 9.4.3.11.

9.5.3.11 General Anesthesia

In refractory bronchospasm, it may be necessary to resort to general anesthesia. The use of helium–oxygen mixtures as a strategy to reduce airway pressures in obstructive lung disease has been discussed section 17.9.

9.5.4 Bronchopleural Fistula

The development of a pneumothorax in patients on positive pressure ventilation is a medical urgency. Even a small pneumothorax occurring in a mechanically ventilated patient must be treated as a potential emergency because of its propensity to evolve into a tension pneumothorax. A chest drain must promptly be inserted. Most frequently, pneumothoraces in the setting of mechanical ventilation are due to alveolar overdistension by inappropriately high tidal volumes, but may also be predisposed to by the underlying lung pathology like pneumonia or ARDS. Also, mechanically ventilated patients are frequently subjected to numerous interventions like central venous catheter placement, thoracentesis, and transbronchial biopsies, all of which have the potential to disrupt the visceral pleura.

Since alveolar overdistension seems to be in large part responsible for pneumothorax, an attempt must be made to minimize air trapping by the use of smaller tidal volumes and low overall minute volumes, and by reduction in PEEP.

Positive pressure breathing is capable of causing large air leaks through a bronchopleural fistula (BPF), though most leaks are trivial. A BPF can be quantified from ventilator graphics as volume that is "lost" – that is, the difference between the inspiratory and expiratory tidal volumes Figs. 8.13 & 8.39.

A small BPF will bubble through the water seal only during inspiration, whereas a larger leak will bubble during expiration as well. When the inspiratory tidal volume exceeds the expiratory tidal volume by a significant amount (e.g., about 150 mL), an air leak through the BPF can be anticipated. Although in theory, a large air leak through the BPF could be expected to reduce effective alveolar ventilation (because of the loss of delivered tidal volumes through the chest drain), in practice, this is not usually the case.[16]

In general, a BPF is not expected to produce special derangements in pulmonary physiology over and above those produced by the underlying pathology; in fact, the BPF usually resolves *parri passu* with improvement in the inciting lung pathology.[145]

For these reasons, specific measures directed at reducing the leak per se are probably unnecessary, though attempts must certainly be made to contain the alveolar distension that might have resulted in the BPF.

The literature is replete with a large number of methods that have been targeted at reducing the air leaks: high frequency jet ventilation, independent lung ventilation, occlusion of the chest drain during the inspiratory cycle of ventilator, and the application of PEEP to the chest drain.[144] When identification of the bronchial segment – within which the BPF exists – has been possible, occlusion of that segment has been undertaken by a variety of methods such as a balloon of a Fogarty or a Swan–Ganz catheter. Alternatively, successful attempts to seal off the relevant bronchopulmonary segment by gelfoam, fibrin, or laser coagulation have been reported.[129,168,192]

9.6 Neuromuscular Disease

Ventilation is determined by bulk airflow in and out of the lungs. Oxygenation is determined by bulk flow as well as the integrity of the lung parenchyma and vasculature.

In neuromuscular disease, ventilatory failure can occur on account of the processes that impair transmission of neural input from the respiratory center to the respiratory muscles, or those that prevent proper contraction of respiratory muscles themselves. Typically, the respiratory center itself is unaffected and so the respiratory drive is intact.[166] The common conditions that cause neuromuscular dysfunction are Guillian–Barre syndrome, amyotrophic lateral sclerosis, poliomyelitis, and myasthenia gravis (see Fig 3.16).

Since the lungs are essentially normal, the gas exchange mechanisms are by and large unaffected. Rather, the situation is one of type II respiratory failure with the fall in PaO_2 being matched by a rise in $PaCO_2$. The A-a DO_2 gradient is normal unless significant atelectasis occurs (see section 7.1).

The principles underlying the ventilation of patients with spinal injury will be included within this section, in view of the issues that such patients have in common with neuromuscular patients.

The diaphragm is the principal muscle of inspiration; it is innervated by the phrenic nerve which arises from the third to fifth cervical roots (C3–C5). A cervical spine injury sustained above the level of the C3 root results in an immediate cessation of breathing. Diaphragmatic pacing or chronic ventilatory support is necessary, though enough muscular function might eventually return if the injury is incomplete (Fig. 9.12).

With cord lesions between C3 and C5, urgent – and probably chronic – ventilatory support is required as well, because of complete paralysis of both the phrenic and intercostal nerves.[31] Though ventilatory support is invariably required initially, a functional descent of the level of neurologic injury during the healing phase often results in a spontaneous return of enough respiratory muscle function to permit the discontinuance of ventilatory support.[10,93,194]

In many cases, a compensatory increase in the neural output to the diaphragm will occur (operational length compensation), and this often suffices for adequate ventilation. Compensatory mechanisms also operate at the muscular level. Increased recruitment of the accessory muscles of ventilation will eventually occur, and the gradual transition from flaccid to spastic paralysis also aids recovery.[69] The increased muscle tonicity can disadvantage the upper airway somewhat by the spastic contraction of the pharyngeal musculature, but now the chest does not subside during inspiration, as it would during the flaccid stage.[13] Some patients in this group may gradually progress much later – with an age-related decline in pulmonary function – to chronic type II respiratory failure.[11]

Between C6 and C8, patients usually exhibit normal diaphragmatic and accessory respiratory muscle function, though mechanical ventilation can still be required if the injury extends upward across C5 due to hemorrhage or edema.

Lesions of the thoracic spine are rather less likely to result in respiratory embarrassment – unless other thoracic injuries complicate the issue. The preservation of an effective cough

Above C3	C3–C5
• Complete absence of ventilation: requirement for mechanical ventilatory support • High incidence of lung problems (pneumonia, atelectasis)	• Mechanical ventilation required initally • Later, recovery usually permits unassisted breathing • Some patients progress to chronic type II respiratory failure after many years

C6–C8	Thoracic spine
• There is usually normal diaphragm and accessory respiratory muscle function • Mechanical ventilation is required if the spinal lesion extends upwards across C5 due to hemorrhage or edema.	• Cough reflex and pulmonary mechanics relatively preserved • Comorbidities may complicate issues (see text) • Relatively low incidence of lung infections

FIGURE 9.12. Respiratory compromise correlated with the level of spinal injury.

ensures better defense of the airways, and lung infections are unusual.

Most of the complications following spinal cord injury involve the respiratory system.[50,98] The mortality and morbidity is higher the more cephalad the injury: such patients are prone to a greater incidence of pneumonia, atelectasis, and respiratory failure (Fig. 9.13).

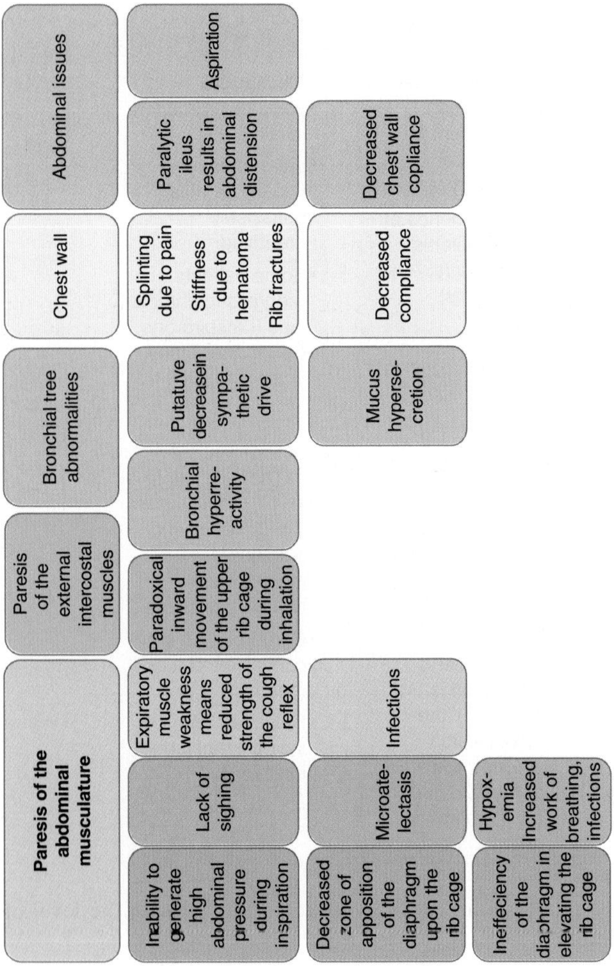
Paresis of the abdominal musculature
Paresis of the external intercostal muscles
Bronchial tree abnormalities
Chest wall
Abdominal issues
Inability to generate high abdominal pressure during inspiration
Lack of sighing
Expiratory muscle weakness means reduced strength of the cough reflex
Paradoxical inward movement of the upper rib cage during inhalation
Bronchial hyperre-activity
Putatuve decreasein sympa-thetic drive
Splinting due to pain
Stiffness due to hematoma
Rib fractures
Paralytic ileus results in abdominal distension
Aspiration
Decreased zone of apposition of the diaphragm upon the rib cage
Microate-lectasis
Infections
Mucus hyperse-cretion
Decreased compliance
Decreased chest wall copliance
Ineffeciency of the diaphragm in elevating the rib cage
Hypox-emia
Increased work of breathing, infections

FIGURE 9.13. Respiratory derangements with spinal cord injury.[185???]

9.6.1 Lung Function

Acutely, in high lesions, the vital capacity can fall to less than 30%.[93] With more caudal injury, the impairment in lung function is less, but significant compromise can nevertheless occur as a result of atelectasis, ineffectual handling of airway secretions, infection, and decreased muscular power.[153] For reasons that are unclear, patients with low cervical lesions – especially when these are diffuse or severe – are susceptible to apneic spells and even respiratory arrest: this can occur as late as a fortnight after the inciting injury.[99]

Lesions at the level of the thoracic spine have a lesser impact on pulmonary mechanics. Presumably due to a decreased sympathetic output, many patients have smaller[68] and more hyperreactive airways.[169]

Quadriplegic patients prefer the supine position. An upright posture allows the abdominal content to fall off the diaphragm. The decreased zone of apposition in the upright patient results in loss of mechanical advantage, since the shortened diaphragm fibers can no longer develop a satisfactory force of contraction.[119] Also, the decrease in the residual volume that the supine posture induces, appears to help.[46] In contrast, patients with generalized muscular weakness due to neuromuscular disease (see below) prefer the seated posture owing to the mechanical advantages that this position affords. In this group of patients, weakness of the muscles of inspiration limits inspired tidal volumes.

Box 9.5 Respiratory Morbidity Associated with Chest Trauma

Pneumonia
Atelectasis
Pneumothorax
Hemothorax, chylothorax
Flail chest
Lung contusion
Myocardial contusion
Tracheobronchial [rupture]
Esophageal injury
Injury to the great vessels
Fat embolism
Paralytic ileus

9.6.2 Inspiratory Muscle Recruitment in Neuromuscular Disease

To preserve alveolar ventilation, the accessory muscles of ventilation (the external intercostals, sternocleidomastoids, scalenes, and trapezii) are increasingly recruited to assist the principal muscle of inspiration, the diaphragm. The shortfall in minute volume is made up by an increase in the respiratory rate. The low tidal volumes and the ineffectual sighs that accompany neuromuscular dysfunction frequently produce microatelectasis, which decreases the compliance; this increases the work of breathing (Fig. 9.14).

9.6.3 Expiratory Muscle Recruitment in Neuromuscular Disease

With increasing inspiratory muscle insufficiency, the expiratory muscles (rectus abdominis, transverse abdominis, internal and external obliques, and internal intercostals) are progressively engaged. Their active contraction pushes the diaphragms well above the usual resting position. During the

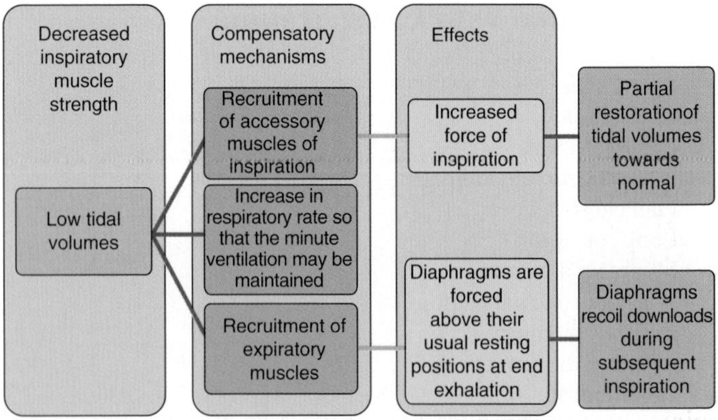
Decreased inspiratory muscle strength
Low tidal volumes
Compensatory mechanisms
Recruitment of accessory muscles of inspiration
Increase in respiratory rate so that the minute ventilation may be maintained
Recruitment of expiratory muscles
Effects
Increased force of inspiration
Diaphragms are forced above their usual resting positions at end exhalation
Partial restorationof tidal volumes towards normal
Diaphragms recoil downloads during subsequent inspiration

FIGURE 9.14. Consequences of decreased inspiratory muscle strength.

Box 9.6 Assessing the Adequacy of Cough

Maximal expiratory pressure (MEP) is a measure of the strength of the expiratory muscles. A MEP of less than 60 cm H_2O implies a weak cough[175]; with a MEP less than 40 cm H_2O, clearance of airway secretions is generally poor, and this often presages infection.[90]

The cough force can also be gauged by the peak cough flow (PCF). A PCF less than 160 L/min identifies the patients with an ineffective cough. Patients with a low PCF are at a risk for respiratory tract infections, which can further reduce muscle strength.

succeeding inspiration, the upwardly displaced diaphragms passively recoil downward, expanding the thoracic cavity – this aids inspiration.

It now appears that the abdominal muscles – the "cough muscles" – may play a more important role in respiration than previously realized, and may be capable of augmenting minute ventilation, even in normal subjects.[39]

9.6.4 Bulbar Muscles Involvement in Neuromuscular Disease

Dysfunction of the bulbar muscle (muscles of the lips, tongue, palate, pharynx, and larynx) predisposes to aspiration; aspirational tracheobronchitis and atelectasis can worsen airway mechanics and gas exchange. Fulminant aspiration pneumonia can develop as a consequence of the loss of the cough reflex [62,180]; respiratory infections are common precipitants of acute on chronic respiratory failure. Patients with spinal injuries can have associated ileus which in itself is a risk factor for aspiration.[64]

Bulbar muscle involvement, by narrowing the upper airways, can also contribute to alveolar hypoventilation during sleep.

9.6.5 Assessment of Lung Function

Although difficult to measure in the ICU patient, the FVC can provide a passable estimate of *inspiratory* muscle strength; decreased *expiratory* muscle strength can also diminish the FVC. Normally, supine FVCs are lower by about 10% than those obtained when erect: allowance must be made for this. A normal supine FVC will virtually exclude significant inspiratory muscle weakness.[4] When the FVC falls below 50% of the predicted value, ventilatory support is generally required.[30]

The maximal inspiratory pressure (MIP) is a measure of the strength of the inspiratory muscles – principally the diaphragm. A reduced MIP often heralds alveolar hypoventilation; an MIP value of at least minus 30 cm H_2O is usually required to stave off the need for some form of mechanical ventilation.[90] In some neurologic conditions like Guillian–Barre syndrome, the MIP does not appear to be a reliable indicator of weaning.

9.6.6 Mechanical Ventilation in Neuromuscular Disease

About 20% of all patients who require mechanical ventilation do so as a result of neurological dysfunction.[44]

In spite of the pathological pathways operative in neuromuscular disease (Fig. 9.15), pulmonary mechanics can be considered to be more or less normal. The limitations for using large tidal volumes do not apply here – as they do, for instance, in obstructive or restrictive lung diseases. For the same reason, patients are less likely to develop barotrauma. Because their ventilatory drive is normal, patients actually show a preference for large tidal volumes (12–15 mL/kg body weight) and

Inspiratory muscle (diaphragm, external intercostals, sternocleidomastoids, scalenes, and trapezii) dysfunction results in decreased tidal volumes

- **To maintain alveolar ventilation the following adaptations occur:**
  - Accessory muscles are recruited.
  - Parients adopt an upright position to gravitationally aid diaphragm
  - Respiratory frequency increases
  - Beyond a point, falling tidal volumes result in alveolar hypoventilation, and the PCO_2 begins to rise
- **Altered compliance**
  - Low tidal volumes, and the ineffective sighs that (accompany) neuromuscular disease result inbasal atelectasis
  - Decreased compliance and increased work of breathing results in respiratory musclefatigue
- **Cough reflex**
  - Limitation of tidal volume during the inspiratory phase of the cough reflex results in lower expiratory tidal volumes and decreases peak airflow during cough
  - Lower inspiratory tidal volumes mean decreased stretching and lenghthening of the expiratory muslces (and therefore decreased expiratory force) during coughing

Expiratory muscle (rectus abdominis, transverse abdominis, internal and external obliques, and internal intercostals) dysfunction

- **Cough**
  - Decrease in the strength of cough
- **Ventilation**
  - When the inspiratory muscles are weak, the expiratory muscles assist them by pushing the diaphragms above their usual resting position. During the subsequent inspiration. The displaced diaphragms recoil downwards, expanding the thoracic cavity and so aiding inspiration (see text)

Bulbar muscle (muscles of the lips, tongue, palate, pharynx, and larynx) dysfunction

- **Cough reflex**
  - Glottic dyfunction and inadequate closure during compressive phase of cough reflex
- **Aspiration**
  - Poor handling of food boluses predisposes to aspiration
- **Nocturnal hypoventilation**
  - Upper airway narrowing during sleep leads to worsening alveolar ventilation

FIGURE 9.15. Pathological pathways in neuromuscular disease by muscle group.

high flow rates.[166] When adequate tidal volumes are not dispensed, these patients are prone to develop atelectasis.

Partial or complete mechanical ventilatory support may be provided as needed. Either positive or negative pressure ventilation can be used – at the present time, it appears that there is not much to choose between the two. Noninvasive positive pressure support has been used with success for the long-term ventilation of patients with neuromuscular injury.

In view of their propensity to aspirate, patients with spinal injury should be nursed well propped up.[182] An obvious concern is that neck hyperextension during intubation can aggravate the cord lesion. Fiberoptic guidance is frequently required; sometimes even nasotracheal intubation will be needed.

In many cases, prolonged ventilation can be anticipated, and early conversion to tracheostomy is preferable for the ease of access to airway secretions it affords, as also for the need to forestall endotracheal tube-related complications. Tracheostomy has special advantages when used with negative pressure ventilation: it circumvents the problematic upper airway collapse that negative airway pressure can produce.

Pulmonary infection should be treated aggressively.

9.7 Nonhomogenous Lung Disease

When there is a gross discrepancy between the extent of disease in the two lungs, mechanics are likely to differ considerably on both sides. The healthier and more compliant side is likely to receive the bulk of the ventilation. If tidal volumes are not decreased in proportion to the loss of functional lung volume, alveolar overdistension is likely to occur in the relatively unaffected regions, and barotrauma can occur. What should constitute the ideal ventilatory strategy in such situations is presently unclear. Although differential lung ventilation has been adopted on occasion, that it reliably improves the outcome has not been proven.[1,134]

At the present time therefore, the problem may initially be approached conservatively, and the patient ventilated in the conventional manner, regardless of the presence of unilateral involvement. If hypoxemia should then prove difficult to manage, a change in position of the patient (such as in the decubitus position, with the affected lung superior), may be attempted. This would cause preferential perfusion of the relatively healthy dependent lung, thereby achieving better *V/Q* matching.

9.8 Mechanical Ventilation in Flail Chest

Flail chest most commonly occurs as a result of blunt trauma to the chest (usually after falls, road traffic accidents, or following cardiopulmonary resuscitation). Pathologic fractures as are seen to occur with multiple myeloma can also rarely result in flail chest. When two or more ribs or the sternum are fractured in two different places, a flail segment is created; the segment is uncoupled from the chest wall and passively collapses inward during inspiration, secondary to the negative intrathoracic pressure.

The inward buckling of the flail segment causes the vital capacity to decrease. The deranged chest mechanics necessitate a greater shortening of the inspiratory muscles for a given tidal volume; also the lung is stiff if any significant degree of parenchymal contusion is present. This results in increased work of breathing with consequent predisposition to respiratory muscle fatigue.

Pulmonary derangements with flail chest may extend for a prolonged period of time. The reduced FRC may take up to 6 months to return to normal,[82] sometimes much longer when associated pulmonary contusion is present.

Although flail chest per se is capable of producing respiratory failure, the gas derangements produced by chest trauma are more likely to be caused by underlying pulmonary contusion than by the flail segment itself.[3] The occurrence of flail chest appears to increase the mortality associated with chest trauma.[53]

Mechanical ventilation with PEEP can help by providing internal splinting to the flail segment. The indication for invasive mechanical ventilation in chest trauma is not the presence of a flail segment itself, but the occurrence of respiratory failure.[164,183] CPAP stabilizes the chest wall and improves respiratory system mechanics; it has been shown to be associated with a better outcome.[19] Noninvasive ventilation may help in less severe cases.

Selected patients with major chest wall resection following trauma may be offered negative pressure ventilation with cuirass,[72] or external fixation with acrylic frames,[3] but it is unclear as to what extent these help. Occasionally, recourse has to be taken to surgical stabilization with wires or external plates, but this is generally rarely required.

References

1. Adoumie R, Shennib H, Brown R, et al Differential lung ventilation. Applications beyond the operating room. *J Thorac Cardiovasc Surg*. 1993;105:229–233
2. Albert RK, Leasa D, Sanderson M, et al The prone position improves arterial oxygenation and reduces shunt in oleic-acid-induced acute lung injury. *Am Rev Respir Dis*. 1987;135:628
3. Ali J, Harding B, de Niord R. Effect of temporary external stabilisation on ventilator weaning after sternal resection. *Chest*. 1989;95:472–473
4. Allen SM, Hunt B, Green M. Fall in vital capacity with posture. *Br J Dis Chest*. 1985;79:267–271
5. American Thoracic Society, European Thoracic Society Task Force. Standards for the diagnosis and management of patients with COPD [internet]. Version 1.2. New York: American Thoracic Society; 2004 [updated 8 Sep 2005]
6. Anrep GV, Pascual W, Rossler R. Respiratory variations in the heart rate. I. The reflex mechanism of the respiratory arrhythmia. *Proc R Soc Lond B Biol Sci*. 1936;119:191–217
7. ARDS Network. Ventilation with lower tidal volumes as compared with traditional tidal volumes for acute lung injury and the acute respiratory distress syndrome. *New Engl J Med*. 2000;342:1301–1308
8. Armstrong BW Jr, MacIntyre NR. Pressure-controlled, inverse ratio ventilation that avoids air trapping in the adult respiratory distress syndrome. *Crit Care Med*. 1995;23:279

9. Asostoni E. Mechanics of the pleural space. In: Macklem P, Mead J, eds. *Handbook of Physiology*. Bethesda: American Physiologic Society; 1986:531–558
10. Axen K, Pineda H, Shunfenthal I, Haas F. Diaphragmatic function following cervical cord injury: neurally mediated improvement. *Arch Phys Med Rehabil*. 1985;66:219
11. Bach JR. Inappropriate weaning and late onset ventilatory failure of individuals with traumatic spinal cord injury. *Paraplegia*. 1993;31:430
12. Baillard C, Boussarsar M, Fosse JP, et al Cardiac troponin I in patients with severe exacerbation of chronic obstructive pulmonary disease. *Intensive Care Med*. 2003;29:584–589
13. Ball PA. Critical care of spinal cord injury. *Spine*. 2001;26(24 suppl):S27
14. Baumann WR, Ulmer JL, Ambrose PS, et al Closure of a bronchopleural fistula using decalcified human spongiosa and a fibrin sealant. *Ann Thorac Surg*. 1997;64:2301
15. Ben-Haim SA, Amar R, Shofty R, et al The effect of positive end-expiratory pressure on the coronary blood flow. *Cardiology*. 1989;76:193–200
16. Bishop MJ, Benson MS, Pierson DJ. Carbon dioxide excretion via bronchopleural fistulas in adult respiratory distress syndrome. *Chest*. 1987;91:400
17. Blanch L, Mancebo J, Perez M, et al Short-term effects of prone position in critically ill patients with acute respiratory distress syndrome. *Intensive Care Med*. 1997;23:1033
18. Boix JH, Marin J, Enrique E, Monferrer J, Bataller A, Servera E. Modifications of tissular oxygenation and systemic hemodynamics after the correction of hypocapnia induced by mechanical ventilation. *Rev Esp Fisiol*. 1994;50:19–26
19. Bolliger CT, van Eeden SF. Treatment of multiple rib fractures: randomized control trial comparing ventilatory and nonventilatory management. *Chest*. 1990;97:943–948
20. Broccard AF. Respiratory acidosis and acute respiratory distress syndrome: time to trade in a bull market? *Crit Care Med*. 2006;34:229
21. Brochard L. Intrinsic (or auto-) positive end-expiratory pressure during spontaneous or assisted ventilation. *Intensive Care Med*. 2002;28:1552–1554
22. Brochard L, Mancebo J, Wysocki M, et al Noninvasive ventilation for acute exacerbations of chronic obstructive pulmonary disease. *N Engl J Med*. 1995;333:817

23. Brower RG, Lanken PN, MacIntyre N, et al Higher versus lower positive end-expiratory pressures in patients with the acute respiratory distress syndrome. *N Engl J Med*. 2004;351:327
24. Calandrino FS Jr, Anderson DJ, Mintun MA, et al Pulmonary vascular permeability during the adult respiratory distress syndrome: a positron emission tomographic study. *Am Rev Respir Dis*. 1988;138:421
25. Caricato A, Conti G. Della Corte F, Mancino A, Santilli F, Sandroni C, et al Effects of PEEP on the intracranial system of patients with head injury and subarachnoid hemorrhage: the role of respiratory system compliance. *Trauma*. 2005;58(3):571–576
26. Casetti AV, Bartlett RH, Hirschl RB. Increasing inspiratory time exacerbates ventilator-induced lung injury during high pressure/high-volume mechanical ventilation. *Crit Care Med*. 2002;30:2295–2299
27. Cassidy SS, Eschenbacher WI, Johnson RL Jr. Reflex cardiovascular depression during unilateral lung hyperinflation in the dog. *J Clin Invest*. 1979;64:620–626
28. Cereda M, Foti G, Musch G, et al Positive end-expiratory pressure prevents the loss of respiratory compliance during low tidal volume ventilation in acute lung injury patients. *Chest*. 1996;109:480
29. Chatte G, Sab JM, Dubois JM, et al Prone position in mechanically ventilated patients with severe acute respiratory failure. *Am J Respir Crit Care Med*. 1997;155:473
30. Chaudri MB, Liu C, Hubbard R, et al Relationship between supramaximal flow during cough and mortality in motor neurone disease. *Eur Respir J*. 2002;19:434
31. Como JJ, Sutton ER, McCunn M, et al Characterizing the need for mechanical ventilation following cervical spinal cord injury with neurologic deficit. *J Trauma*. 2005;59(4):912–916
32. Connors AF, Coussa ML, Guerin C, Eissa NT, et al Partitioning of work of breathing in mechanically ventilated COPD patients. *J Appl Physiol*. 1993;75:1711
33. Connors AF, McCaffree DR, Gray BA. Effect of inspiratory flow rate on gas exchange during mechanical ventilation. *Am Rev Respir Dis*. 1981;124:537
34. Coussa ML, Guerin C, Eissa NT, et al Partitioning of work of breathing in mechanically ventilated COPD patients. *J Appl Physiol*. 1993;75:1711
35. Crotti S, Pelosi P, Mascheroni D, et al The effect of extrinsic PEEP on lung inflation and regional compliance in mechanically

ventilated patients: a CT scan study. *Intensive Care Med.* 1995;21:S135

36. Cujec B, Polasek P, Mayers I, et al Positive end-expiratory pressure increases the right-to-left shunt in mechanically ventilated patients with patent foramen ovale. *Ann Intern Med.* 1993;119:887
37. Dambrosio M, Roupie E, Mollet JJ, et al Effects of positive end-expiratory pressure and different tidal volumes on alveolar recruitment and hyperinflation. *Anesthesiology*. 1997;87:495
38. de Durante G, del Turco M, Rustichini L, et al ARDSNet lower tidal volume ventilatory strategy may generate intrinsic positive end-expiratory pressure in patients with acute respiratory distress syndrome. *Am J Respir Crit Care Med.* 2002;165:1271
39. De Troyer A. Mechanical role of the abdominal muscles in relation to posture. *Respir Physiol.* 1983;53:311–353
40. Deem S. Management of acute brain injury and associated respiratory issues. *Respir Care*. 2006;51(4):357–367
41. Diamond S, Goldbweber R, Katz S. Use of D-dimer to aid in excluding deep venous thrombosis in ambulatory patients. *Am J Surg*. 2005;189:23–26
42. Dreyfuss D, Saumon G. Should the lung be rested or recruited? The Charybdis and Scylla of ventilator management. *Am J Respir Crit Care Med*. 1994;149:1066
43. Eisner MD, Thompson T, Hudson LD, et al Efficacy of low tidal volume ventilation in patients with different clinical risk factors for acute lung injury and the acute respiratory distress syndrome. *Am J Respir Crit Care Med*. 2001;164(2):231–236
44. Esteban A, Alia I, Gordo F, et al Prospective, randomized trial comparing pressure-controlled ventilation and volume-controlled ventilation in ARDS. *Chest*. 2000;117:1690–1696
45. Esteban A, Anzueto A, Alia I, et al How is mechanical ventilation employed in the intensive care unit? An international utilization review. *Am J Respir Crit Care Med*. 2000;161(5):1450–1458
46. Estenne M, De Troyer A. Mechanism of the postural dependence of vital capacity in tetraplegic subjects. *Am Rev Respir Dis*. 1987;135:367–371
47. Feihl F, Perret C. Permissive hypercapnia: how permissive should we be? *Am J Respir Crit Care Med*. 1994;150:1722
48. Ferguson ND, Frutos-Vivar F, Esteban A, et al Airway pressures, tidal volumes, and mortality in patients with acute respiratory distress syndrome. *Crit Care Med*. 2005;33(1):21–30
49. Fernandez-Mondejar E, Vazquez-Mata G. PEEP: more than just support? *Intensive Care Med*. 1998;24:1

50. Fishburn MJ, Marino RJ, Ditunno JF. Atelectasis and pneumonia in acute spinal cord injury. *Arch Phys Med Rehabil*. 1990;71:197
51. Fleury B, Murciano D, Talamo C, et al Work of breathing in patients with obstructive pulmonary disease in acute respiratory failure. *Am Rev Respir Dis*. 1985;131:822–827
52. Fridrich P, Krafft P, Hochleuthner H, et al The effects of long-term prone positioning in patients with trauma-induced adult respiratory distress syndrome. *Anesth Analg*. 1996;83:1206
53. Gailard M, Herve C, Mandin L, Raynaud P. Mortality prognostic factors in chest injury. *J Trauma*. 1990;30:93–96
54. Gamberoni C, Colombo G, Aspesi M, et al Respiratory mechanics in brain injured patients. *Minerva Anestesiol*. 2002;68(4):291–296
55. Gattinoni L, Mascheroni D, Torresin A, et al Morphological response to positive end expiratory pressure in acute respiratory failure. Computerized tomography study. *Intensive Care Med*. 1986;12:137
56. Gattinoni L, Pelosi A, Avalli L, et al Pressure-volume curve of total respiratory system in acute respiratory failure: a CT scan study. *Am Rev Respir Dis*. 1987;136:730
57. Gattinoni L, Pelosi P, Crotti S, et al Effects of positive end-expiratory pressure on regional distribution of tidal volume and recruitment in adult respiratory distress syndrome. *Am J Respir Crit Care Med*. 1995;151:1807
58. Georgiadis D, Schwarz S, Baumgartner RW, Veltkamp R, Schwab S. Influence of positive end-expiratory pressure on intracranial pressure and cerebral perfusion pressure in patients with acute stroke. *Stroke*. 2001;32(9):2088–2092
59. Georgopoulos D, Brochard L. Ventilator strategies in acute exacerbations of COPD. *Eur Resp Monogr*. 1998;8:12–44
60. Georgopoulos D, Rossi A, Moxham J. Ventilatory support in COPD. *Eur Resp Monogr*. 1998;7:189–208
61. Gibney RTN, Wilson RS, Pontoppidan H. Comparison of work of breathing on high gas flow and demand valve continuous positive airway pressure systems. *Chest*. 1982;82:692
62. Gibson GJ, Pride NB, Davis JN, et al Pulmonary mechanics in patients with respiratory muscle. *JAMA*. 1976;235:733
63. Glenny RW, Lamm WJ, Albert RK, et al Gravity is a minor determinant of pulmonary blood flow distribution. *J Appl Physiol*. 1991;71:620
64. Gore RM, Mintzer RA, Calenoff L. Gastrointestinal complications of spinal cord injury. *Spine*. 1981;6(6):538–544

65. Gottesman RF, Komotar R, Hillis AE. Neurologic aspects of traumatic brain injury. *Int Rev Psychiatry*. 2003;15(4): 302–309
66. Gottfried SB. The role of PEEP in the mechanically ventilated COPD patient. In: Marini JJ, Roussos C, eds. *Ventilatory Failure*. Springer: New York; 1991:392–418
67. Grasso S, Mascia L, Del Turco M, et al Effects of recruiting maneuvers in patients with acute respiratory distress syndrome ventilated with protective ventilatory strategy. *Anesthesiology*. 2002;96:795–802
68. Grimm DR, Chandy D, Almenoff PL, et al Airway hyper-reactivity in subjects with tetraplegia is associated with reduced baseline airway caliber. *Chest*. 2000;118:1397
69. Haas F, Axen K, Pineda H, et al Temporal pulmonary function changes in cervical cord injury. *Arch Phys Med Rehabil*. 1985; 66:139
70. Hager DN, Krishnan JA, Hayden DL, Brower RG. Tidal volume reduction in patients with acute lung injury when plateau pressures are not high. *Am J Respir Crit Care Med*. 2005; 172:1241
71. Haluszka J, Chartrand DA, Grassino AE, et al Intrinsic PEEP and arterial CO_2 in stable patients with chronic obstructive pulmonary disease. *Am Rev Respir Dis*. 1990;141:1194–1197
72. Hartke RH Jr, Block AJ. External stabilisation of flail chest using continuous negative extrathoracic pressure. *Chest*. 1992;102:1283–1285
73. Harvey MG, Hancox RJ. Elevation of cardiac troponins in exacerbation of chronic obstructive pulmonary disease. *Emerg Med Australas*. 2004;16:212–215
74. Helmy A, Vizcaychipi M, Gupta AK. Traumatic brain injury: intensive care management. *Br J Anaesth*. 2007;99(1):32–42.
75. Hess DR, Kacmarek RM. Cardiovascular failure. *Essentals of Mechanical Ventilation*. London: McGraw-Hill; 2002
76. Ikeda Y, Long DM. The molecular basis of brain injury and brain edema: the role of oxygen free-radicals. *Neurosurgery*. 1990;27:1–11
77. Imsand C, Feihl F, Perret C, Fitting JW. Regulation of inspiratory neuromuscular output during synchronized intermittent mechanical ventilation. *Anesthesiology*. 1994;80:13
78. Jubran A, Tobin MJ. Mechanical ventilation in acute respiratory failure complicating chronic obstructive pulmonary disease. UpToDate • www.uptodate.com (800):998–6374;(781): 237–4788

79. Jubran A, Van de Graaff WB, Tobin MJ. Variability of patient-ventilator interaction with pressure support ventilation in patients with COPD. *Am J Respir Crit Care Med*. 1995;152:129
80. Kacmarek RM, Schwartz DR. Lung recruitment. *Respir Care Clin N Am*. Dec 2000;6(4):597–623
81. Kimball WR, Leith DE, Robins AG. Dynamic hyperinflation and ventilatory dependence in chronic obstructive pulmonary disease. *Am Rev Respir Dis*. 1982;126:991–995
82. Kishikawa M, Yoshioka T, Shimazu T, et al Pulmonary contusion causes long-term respiratory dysfunction with decreased functional residual capacity. *J Trauma*. 1991;31:1203–1210
83. Kregenow DA, Rubenfeld GD, Hudson LD, Swenson ER. Hypercapnic acidosis and mortality in acute lung injury. *Crit Care Med*. 2006;34:1
84. Laghi F, Segal J, Choe WK, Tobin MJ. Effect of imposed inflation time on respiratory frequency and hyperinflation in patients with chronic obstructive pulmonary disease. *Am J Respir Crit Care Med*. 2001;163:1365–1370
85. Lai-Fook SJ, Rodarte JR. Pleural pressure distribution and its relationship to lung volume and interstitial pressure. *J Appl Physiol*. 1991;70:967
86. Lamb VJ. The inspiratory workload of patient-initiated mechanical ventilation. *Am Rev Respir Dis*. 1986;134:902
87. Lamm WJ, Graham MM, Albert RK. Mechanism by which the prone position improves oxygenation in acute lung injury. *Am J Respir Crit Care Med*. 1994;150:184
88. Langer M, Mascheroni D, Marcolin R, et al The prone position in ARDS patients. A clinical study. *Chest*. 1988;94:103
89. Larson RP, Capps JS, Pierson DJ. A comparison of three devices used for quantitating bronchopleural air leak. *Respir Care*. 1986;31:1065
90. Lawn ND, Fletcher DD, Henderson RD, et al Anticipating mechanical ventilation in Guillain-Barré syndrome. *Arch Neurol*. 2001;58:893
91. Leatherman JW, McArthur C, Shapiro RS. Effect of prolongation of expiratory time on dynamic hyperinflation in mechanically ventilated patients with severe asthma. *Crit Care Med*. 2004;32:1542–1545
92. Leatherman JW. Mechanical ventilation in severe asthma. In: Marini JJ, Slutsky AS, eds. *Physiological Basis of Ventilatory Support*. New York: Marcel Dekker; 1998:1155–1185
93. Ledsome JR, Sharp JM. Pulmonary function in acute cervical cord injury. *Am Rev Respir Dis*. 1981;124(1):41–44

94. Lesage A, Ramakers M, Daubin C, et al Complicated acute myocardial infarction requiring mechanical ventilation in the intensive care unit: prognostic factors of clinical outcome in a series of 157 patients. *Crit Care Med.* 2004;32:100–105
95. Lessard MR, Lofaso F, Brochard L. Expiratory muscle activity increases intrinsic positive end-expiratory pressure independently of dynamic hyperinflation in mechanically ventilated patients. *Am J Respir Crit Care Med.* 1995;151:562–569
96. Lim CM, Jung H, Koh Y, et al Effect of alveolar recruitment maneuver in early acute respiratory distress syndrome according to antiderecruitment strategy, etiological category of diffuse lung injury, and body position of the patient. *Crit Care Med.* 2003;31:411–418
97. Lim SC, Alexander B, Simonson DA, et al Transient hemodynamic effects of recruitment maneuvers in three experimental models of acute lung injury. *Crit Care Med.* 2004;32:2378–2384
98. Linn WS, Adkins RH, Gong H Jr, Waters RL. Pulmonary function in chronic spinal cord injury: a cross-sectional survey of 222 southern California adult outpatients. *Arch Phys Med Rehabil.* 2000;81:757
99. Lu K, Lee TC, Liang CL, et al Delayed apnea in patients with mid- to lower cervical spinal cord injury. *Spine.* 2000;25(11): 1332–1338
100. Lutch JS, Murray JF. Continuous positive-pressure ventilation: effects on systemic oxygen transport and tissue oxygenation. *Ann Intern Med.* 1972;76:193
101. Mackersie RC. Ventilatory support following major trauma. In: Stock MC, Perel A, eds. *Handbook of Mechanical Ventilatory Support.* Baltimore: Williams & Wilkins; 1992
102. Malbouisson LM, Muller JC, Constantin JM, et al Computed tomography assessment of positive end-expiratory pressure-induced alveolar recruitment in patients with acute respiratory distress syndrome. *Am J Respir Crit Care Med.* 2001; 163:1444
103. Maltais F, Reissmann H, Navalesi P, et al Comparison of static and dynamic measurements of intrinsic PEEP in mechanically ventilated patients. *Am J Respir Crit Care Med.* 1994;150: 1318–1324
104. Mancebo J. PEEP, ARDS and alveolar recruitment. *Intensive Care Med.* 1992;18:383
105. Marcy TW, Marini JJ. Inverse ratio ventilation in ARDS. Rationale and implementation. *Chest.* 1991;100:494

106. Marcy TW. Inverse ratio ventilation. In: Tobin MJ, ed. *Principles and Practice of Mechanical Ventilation*. New York: McGraw-Hill; 1994:319
107. Marik PE, Varon J, Trask T. Management of head trauma. *Chest*. 2002;122(2):699–711
108. Marini JJ, O'Quin R, Culver BH, et al Estimation of transmural cardiac pressures during ventilation with PEEP. *J Appl Physiol*. 1982;53:384
109. Marini JJ. Lung mechanics in the adult respiratory distress syndrome. Recent conceptual advances and implications for management. *Clin Chest Med*. 1990;11:673
110. Marini JJ. Should PEEP be used in airflow obstruction? *Am Rev Respir Dis*. 1989;140:1–3
111. Marini JJ, Rodriguez RM, Lamb VJ. The inspiratory workload of patient-initiated mechanical ventilation. *Am Rev Respir Dis*. 1986;134:902
112. Marini JJ, Smith TC, Lamb VJ. External work output and force generation during synchronized intermittent mechanical ventilation: effect of machine assistance on breathing effort. *Am Rev Respir Dis*. 1988;138:1169
113. Maron MB, Dawson CA. Pulmonary venoconstriction caused by elevated cerebrospinal fluid pressure in the dog. *J Appl Phsiol*. 1980;49:73
114. Mathru M, Rao TL, El-Etr AA, et al Hemodynamic response to changes in ventilatory patterns in patients with normal and poor left ventricular reserve. *Crit Care Med*. 1982;10:423–426
115. Matthay MA. Acute hypoxemic respiratory failure: Pulmonary edema and ARDS. In: George RB, Light RW, Matthay MA, et al, eds. *Chest Medicine. Essentials of Pulmonary and Critical Care Medicine*. 3rd ed. Baltimore: Williams & Wilkins; 1995:593
116. Mazzara JT, Ayres SM, Grace WJ. Extreme hypocapnia in the critically ill patient. *Am J Med*. 1974;56:450–456
117. McCaffree DR, Gray BA. Effect of inspiratory flow rate on gas exchange during mechanical ventilation. *Am Rev Respir Dis*. 1981;124:5379
118. McClintock D, Zhuo H, Wickersham N, et al Biomarkers of inflammation, coagulation and fibrinolysis predict mortality in acute lung injury. *Crit Care*. 2008;12:R41
119. McCool FD, Brown R, Mayewski RJ, Hyde RW. Effects of posture on stimulated ventilation in quadriplegia. *Am Rev Respir Dis*. 1988;138:101
120. Meade MO, Cook DJ, Guyatt GH, et al Ventilation strategy using low tidal volumes, recruitment maneuvers, and high

positive end-expiratory pressure for acute lung injury and acute respiratory distress syndrome: a randomized controlled trial. *JAMA*. 2008;299:637

121. Medoff BD, Harris RS, Kesselman H, et al Use of recruitment maneuvers and high-positive end-expiratory pressure in a patient with acute respiratory distress syndrome. *Crit Care Med*. 2000;28:1210–1216
122. Menitove SM, Goldring RM. Combined ventilator and bicarbonate strategy in the management of status asthmaticus. *Am J Med*. 1983;74:898
123. Mercat A, Titiriga M, Anguel N, et al Inverse ratio ventilation (I/E=2/1) in acute respiratory distress syndrome. *Am J Respir Crit Care Med*. 1997;155:1637
124. Michard F, Chemla D, Richard C, et al Clinical use of respiratory changes in arterial pulse pressure to monitor the hemodynamic effects of PEEP. *Am J Respir Crit Care Med*. 1999; 159:935
125. Modelska K, Pittet JF, Folkesson HG, et al Acid-induced lung injury. Protective effect of anti-inter-leukin-8 pretreatment on alveolar epithelial barrier function in rabbits. *Am J Respir Crit Care Med*. 1999;160(5 Pt 1):1450–1456
126. Moss M, Mannino DM. Race and gender differences in acute respiratory distress syndrome deaths in the United States: an analysis of multiple-cause mortality data (1979–1996). *Crit Care Med*. 2002;30(8):1679–1685
127. Mure M, Martling CR, Lindahl SG. Dramatic effect on oxygenation in patients with severe acute lung insufficiency treated in the prone. *Crit Care Med*. 1997;25:1539
128. Muscadere JG, Mullen JB, Gan K, et al Tidal ventilation at low airway pressures can augment lung injury. *Am J Respir Crit Care Med*. 1994;149:1327
129. Nicholas JM, Dulchavsky SA. Successful use of autologous fibrin gel in traumatic bronchopleural fistula: case report. *J Trauma*. 1992;32:87
130. Nyren S, Mure M, Jacobsson H, et al Pulmonary perfusion is more uniform in the prone than in the supine position: scintigraphy in healthy humans. *J Appl Physiol*. 1999;86: 1135
131. O'Donohue WJ Jr, Baker JP, Bell GM, et al Respiratory failure in neuromuscular disease. *Chest*. 1973;63(5):818–821
132. Oakes DF, Shortall SP, eds. *Ventilator Management: A Bedside Reference Guide*. 2nd ed. Orono: Health Educator Publications; 2005

133. Ognibene FP, Martin SE, Parker MM, et al Adult respiratory distress syndrome in patients with severe neutropenia. *N Engl J Med*. 1986;315(9):547–551
134. Parish JM, Gracey DR, Southorn PA, et al Differential mechanical ventilation in respiratory failure due to severe unilateral lung disease. *Mayo Clin Proc*. 1984;59:822–828
135. Parker JS, deBoisbianc BP. Case report: intermittent, positive pressure ventilation-dependent right bundle branch block. *Am J Med Sci*. 1991;302:380–381
136. Pelosi, P, Cadringer, P, Bottino, N, et al Sigh in acute respiratory distress syndrome. Am J Respir Crit Care Med 1999; 159:872) or Pelosi, P, Bottino, N, Chiumello, D, et al Sigh in supine and prone position during acute respiratory distress syndrome. Am J Respir Crit Care Med 2003; 167:521
137. Pelosi, P, Tubiolo, D, Mascheroni, D, et al Effects of the prone position on respiratory mechanics and gas exchange during acute lung injury. *Am J Respir Crit Care Med*. 1998;157:387
138. Pepe PE, Marini JJ. Occult positive end-expiratory pressure in mechanically ventilated patients with airflow obstruction. *Am Rev Respir Dis*. 1982;126:16611
139. Pepe PE, Hudson LE, Carrico HJ. Early application of positive end-expiratory pressure in patients at risk for the adult respiratory distress syndrome. *N Engl J Med*. 1984;311:281
140. Petrof BJ, Legaré M, Goldberg P, et al Continuous positive airway pressure reduces work of breathing and dyspnea during weaning from mechanical ventilation in severe chronic obstructive pulmonary disease. *Am Rev Respir Dis*. 1990;141:28118
141. Petrucci N, Iacovelli W. Ventilation with lower tidal volumes versus traditional tidal volumes in adults for acute lung injury and acute respiratory distress syndrome. *Cochrane Database Syst Rev*. 2004;(2):CD003844
142. Petty TL. The uses, abuse, and mystique of positive end-expiratory pressure. *Am Rev Respir Dis*. 1988;138:475
143. Piehl MA, Brown RS. Use of extreme position changes in acute respiratory failure. *Crit Care Med*. 1976;4:13
144. Pierson DJ. Barotrauma and bronchopleural fistula. In: Tobin MJ, ed. *Principles and Practice of Mechanical Ventilation*. New York: McGraw-Hill; 1994:813
145. Pierson DJ, Horton CA, Bates PW. Persistent bronchopleural air leak during mechanical ventilation: a review of 39 cases. *Chest*. 1986;90:321

146. Pinsky MR. The effects of mechanical ventilation on the cardiovascular system. *Crit Care Clin*. 1990;6:663–678
147. Prin S, Chergui K, Augarde R, et al Ability and safety of a heated humidifier to control hypercapnic acidosis in severe ARDS. *Intensive Care Med*. 2002;28:1756
148. Quist J, Pontoppidan H, Wilson RS, et al Hemodynamic responses to mechanical ventilation with PEEP. *Anesthesiology*. 1971;42:45
149. Rahn H, Otis AB, Chadwick LE, Fenn WO. The pressure-volume diagram of the thorax and lung. *Am J Physiol*. 1946;146:161–178
150. Ralph DD, Robertson HT, Weaver LJ, et al Distribution of ventilation and perfusion during positive end-expiratory pressure in the adult respiratory distress syndrome. *Am Rev Respir Dis*. 1985;131:54
151. Ranieri VM, Giuliani R, Fiore T, et al Volume-pressure curve of the respiratory system predicts effects of PEEP in ARDS: "occlusion" versus "constant flow" technique. *Am J Respir Crit Care Med*. 1994;149:19
152. Ranieri VM, Giuliani R, Cinnella G, et al Physiologic effects of positive end-expiratory pressure in patients with chronic obstructive pulmonary disease during acute ventilatory failure and controlled mechanical ventilation. *Am Rev Respir Dis*. 1993;147:5
153. Reines HD, Harris RC. Pulmonary complications of acute spinal cord injuries. *Neurosurgery*. 1987;21(2):193–196
154. Rice TW, Wheeler AP, Bernard GR, et al Comparison of the SpO_2/FIO_2 Ratio and the PaO_2/FIO_2 ratio in patients with acute lung injury or ARDS. *Chest*. 2007;132:410
155. Richardson DW, Kontos HA, Raper AJ, Patterson JL Jr. Systemic circulatory responses to hypocapnia in man. *Am J Physiol*. 1972;223:1308–1312
156. Richecoeur J, Lu Q, Vieira SR, et al Expiratory washout versus optimization of mechanical ventilation during permissive hypercapnia in patients with severe acute respiratory distress syndrome. *Am J Respir Crit Care Med*. 1999;160:77
157. Robertson CH, Pagel MA, Johnson RL Jr. The distribution of blood flow, oxygen consumption and work output among the respiratory muscles during unobstructed hyperventilation. *J Clin Invest*. 1977;59:31–42
158. Rossi A, Ranieri M. Positive end-expiratory pressure. In: Tobin MJ, ed. *Principles and Practice of Mechanical Ventilation*. New York: McGraw-Hill; 1994:259

159. Roupie E, Dambrosio M, Servillo G, et al Titration of tidal volume and induced hypercapnia in acute respiratory distress syndrome. *Am J Respir Crit Care Med.* 1995;152:121
160. Sassoon CS, Zhu E, Caiozzo VJ. Assist-control mechanical ventilation attenuates ventilator-induced diaphragmatic dysfunction. *Am J Respir Crit Care Med.* 2004;170:626–632
161. Sassoon CSH, Del Rosario N, Fei R, et al Influence of pressure- and flow-triggered synchronous intermittent mandatory ventilation on inspiratory muscle work. *Crit Care Med.* 1994;22:1933
162. Saulnier FF, Durocher AV, Deturck RA, et al Respiratory and hemodynamic effects of halothane in status asthmaticus. *Intensive Care Med.* 1990;16:104
163. Scharf SM, Iqbal M, Keller C, et al Hemodynamic characterization of patients with severe emphysema. *Am J Respir Crit Care Med.* 2002;166:314–322
164. Shackford SR, Smith DE, Zarins CD, et al The management of flail chest: a comparison of ventilatory and nonventilatory treatment. *Am J Surg.* 1976;132:759–762
165. Shepherd JT. The lungs as receptor sites for cardiovascular regulation. *Circulation.* 1981;63:1–10
166. Slutsky AS. Mechanical ventilation. American College of Chest Physicians' Consensus Conference. *Chest.* 1993;104:1833
167. Smith TC, Marini JJ. Impact of PEEP on lung mechanics and work of breathing in severe airflow obstruction. *J Appl Physiol.* 1988;65:1488
168. Sprung J, Krasna MJ, Yun A, et al Treatment of a bronchopleural fistula with a Fogarty catheter and oxidized regenerated cellulose (surgicel). *Chest.* 1994;105:1879
169. Spungen AM, Dicpinigaitis PV, Almenoff PL, Bauman WA. Pulmonary obstruction in individuals with cervical spinal cord lesions unmasked by bronchodilator administration. *Paraplegia.* 1993;31:404
170. Steltzer H, Krafft P, Fridrich P, et al Right ventricular function and oxygen transport patterns in patients with acute respiratory distress syndrome. *Anaesthesia.* 1994;49:1039
171. Stocchetti N, Maas AI, Chieregato A, van der Plas AA. Hyperventilation in head injury: a review. *Chest.* 2005;127(5):1812–1827
172. Stocker R, Neff T, Stein S, et al Prone positioning and low-volume pressure-limited ventilation improve survival in patients with severe ARDS. *Chest.* 1997;111:1008

173. Sugiura M, McCulloch PR, Wren S, et al Ventilator pattern influences neutrophil influx and activation in atelectasis-prone rabbit lung. *J Appl Physiol*. 1994;77:1355
174. Suter PM, Fairley HB, Isenberg MD. Optimum end-expiratory airway pressure in patients with acute pulmonary failure. *N Engl J Med*. 1975;292:284
175. Szeinberg A, Tabachnik E, Rashed N, et al Cough capacity in patients with muscular dystrophy. *Chest*. 1988;94:1232
176. Takeuchi M, Goddon S, Dolhnikoff M, et al Set positive end-expiratory pressure during protective ventilation affects lung injury. *Anesthesiology*. 2002;97:682–692
177. Terragni PP, Rosboch G, Tealdi A, et al Tidal hyperinflation during low tidal volume ventilation in acute respiratory distress syndrome. *Am J Respir Crit Care Med*. 2007;175:160
178. Theodore J, Robin ED. Speculations on neurogenic pulmonary edema. *Am Rev Respir Dis*. 1976;113:405
179. Tobin MJ, Lodato RF. PEEP, Auto-PEEP and waterfalls. *Chest*. 1989;96:449
180. Tobin MJ. Respiratory muscles in disease. *Clin Chest Med*. 1988;9:263–286
181. Tobin MJ, Jubran A. Pathophysiology of failure to wean from mechanical ventilation. *Schweiz Med Wochenschr*. 1994;124:2139
182. Torres A, Serra-Batlles JS, Ros E, et al Pulmonary aspiration of gastric contents in patients receiving mechanical ventilation: the effect of body position. *Ann Intern Med*. 1992;116:540
183. Trinkle JK, Richardson JD, Franz JL, et al Management of flail chest without mechanical ventilation. *Ann Thorac Surg*. 1975;19:355–363
184. Tzlepis GE, McCool FD, Hoppin FG Jr. Chest wall distortion in patients with flail chest. *Am Rev Respir Dis*. 1989;140:31–37
185. Urmey W, Loring S, Mead J, et al Upper and lower rib cage deformation during breathing in quadriplegics. *J Appl Phys*. 1986;60:618
186. Valadka AB, Robertson CS. Surgery of cerebral trauma and associated critical care. *Neurosurgery*. 2007;61(1 suppl):203–220
187. Varoli F, Roviaro G, Grignani F, et al Endoscopic treatment of bronchopleural fistulas. *Ann Thorac Surg*. 1998;65:807
188. Vender JR. Hyperventilation in severe brain injury revisited. *Crit Care Med*. 2000;28(9):3361–3362
189. Vieillard-Baron A, Jardin F. The issue of dynamic hyperinflation in acute respiratory distress syndrome patients. *Eur Respir J Suppl*. 2003;42:43s-47s

190. Vieillard-Baron A, Prin S, Augarde R, et al Increasing respiratory rate to improve CO_2 clearance during mechanical ventilation is not a panacea in acute respiratory failure. *Crit Care Med.* 2002;30:1407–1412
191. Villar J, Blazquez MA, Lubillo S, et al Pulmonary hypertension in acute respiratory failure. *Crit Care Med.* 1989;17:523
192. Wang KP, Schaeffer L, Heitmiller R, Baker R. Nd YAG laser closure of a bronchopleural fistula. *Monaldi Arch Chest Dis.* 1993;48:301
193. Ware LB, Matthay MA. Clinical practice. Acute pulmonary edema. *N Engl J Med.* 2005;353:2788
194. Wicks AB, Menter RR. Long-term outlook in quadriplegic patients with initial ventilator dependency. *Chest.* 1986;90:406
195. Zink BJ. Traumatic brain injury outcome: concepts for emergency care. *Ann Emerg Med.* 2001;37(3):318–332
196. Brain Trauma Foundation. *Management and Prognosis of Severe Traumatic Traumatic Brain Injury.* New York, NY: The Brain Trauma Foundation; 2000
197. Deem S. Management of acute brain injury and associated respiratory issues. *Respir Care.* 2006;51(4):357–367
198. Pelosi P, Bottino N, Chiumello D, et al Sigh in supine and prone position during acute respiratory distress syndrome. *Am J Respir Crit Care Med.* 2003;167:52

Chapter 10
The Complications of Mechanical Ventilation

Mechanical ventilation, though potentially lifesaving, is capable of producing complications, some of which may in themselves be life threatening. Several of these complications are related to endotracheal intubation. Critically ill patients are often immunosuppressed and are susceptible to nosocomial pneumonia for a number of reasons. Endotracheal intubation may predispose these patients to ventilator-associated pneumonia (VAP), which is a form of nosocomial pneumonia. A large number of complications are a direct result of generation of positive pressure inside the thorax (e.g., barotrauma and hypotension) and these will be dealt with later in this chapter.

It is important to realize that complications in ventilated patients are relatively common, and meticulous monitoring is vital for their prevention. Prompt corrective action may be life saving if some of these complications (such as a pneumothorax or sudden blockage of an endotracheal tube) occur. Complications can not only occur at the time of initiating mechanical ventilatory support, but also at any time during the course of ventilatory support. For purposes of discussion, these have been organized into as follows:

1. Peri-intubation complications
2. Complications that can occur acutely at any stage during mechanical ventilation
3. Delayed complications

A. Hasan, *Understanding Mechanical Ventilation*,
DOI: 10.1007/978-1-84882-869-8_10,

10.1 Peri-Intubation Complications

10.1.1 Laryngeal Trauma

Even elective intubation can be associated with problems. Hurried or difficult intubations in technically demanding situations have been associated with a variety of complications.

Left-sided vocal cord injury is more common than right-sided vocal cord injury, because the endotracheal tube tip is likely to deviated leftward when introduced from the right side of the mouth.[67] Most laryngeal injuries are minor, but vocal cord lacerations, hematomas, and very rarely, arytenoids dislocations can occur. Persistent hoarseness after extubation is a sign of laryngeal injury sustained at the time of intubation.

10.1.2 Pharyngeal Trauma

Blind nasal intubation or intubation with the stylet projecting beyond the tip of the endotracheal tube can produce pharyngeal injury. As would be expected, the incidence of pharyngeal trauma is high in difficult intubations (up to 50% of cases),[26] but this complication has been described with relatively straightforward intubations as well. Lacerations of the pyriform sinuses have been associated with pneumomediastinum and bilateral pneumothoraces.[97] Trauma to the posterior pharyngeal wall can introduce infection into the retropharyngeal space with subsequent mediastinitis. Cardiac arrest can occur with injury to the pyriform sinuses, posterior pharyngeal wall, or hypopharynx. Endoscopy may be required for diagnosis and assessment.

Box 10.1 Complications Related to Pharyngeal Trauma

Mediastinal emphysema
Subcutaneous emphysema
Pharyngeal hematoma
Upper airway obstruction
Pharyngeal abscess
Mediastinitis
Pneumomediastinum
Pneumothorax

10.1.3 Tracheal or Bronchial Rupture

Though rare, this complication can occur when the membranous posterior part of the trachea is transgressed by the tip of the endotracheal tube during vigorous or repeated attempts at intubation. A stylet protruding beyond the tip of the endotracheal tube can increase the chances of this, and patients at extremes of age may be especially prone.[103] The occurrence of subcutaneous or mediastinal emphysema or of gastric distension should prompt.[31,74,99] Chest imaging and endoscopy for diagnosis, surgical repair may be necessary.

10.1.4 Epistaxis

Epistaxis is more frequently seen with nasal rather than oral intubation. Although usually minor and self-limiting, it can on occasion be significant. Relatively large bleeds can occur if areas on the anterior nasal septum or the posterior pharyngeal wall are traumatized. Nasal intubation is relatively contraindicated in uncontrolled hypertension, blood dyscrasias, anticoagulation or aspirin use, or in severe hepatic derangement where the risk of hemorrhage is high. The risk of a bleed can be minimized by prior visualization of the nasal cavity to rule out the presence of nasal polyps, a deviated nasal septum, or other causes of intranasal obstruction, and by lubricating the endotracheal tube well. Instilling nasal decongestants prior to nasal intubation may also help prevent epistaxis. Although minor nasal bleeds are mostly self-limiting, direct nasal pressure and topical vasoconstrictors may help. Occasionally, nasal packing will be necessary.

10.1.5 Tooth Trauma

An approximate incidence of between 1 in 150 and 1 in 1,500 intubations makes tooth injury a relatively common complication of intubation.[61] Understandably, most injuries occur during difficult intubations. Because of the shape of the laryngoscope blade, the two left upper incisors and the right central incisor are liable to suffer damage. Dental protection during intubation safeguards to some extent against tooth trauma, but the extra padding narrows the intubation window and can prevent proper visualization of the vocal cords. All fragments of a broken tooth should be retrieved, X-rays checked, and a dental consultation obtained.

10.1.6 Cervical Spine Injury

Since intubation of the larynx involves manipulation of the head and neck, caution should be exercised when the cervical spine could be unstable, such as after road traffic accidents. In such cases the cervical spine should be assumed to be unstable unless otherwise proven; suitable precautions must be taken and the neck immobilized by a hard collar. When the situation permits, a blind nasal or fibreoptic bronchoscopic intubation can be carried out in the cooperative patient, or a tracheotomy considered. In highly emergent situations, in-line manual traction may be applied during intubation.

10.1.7 Esophageal Intubation

Poor visualization of the glottis is a common problem during intubation and esophageal intubation is always possible when the vocal cords cannot be properly visualized. Unrecognized placement of the endotracheal tube into the esophagus can have catastrophic consequences, resulting in cerebral anoxia – if not in mortality. Despite the fact that checks are routinely performed by the intubating physician to ascertain correct placement of the tube, many of these methods are fallible and may misguide even the most experienced. Although the most reliable of these methods is the actual visualization of the passage of the endotracheal tube through the glottis, esophageal intubations have been known to occur despite claims of satisfactory vocal cord visualization.

Clinical signs by which the position of the tube is gaged are especially misleading in the obese. The chest and the epigastrum should both be for auscultated to check if air is entering the stomach rather than the lungs. Neither of these signs, however, can tell with absolute certainty if the endotracheal tube is correctly placed: the conduction of breath sounds to the chest wall is possible even though the tube may reside in the esophagus. Neither does the exhalation of air from the endotracheal tube rule out esophageal intubation, as some return of the insufflated air is possible even with esophageal intubation. The occurrence of chest wall movement on bagging the patient does not necessarily mean that the endotracheal tube lies within the trachea, as gastric inflation during bagging can result in some movement of the chest wall – and even sustain gas exchange for a while – because of the diaphragmatic movement so produced.[60] A condensate on the surface of the endotracheal tube is not a guarantee of tracheal intubation either. A fall in the oxygen saturation detected by pulse oximetry is often a late sign, and as mentioned earlier, some degree of gas exchange is possible by the diaphragmatic movement induced by gas insufflation into the stomach in esophageal intubation.

As things stand, capnometry may be the most reliable of the available indices – short of bronchoscopic confirmation of tracheal intubation – that distinguish tracheal from esophageal intubation. Carbon dioxide is transported from the pulmonary capillaries into the alveoli and makes its way out of the respiratory tract during expiration. The detection of CO_2 can only mean that the endotracheal tube resides in the tracheobronchial tree. However, if the patient had initially been manually ventilated with bag and mask, some of the exhaled gas may have been forced into the esophagus during bagging; hence, detection of carbon dioxide is possible for the initial few moments following an esophageal intubation that has been preceded by bagging.[50,60,69] In such cases the end-tidal CO_2 quickly falls to a negligible level. This is in contrast to the persistently detectable end-tidal CO_2 seen with tracheal intubation. Colorimetric end-tidal monitors are a cheaper option to formal capnometry, and may be just as effective and provide an alternative to capnometry in emergency rooms.[37]

10.1.8 Esophageal Perforation

The posterior wall of the esophagus can sometimes be perforated by the tip of the endotracheal tube. Anterior esophageal wall perforation is distinctly unusual: it has not yet been reported.[30,48]

10.1.9 Right Main Bronchial Intubation

Ideally, the tip of the endotracheal tube should be located at least 2–2.5 cm above the carina, and yet should be low enough for the cuff of the endotracheal tube to reside below the cricoid cartilage. The right main bronchus is more aligned with the trachea compared to the left bronchus, and a deeply positioned endotracheal tube preferentially enters the right main bronchus. This results in blockage of the left main bronchus by the side of the endotracheal tube, leading to lack of aeration – and ultimate collapse – of the left lung. The tidal volume that is intended for both lungs now enters the right lung alone, resulting in its overdistension; right-sided pneumothorax may occur.

If the endotracheal tube should slip down any further, its tip might actually lie in the intermediate bronchus and consequently the orifice of the right upper lobe bronchus may also be blocked by the wall of the endotracheal tube. This would result in ventilation of the right lower lobe alone with the relatively large tidal volumes intended for both lungs.

The placement of the endotracheal tube tip 23 cm from the incisors in men and 21 cm from the incisors in women almost always results in an acceptable location of the endotracheal tube tip, except if the patient is remarkably tall or short.

Substantial movement of the endotracheal tube may occur with flexion and extension of the neck.[19] Intuitively, it is often assumed that flexion of the neck results in upward movement of the endotracheal tube tip and extension results in its downward migration. But the opposite of this actually occurs. The position of the endotracheal tube must always be checked by a chest radiograph, particularly after intubation or after adjustment of the tube position. Identification of the carina on the chest film provides a reference point for the location of the endotracheal tube. If the carina is not clearly visible on the X-ray, the body of the sixth thoracic vertebrum may be taken as reference point instead (the carina is usually located within a distance of less than the height of a vertebral body from the sixth thoracic vertebrum).[38] The designated location of endotracheal tube tip should accordingly be 2–2.5 cm above this point, which normally lies between D2 and D4.

10.1.10 Arrhythmias

Pharyngeal stimulation during intubation evokes a pressor response. A transient increase in blood pressure and heart rate is common,[25,33,53] and this response can be exaggerated in hypertensive patients[95] and during nasotracheal intubations.[92]

Stimulation of the carina or of other parts of the airway by the endotracheal tube can result in a variety of arrhythmias. Between 0.4–3.1% of patients may suffer fatal cardiac arrest at the time of intubation.[63] Children and young adults have bradyarrhythmias more frequently than older individuals. In the latter, supraventicular tachyarrhythmias and ventricular dysrhythmias are more likely to occur.

10.1.11 Aspiration

Aspiration of gastric contents during intubation may have disastrous consequences. Critically ill patients often have poor gastric emptying times and may require the emptying of the stomach contents by a nasogastric tube prior to intubation. The use of succinylcholine for pharmacological paralysis has been associated with contraction of the gastric smooth muscle, causing vomiting and aspiration.

10.1.12 Bronchospasm

Bronchospasm due to irritation of the airways by the endotracheal tube is not uncommon and this may be more pronounced in the setting of hyperreactive airways.[1]

10.1.13 Neurologic Complications

Difficult intubations with delays in securing airway control can result in anoxic neurologic injury. Intracranial pressure has been shown to transiently rise during intubation.[82]

10.2 Problems Occurring Acutely at any Stage

At any time in mechanical ventilated patients, acute complications are possible. Tube-related complications are common and can occur in as many as two-thirds of all intubated patients.[96]

10.2.1 Endotracheal Tube Obstruction

An obstructed endotracheal tube presents a typical emergency in a mechanical ventilated patient. Endotracheal tube obstruction can occur insidiously, leading to gradually increasing peak inflation pressures. On spontaneous modes of ventilation the patient's breathing may be labored. This can result in patient-exhaustion with failure to wean, or an inability to sustain the desired amount of minute ventilation. A high level of pressure support may be required to maintain tidal volumes that were earlier possible with a lower level of pressure support.

Endotracheal tubes are just as liable to sudden obstruction. An endotracheal tube with its lumen gradually narrowed by the buildup of detritus on its luminal surface may suddenly get completely occluded if a relatively small clot or a plug of inspissated sputum should lodge in its orifice. A medical emergency then presents itself. Rare causes of endotracheal tube obstruction include kinking or external pressure by an overinflated cuff; a cuff can occasionally "herniate" into the lumen of the tube. Distress in an awake patient, coupled with the activation of the high airway pressure alarm and possibly a drop in oxygen saturation, is the clue to the problem. In such situations when the patient is taken off the ventilator and "bagged," the bag appears stiff and unyielding to manual compression. A suction catheter passed down the endotracheal tube may get impeded by the blockage. If the endotracheal tube cannot be immediately unblocked, it must be replaced with a fresh tube on an emergency basis.

10.2.2 Airway Drying

Normally a thin film of moisture should be visible on the inner surface of the endotracheal tube. If the endotracheal tube is dry, this implies that local airway hydration may be less than optimal. Lack of airway hydration leads to inspissation of airway secretions and predisposes to blockage of the endotracheal tube. Keeping the inspired air humid safeguards against occlusion, but obstruction can nonetheless occur. When a partial blockage of the endotracheal tube is suspected, the tube should be replaced in the interest of safety. Attempts to unblock the tube by instilling copious quantities of fluid down its lumen may be rewarded by the subsequent occurrence of ventilator-associated pneumonia. Where heat-moisture exchangers are used, their contamination with expectorated secretions may increase airway resistance substantially, thereby increasing the work of breathing.

10.2.3 Upward Migration of the Endotracheal Tube

The downward migration of the endotracheal tube has been discussed above. The endotracheal tube can also migrate upward. Ventilator circuitry and HME filters exert considerable traction on the endotracheal tube and tend to drag it up and out. Surprisingly, a high tube location may sometimes go undetected. This could happen even with the endotracheal tube tip lying in the pharynx because some ventilation can still occur. The movements of a poorly sedated or agitated patient can result in tube migration, and even in extubation.

10.2.4 Self-Extubation

The frequency of self-extubation is surprisingly high.[87] Unplanned extubation is usually deliberate on the part of the patient.[15] The removal of the endotracheal tube by a physiologically unstable patient can have catastrophic results. When self-extubation occurs during weaning, the need for reintubation is predictably less.[9] The consequences of unplanned extubation and reintubation are an increased risk for ventilator-associated pneumonia, a protracted ICU stay,[30] a longer time spent on the ventilator,[30] and overall, a longer hospitalization. Patients who are uncooperative due to disorientation or other factors must be restrained or sedated as appropriate to prevent this dangerous complication. Keeping the patient as comfortable as possible, and matching ventilator settings to the patient's needs, may go a long way toward preventing self-extubation.

10.2.5 Cuff Leak

The cuff of an endotracheal tube can sometimes leak. Apart from allowing pooled secretions to trickle down into the lower airways (and thereby increasing the risk of ventilator-associated pneumonia), a cuff leak can result in sudden loss of airway pressures, especially when PEEP is used, causing autocycling of the ventilator. A cuff leak may manifest itself by the sudden ability of an intubated patient to vocalize.

10.2.5.1 Dynamic Hyperinflation

Inspiration during positive pressure breathing is followed by passive exhalation, at the end of which the thorax returns to its resting state. At this point the elastic recoil that tends to collapse the lung is counterbalanced by the forces that tend to pull the thoracic wall outward. The volume of air contained in the lung at this point is termed the functional residual capacity (FRC). Delivery of a premature inspiratory breath before the exhaling lung has reached its FRC results in air trapping. In practice, this occurs if there is delayed lung emptying due to some reason.

The failure of the lung to empty to a FRC that is appropriate for the level of set PEEP is termed dynamic hyperinflation (DH). Although the terms DH and auto-PEEP (also known as intrinsic PEEP, $PEEP_i$) are often used synonymously, auto-PEEP is really the consequence of DH and is the buildup of alveolar pressure relative to atmospheric pressure. Under normal circumstances at end-expiration (in the absence of DH and PEEPi), the alveolar pressure must equal the atmospheric pressure, since at end-expiration there is no flow of air through the bronchial tree. However, in the presence of auto-PEEP, despite the cessation of airflow at end-expiration, there is no equalization of pressure between the alveoli and the mouth and alveolar pressure continues to be positive, relative to the central airway pressure.

It is important to realize that auto-PEEP does not always reflect DH. In a well-sedated and/or paralyzed patient who is not making active respiratory effort, auto-PEEP can only result from DH. However, in a patient who is making active attempts at exhalation, either because of a high respiratory drive or on account of increased expiratory resistance (because the expiratory muscles are trying to squeeze out the air through narrowed airways), a measurable auto-PEEP may occur even in the absence of DH.

DH may be the consequence of any factor that prevents exhalation in the allotted time (See Fig. 10.1).

When auto-PEEP occurs in the absence of DH, the resting position of the lung is actually below its usual FRC, since the expiratory muscles are actively engaged in squeezing the thorax to a smaller volume. In this case, the cycling of the tidal volume is not near the total lung capacity (the lung is not overinflated) and the work of breathing is not unduly high.

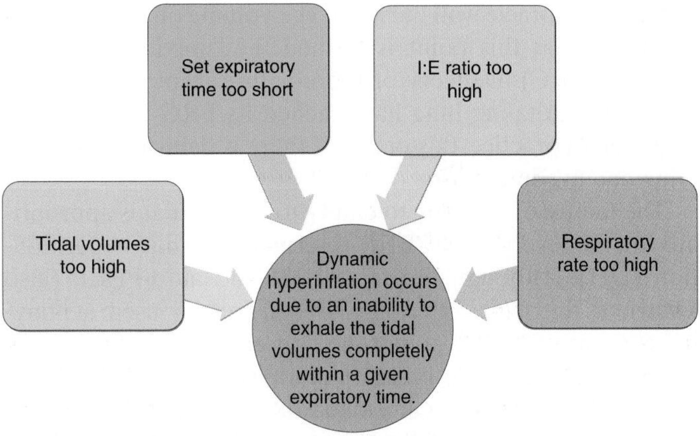
Set expiratory time too short
I:E ratio too high
Tidal volumes too high
Respiratory rate too high
Dynamic hyperinflation occurs due to an inability to exhale the tidal volumes completely within a given expiratory time.

FIGURE 10.1. Dynamic hyperinflation: mechanisms of causation.

Machine related causes

- A partially blocked or kinked endotracheal tube
- Clogging of the circuits by water or secretions
- A poorly functioning expiratory valve

Patient related causes

- Bronchospasm
- Mucosal edema
- Airway inflammation
- Profuseness of airway secretions

FIGURE 10.2. Causes of dynamic hyperinflation.

When DH exists, however, work of breathing is high, and triggering of the ventilator becomes difficult. To trigger the ventilator, the patient has to first generate a negative pressure to overcome the auto-PEEP that DH has produced. In contrast, when auto-PEEP occurs in the absence of DH, there is no difficulty in triggering the ventilator. Finally, DH, by increasing mean airway pressure, also has an unfavorable impact on the systemic circulation.

Treatment strategies for DH are directed at improving lung emptying. Decreasing the I:E ratio increases the time available for expiration. Reducing the minute volume also decreases the air trapping (when the tidal volume is reduced, a lesser amount of air has to be expired in the available expiratory time. If the respiratory rate is decreased, both the inspiratory and expiratory times increase as a result of prolongation of the entire respiratory cycle. The increased expiratory time permits more complete exhalation).

Ventilation with a low minute ventilation often involves the acceptance of a $PaCO_2$ in the higher ranges (permissive hypercapnia), which is the price of preventing lung injury. Finally, to offset the high work of breathing imposed by auto-PEEP that is due to DH, a small amount of external PEEP can be added (equal to 75% of the auto-PEEP). This reduces the pressure gradient against which the patient must inspire and makes for more comfortable breathing on the spontaneous modes. When auto-PEEP is present in the absence of DH, such a measure is unnecessary and the addition of external PEEP serves no purpose.

Box 10.2 Too Little Time to Exhale

'I shall describe a sign which promises to be of the greatest importance in diagnosis. By making the patient perform a number of forced inspirations rapidly...the repetition of the inspiratory efforts cause such an accumulation of air in the diseased portion of the lung as ultimately to prevent its further expansion. The results of this experiment are easily explained by referring to the difficulty of expiration which occurs in this disease'.

William Stokes in *Diseases of the Lung and Windpipe, 1837*

10.2.6 Ventilator-Associated Lung Injury (VALI) and Ventilator-Induced Lung Injury (VILI)

An injured lung is susceptible to further injury. Mechanical ventilation is itself capable of producing or exacerbating acute lung damage. The term VALI is used to describe acute lung injury that develops during the course of mechanical ventilation. VALI is termed VILI if that mechanical ventilation per se can be causally linked to the ALI. Since VILI can be practically impossible to prove at the bedside, the term VALI is the more commonly used.[49] VALI presents in a manner identical to ARDS, with radiologic deterioration and worsening oxygenation (Section 9.4).[49]

10.2.6.1 Barotrauma

When the alveolar pressure rises excessively relative to the pressure in the interstitial space, alveolar rupture can occur. Air can then enter the pulmonary interstitium from where it can dissect along the perivascular sheaths and make its way to the mediastinum (pneumomediastinum). In such cases, the mediastinal pleura may eventually rupture, resulting in a pneumothorax (Fig. 10.3).[35,66]

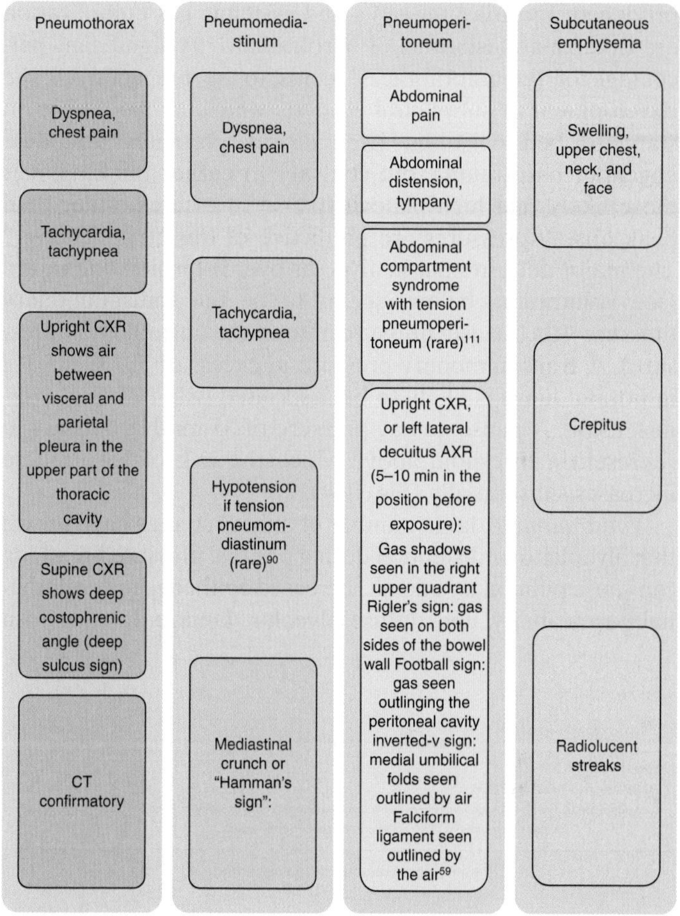
Pneumothorax
Dyspnea, chest pain
Tachycardia, tachypnea
Upright CXR shows air between visceral and parietal pleura in the upper part of the thoracic cavity
Supine CXR shows deep costophrenic angle (deep sulcus sign)
CT confirmatory
Pneumomedia-stinum
Dyspnea, chest pain
Tachycardia, tachypnea
Hypotension if tension pneumom-diastinum (rare)90
Mediastinal crunch or "Hamman's sign":
Pneumoperi-toneum
Abdominal pain
Abdominal distension, tympany
Abdominal compartment syndrome with tension pneumoperi-toneum (rare)111
Upright CXR, or left lateral decuitus AXR (5–10 min in the position before exposure): Gas shadows seen in the right upper quadrant Rigler's sign: gas seen on both sides of the bowel wall Football sign: gas seen outlinging the peritoneal cavity inverted-v sign: medial umbilical folds seen outlined by air Falciform ligament seen outlined by the air59
Subcutaneous emphysema
Swelling, upper chest, neck, and face
Crepitus
Radiolucent streaks

FIGURE 10.3. The manifestations of barotrauma.

A pneumothorax in a patient on a mechanical ventilator must always be presumed to be a tension pneumothorax and prompt action should be taken.

If the air from a pneumomediastinum dissects up the subcutaneous tissues of the neck and elsewhere, subcutaneous emphysema occurs. If the air dissects through the fascial planes down to the peritoneum, a pneumoperitoneum is produced. Tension lung cysts and systemic gas embolization are other manifestations of barotrauma.[68] A significant percentage of pneumothoraces seems to be preceded by the development of subpleural air cysts which can be visible on standard bedside films. High airway pressures doubtless engender barotrauma, but contrary to earlier thinking, it is more likely that high plateau (pause) pressures rather than peak airway pressures are predictive of this complication.[65] The major determinant in alveolar overdistension and injury (see volutrauma below) seems to be the transpulmonary pressure (the pause pressure minus the intrapleural pressure). A transpulmonary pressure in excess of 30–35 mmHg in normal lungs is likely to be associated with alveolar overdistension. A pause airway pressure of 35 mmHg appears to represent a threshold above which the risk of barotrauma increases substantially (Fig. 10.4).[12]

Volutrauma: A large number of animal studies have shown that alveolar overdistention during positive pressure breathing can cause pulmonary edema, increased epithelial and endothelial permeability, and diffuse alveolar damage, leading to a

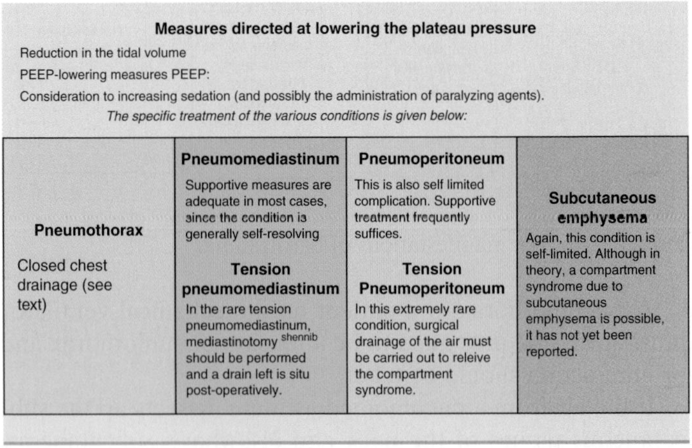
Measures directed at lowering the plateau pressure
Reduction in the tidal volume
PEEP-lowering measures PEEP:
Consideration to increasing sedation (and possibly the administration of paralyzing agents).
The specific treatment of the various conditions is given below:
Pneumothorax
Closed chest drainage (see text)
Pneumomediastinum
Supportive measures are adequate in most cases, since the condition is generally self-resolving
Tension pneumomediastinum
In the rare tension pneumomediastinum, mediastinotomy shennib should be performed and a drain left is situ post-operatively.
Pneumoperitoneum
This is also self limited complication. Supportive treatment frequently suffices.
Tension Pneumoperitoneum
In this extremely rare condition, surgical drainage of the air must be carried out to releive the compartment syndrome.
Subcutaneous emphysema
Again, this condition is self-limited. Although in theory, a compartment syndrome due to subcutaneous emphysema is possible, it has not yet been reported.

FIGURE 10.4. Possible actions directed at lowering the plateau pressure.

condition indistinguishable from the acute respiratory distress syndrome.[75, 76] Experimentally, this form of lung injury can be limited if the lung is prevented from overdistending even in the face of high airway pressures.[27, 28] The term volutrauma has therefore been used to describe this form of lung injury to distinguish it from barotrauma, because the inciting event appears to be alveolar overstretching at end-inspiration, rather than high airway pressure.

In other words, large tidal volumes have a damaging effect independent of the positive pressures that they produce. Consequently, there has been a paradigm shift in strategy, from ventilation of patients with relatively high tidal volumes (10 mL/kg) to low tidal volumes (6 mL/kg), especially in the setting of ARDS (where the patient must be visualized as having "baby lungs"). In ARDS, volutrauma may be minimized by using low tidal volumes (to the order of 6 mL/kg or even lower). The simultaneous application of PEEP to keep the alveoli from collapsing prevents the need for excessively large pressures for opening up collapsed alveoli. PEEP by obviating the need to repetitively open up collapsed alveoli during each inspiration (tidal atelectasis) reduces the shearing forces that operate at the interface between collapsed and patent alveoli. Atelectrauma, as it is called, is thus prevented.[43,55] For further discussion on VALI see ARDS section 9.4.

The use of these two strategies together – the application of PEEP together with low tidal volumes – may be successful in minimizing lung injury in ARDS. The low tidal volumes are liable to produce hypoventilation, but the $PaCO_2$ may be allowed to rise in a controlled manner in order to avoid dangerously high airway pressures: this is called permissive hypercapnia (section 9.4).

Biotrauma: Biotrauma is a relatively recently recognized form of lung injury.[105] Inflammatory cytokines are released from the lung in response to alveolar overdistension.[79] Deformation of cells or of cellular receptors may induce biochemical responses through mechanisms that are as yet obscure, a phenomenon that has been termed mechanotransduction.

These cytokines, which appear to be predominantly produced by the alveolar macrophages,[79] are thought to seep from the lungs into the systemic circulation. This provides a possible explanation of how mechanical ventilation can itself contribute to end organ failure.[11,93]

Strategies of mechanical ventilation modes that employ high tidal volumes with low PEEP have been shown in experimental animals to increase the risk of bacterial translocation from the lung to the systemic circulation; the predisposition to this seems to be reduced by the addition of PEEP.[71,107] This, in the clinical context, could mean higher chances of bacteremia from a pneumonic lung if a "high-tidal-volume low-PEEP" strategy is used to ventilate the patient. Another drawback of a no-PEEP strategy can be the potential occurrence of cyclical atelectasis, or repetitive alveolar closure with each respiratory cycle, as set out above. For further discussion see section 9.4.

It appears, therefore, that the best strategy is to open up the lung (recruit alveolar units) and hold it open, using low tidal volumes and generous amounts of PEEP. Such an approach, called the open lung strategy, envisages PEEP as an internal splint for the unstable alveoli to prevent collapse of unstable alveolar units at end-expiration.

Lung injury can be compounded by the administration of high concentration of O_2. This has been discussed at a later stage section 10.4.

10.3 Delayed Complications (Fig. 10.5)

10.3.1 Sinusitis

Sinusitis is a relatively recently recognized complication of endotracheal intubation. Nasotracheal intubation is especially likely to result in sinusitis. Sinusitis can also occur as a consequence of the mucosal inflammation that nasogastric tubes produce. Bacterial sinusitis may be an important cause of nosocomial pneumonia, though the evidence for this is as

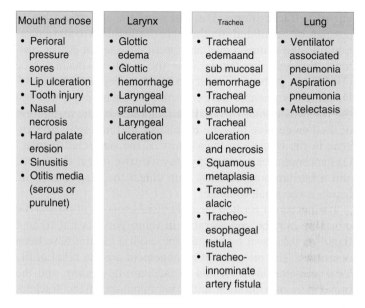

Mouth and nose	Larynx	Trachea	Lung
• Perioral pressure sores • Lip ulceration • Tooth injury • Nasal necrosis • Hard palate erosion • Sinusitis • Otitis media (serous or purulnet)	• Glottic edema • Glottic hemorrhage • Laryngeal granuloma • Laryngeal ulceration	• Tracheal edemaand sub mucosal hemorrhage • Tracheal granuloma • Tracheal ulceration and necrosis • Squamous metaplasia • Tracheom-alacic • Tracheo-esophageal fistula • Tracheo-innominate artery fistula	• Ventilator associated pneumonia • Aspiration pneumonia • Atelectasis

FIGURE 10.5. Delayed complications of mechanical ventilation.

yet circumstantial. A more detailed discussion on sinusitis can be found in Chap. 11

10.3.2 Tracheoesophageal Fistula

Tracheoesophageal fistula occurs in less than 1% patients, but carries with it an extremely high mortality.[24,96]

High endotracheal tube cuff pressure can compromise the capillary perfusion of the tracheal mucosa and lead to ischemic necrosis. Tracheal mucosal injury can be quite insidious and a fistula can go unrecognized until it is quite large.

Air leakage around the cuff or a substantial increase in tracheal secretions may be the first sign of development of a tracheoesophageal fistula. Seepage of feeds through the fistula into the trachea can lead to bouts of coughing during feeding and sometimes to the emergence of the food material out of a tracheostomy. Distension of the abdomen due to passage of ventilated air through the fistulous communication into the stomach may also occur. Passage of gastric contents through the fistula into the tracheobronchial tree resulting in pulmonary injury is a recognized complication.[41] Diagnosis is possible by performing bronchoscopy through the tracheal stoma. This may be facilitated by the instillation of methylene blue into the esophagus and noting its appearance in the trachea in the vicinity of the suspected fistula.[40] Gastroesophageal endoscopy may likewise reveal the defect, and a barium contrast may help clinch the diagnosis if the fistula is too small to detect.

Formal repair is often the only satisfactory solution and the mortality may be considerable in those patients not treated thus.[102] A variety of techniques for surgical closure have been described.[5] The priorities of management are the relief of the local pressure on the fistula to facilitate its healing, and the prevention of aspiration and contamination of the tracheobronchial tree. Positioning the cuff distal to the fistula may enable the fistula to heal. Jet ventilation has been resorted to on occasion, the rationale being that it may help diminish airway pressure and decrease the air loss through the fistula.[77] Delaying repair until the patient has been weaned off the ventilator may have better results.[5,101] A small fistula involving the membranous wall of the trachea can be closed directly, but extensive circumferential tracheal injury necessitates resection and reconstruction. Creation of a feeding jejunostomy ensures a functional valve behind the feeds and diminishes the risk of aspiration. A gastrostomy facilitates gastric drainage.[41] Keeping the patient propped up wherever possible may diminish the risk of aspiration due to reflux of the stomach contents.

Since a tracheoesophageal fistula in itself can produce considerable morbidity and its treatment is no less debilitating, all due care must be taken to present its occurrence. This involves using endotracheal tubes with low-pressure high-volume cuffs, rather than the older high-pressure low-volume cuffs. Even so, cuff pressure needs to be meticulously monitored and its optimization can go a long way toward preventing the subsequent development of a tracheoesophageal fistula.

10.3.2.1 Cuff Pressures

An adequate seal between the ET cuff and the tracheal wall may be accomplished either with the minimal occlusion technique or with the minimal leak technique. In the minimal occlusion technique, the chest piece of the stethoscope is held against the patient's larynx as the pilot bulb of the endotracheal tube cuff is first deflated (with prior thorough throat suctioning) and then gradually inflated with a dry syringe. With increasing inflation of the pilot bulb, the harsh sound of the air leakage during the inspiratory cycle of the ventilator should disappear at some point. The point of disappearance of this sound indicates that just enough air has been inflated into the endotracheal tube cuff to provide minimal occlusion.[8] Alternatively, once the endotracheal tube cuff has been inflated to a point beyond the disappearance of the sound of the air leak, air is very gradually let out from the pilot bulb until the sound of the inspiratory leak is just audible.[73]

Increased cuff pressures should be suspected when the tracheal air column appears widened on the chest film.[54] Objective information of the endotracheal tube cuff pressure is provided by special manometers for the pilot bulb. Cuff pressure should be checked frequently – ideally once during each nursing shift[30] – and restricted to below 20 mmHg (27 cm H_2O). When peak airway pressures are high, a higher cuff pressure is required to achieve an adequate seal. For instance, one study found that it took a cuff pressure of 25 cm H_2O to prevent a leak with peak pressures around 35 mmHg (48 cm H_2O).[42] The requirement of high cuff pressures to prevent air-leak should prompt consideration of foam-cuffed endotracheal tubes.[30]

Very low cuff pressures (below 15 mmHg) can make the patient vulnerable to microaspiration around the cuff and predispose to ventilator-associated pneumonia.[7,81]

10.3.3 Tracheoinnominate Artery Fistula

This dangerous condition is fortunately a rare complication in ventilated patients.[52] It occurs in tracheostomized patients when the pressure of the elbow of the tracheostomy tube produces a full thickness necrosis of the tracheal wall, with erosion into the innominate artery.[21] For this to occur, the elbow of the tracheostomy tube must lie at a level of the innominate artery and the erosion should involve the anterior wall of the trachea. Although this is not usual owing to the normal anatomical disposition of the innominate artery, it becomes possible when the tracheostomy stoma is created at a level below the fourth tracheal ring.[21,52]

Traction on the tracheostomy tube by bulky ventilator circuitry, and heat-moisture exchangers, can cause the tracheostomy stoma to migrate downwards and result in the anatomical adjacence of the elbow of the tracheostomy tube to the innominate artery.

Tracheoinnominate fistulae generally take 48 h or more to develop. Sometimes the development of a large exsanguinating bleed may be preceded by a warning hemorrhage of bright red blood, and disregard for this important sign can lead to a catastrophic bleed later on. Thus, if occurring more than 48 h after a tracheostomy has been done, even a mild bleed should be taken cognizance of and a diagnostic bronchoscopy performed.[21,46]

Once a tracheoinnominate fistula develops, the bleed is frequently devastating and often results in mortality.[72] For immediate control, hyperinflation of the cuff of the tracheostomy tube may be tried, failing which, replacement of the tracheostomy tube by a orotracheally passed endotracheal tube should be done to permit manual compression of the innominate artery by a finger inserted through the tracheostomy stoma; pressure exerted in an anterior direction enables the compression of the innominate artery against the posterior part of the sternum until the patient can be taken to the operating theater for urgent surgical control of the bleed.

10.3.4 Tracheocutaneous Fistula

This too is a rare complication, usually following protracted use of a tracheostomy tube, which causes the tracheostomy stoma to become epithelialized.[58]

Dermal inflammation with the chronic discharge is often troublesome; difficulty in phonation may also occur. The patient may show vulnerability to recurrent lower respiratory tract infection.

10.4 Oxygen-Related Lung Complications

For reasons mentioned below, a high fraction of inspired oxygen (FIO_2) can be detrimental. Indeed, the fact that oxygen could be potentially destructive was recognized soon after its acceptance as a major therapeutic drug. The lung is the organ that by its very purpose is constantly exposed to the highest concentrations of oxygen in the body. As a result, the tracheobronchial and alveolar epithelial cells are at the greatest risk for injury, should they be constantly exposed to a high concentration of oxygen[45] (Fig 10.6).

Oxygen-related lung problems encompass a wide range of respiratory syndromes. The common denominator underlying

Clinical syndromes	Physiological derangements	Cytological changes
• Tracheobronchitis • Adsorptive atelectasis • Hyperoxic hypercabia • Diffuse alveolar damage (DAD) • Bronchopulmonary dysplasia	• Decreased vital capacity • Decreased lung compliance • Decreased D_{LCO}	• Decreased tracheal mucus flow velocity • Decreased alveolar macrophage function[4] • Decreased capillary blood volume • Capillary injury; platelet aggregation within pulmonary capillaries • Endothelial cell damage • Decreased surfactant production

FIGURE 10.6. Oxygen-related lung injury.

many of the manifestations of oxygen-induced injury seems to be toxic oxygen radical-induced cellular damage (see below). Oxygen species such as the superoxide anion, the hydroxyl radical, and hydrogen peroxide have been shown to interfere with the functioning of intracellular macromolecules. Oxygen by its propensity to be rapidly absorbed through the alveolocapillary membrane is capable of causing collapse of the portion of lung behind a blocked bronchus. Also oxygen may possibly suppress the respiratory drive in a certain subset of patients, resulting in ventilatory depression.

10.4.1 Tracheobronchitis

Oxygen therapy in healthy volunteers can lead to substernal discomfort, dry cough, and a pleuritic pain on inspiration, especially if the oxygen being respired is not adequately humidified.[13] Together, these symptoms lead to a sense of dyspnea. These symptoms, which normally occur within 24 h of commencing supplemental oxygen, have been ascribed to a combination of several factors. Bronchoscopically, airway mucosal changes have been observed to develop within hours of administering a high concentration of oxygen.[85] "Hyperoxic tracheobronchitis," along with a variable component of adsorptive atelectasis, has been regarded as being responsible for many of the nonspecific symptoms that can occur at early stages of oxygen therapy (Fig. 10.6).[18]

10.4.2 Adsorptive Altelectasis

The partial pressure of oxygen is lower in the alveoli than in the pulmonary capillary blood. As a result, if a portion of the lung parenchyma gets sequestered from its connections with the tracheobronchial tree due to obstruction in the airways (such as a mucus plug), the oxygen contained within the obstructed segment of the lung is rapidly absorbed into the pulmonary circulation. This results in a loss of volume of the obstructed lung or lobe.

Oxygen is absorbed much more rapidly than nitrogen. Therefore, if bronchial obstruction occurs in a patient breathing high fractions of oxygen, absorption is much faster and collapse of the obstructed segment much more rapid. It has been shown that air from the obstructed portion of a normally healthy lung takes 18–24 h to get absorbed, but when a patient is breathing high fractions of oxygen, collapse may be up to 60 times more rapid[80]; indeed, atelectasis may be radiologically apparent within the hour.[56]

Regions of low-V/Q mismatch are more prone to absorptive atelectasis, since it is in these regions that ventilation is poor, and the oxygen enriched air in the alveoli that is absorbed by alveolar capillaries is not replenished. The administration of low tidal volumes also promotes early alveolar closure. Similarly, a high metabolic rate can theoretically facilitate oxygen absorption from the alveoli.[64]

Closure of perfused alveoli leads to the development of a right to left shunt. The degree of this shunt can be quite variable, but may be substantial, especially in the elderly[108]; the shunt can also be slow to respond to the corrective measures.[88]

10.4.3 Hyperoxic Hypercarbia

In normal individuals breathing supplemental oxygen, a slight stimulation of ventilation occurs due to the Haldane effect[62,100] (Fig. 10.7).

Traditional teaching has it that the respiratory center of the COPD patients is accustomed to the relatively high level of $PaCO_2$ that such patients frequently accumulate; the respiratory drive having been blunted by its constant exposure to the elevated $PaCO_2$, the respiratory center relies on a degree of hypoxia to stimulate it. It has been widely advocated that COPD patients be guarded from high levels of supplemental oxygen, which could theoretically abolish the hypoxic drive that is necessary for them to breathe.

Although hypercapnia undoubtedly does occur in situations where COPD patients are administered high-flow oxygen, there has been considerable rethinking about the

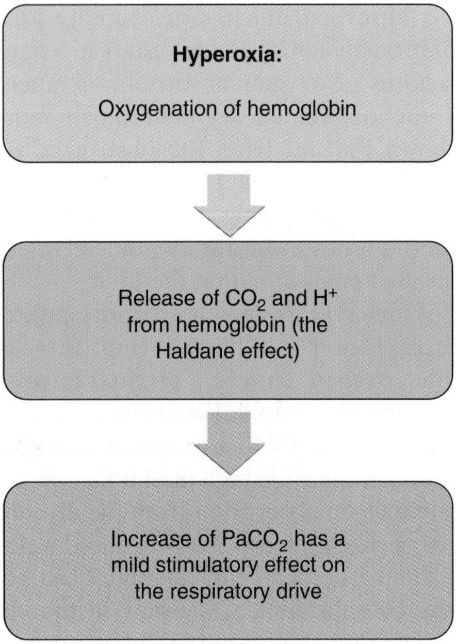
Hyperoxia:
Oxygenation of hemoglobin
Release of CO2 and H+ from hemoglobin (the Haldane effect)
Increase of PaCO2 has a mild stimulatory effect on the respiratory drive

FIGURE 10.7. Hyperoxia in normal individuals stimulates the respiratory drive.

possible underlying mechanisms.[2,83] Ventilatory responses of COPD patients to supplemental oxygen may also depend on whether or not the COPD is in acute exacerbation.[84]

It now appears that a reduction in ventilation contributes to a relatively small degree to the hypercapnia provoked by high levels of supplemental oxygen.[2] The major mechanism that produces hypercapnia in these circumstances appears to be an increase in dead space ventilation. When regional hypoxia occurs, there is a reflex shutdown of the areas of the pulmonary microcirculation that supply the hypoxic alveolar units. This protective reflex ensures that an inappropriate perfusion of unventilated units does not occur. The blood circulation is, thus, preferentially directed to the relatively better ventilated units, reducing the dead space ratio. This results in better *V/Q* matching, which has a favorable effect on the

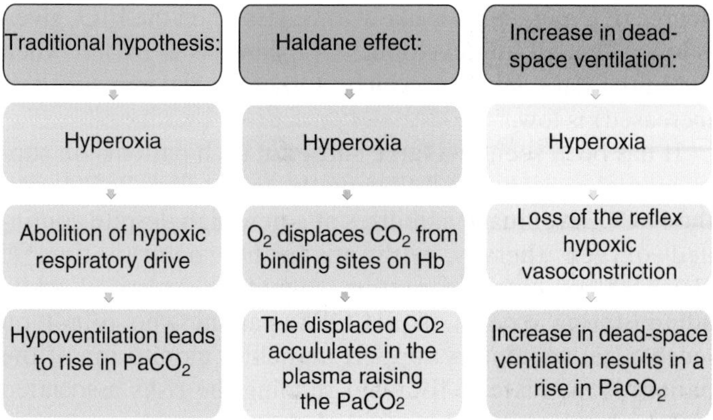
Traditional hypothesis:
Haldane effect:
Increase in dead-space ventilation:
Hyperoxia
Hyperoxia
Hyperoxia
Abolition of hypoxic respiratory drive
O2 displaces CO2 from binding sites on Hb
Loss of the reflex hypoxic vasoconstriction
Hypoventilation leads to rise in PaCO2
The displaced CO2 acculculates in the plasma raising the PaCO2
Increase in dead-space ventilation results in a rise in PaCO2

FIGURE 10.8. Mechanisms of hyperoxic hypercarbia in COPD patients.

blood oxygen levels. When an inappropriately high fraction of oxygen is administered to such patients, it is likely that there is loss of the reflex hypoxic vasoconstriction. Physiological dead space increases with worsening hypercapnia (Fig. 10.8).[2]

A small component of the hypercapnia also comes from the Haldane effect. This effect is due to the relatively poor affinity that CO_2 has for oxyhemoglobin. When the hemoglobin is well saturated with oxygen, the CO_2 that cannot now bind with the hemoglobin accumulates in the plasma, raising the $PaCO_2$ level.[22] When the COPD patient is hypoxic, he is operating on the steep part of the oxyhemoglobin dissociation curve. When supplemental oxygen is administered, the hemoglobin saturation quickly rises, for on the steep part of the oxyhemoglobin dissociation curve, even a small increase in PaO_2 can translate into a large increment in oxygen saturation. When such a large increase in saturation occurs, the increase in the $PaCO_2$ level will be commensurately large. In healthy volunteers who are administered high concentrations of oxygen, the rise in $PaCO_2$ produced by the Haldane effect would cause them to hyperventilate, but a similar effect would be unlikely to occur in COPD patients who are very tolerant to high $PaCO_2$ levels.

Although the relative importance of the above mechanisms has been well elucidated by sophisticated methods, the degree of hypercapnia is likely to be less when the FIO_2 given is low.[23] The risk of developing CO_2 narcosis is greater when the initial PaO_2 level (at which O_2 therapy is commenced or increased) is low.[10,14]

It has been seen in a large subset of such patients on supplemental oxygen that following the initial slow $PaCO_2$ rise, the $PaCO_2$ eventually stabilizes at a new high despite continued oxygen therapy, with no further deterioration.[32,84] Nevertheless, extreme caution should be exercised while administering oxygen to a COPD patient who is not on mechanical ventilatory support and close monitoring of the patient is mandatory. To avoid running the risks associated with high concentrations of inhaled O_2, it may be necessary to target the PaO_2 to just above 60 mm Hg (at which level hemoglobin is usually adequate), rather than try to achieve a more "physiological" PaO_2 (around 100 mm Hg) at the cost of oxygen-related complications. Remedial action for a progressive rise in $PaCO_2$ should not include abrupt cessation of oxygen with the intention of kicking up the respiratory drive in order to forestall intubation and ventilation. Such an action is likely to result in a precipitous fall in PaO_2, with potentially disastrous consequences (see case example 11 in chapter 18). Rather, the FIO_2 should be reduced to 0.24–0.28, in order to keep the oxygen saturation at a reasonable level.

10.4.4 Diffuse Alveolar Damage

Molecular O_2 by itself is relatively innocuous, but when reduced to reactive oxygen radicals, such as the superoxide anion (O_2), the hydrogen peroxide (H_2O_2), and the hydroxyl radical (OH^-), can cause tissue injury (see Fig 10.9). Because

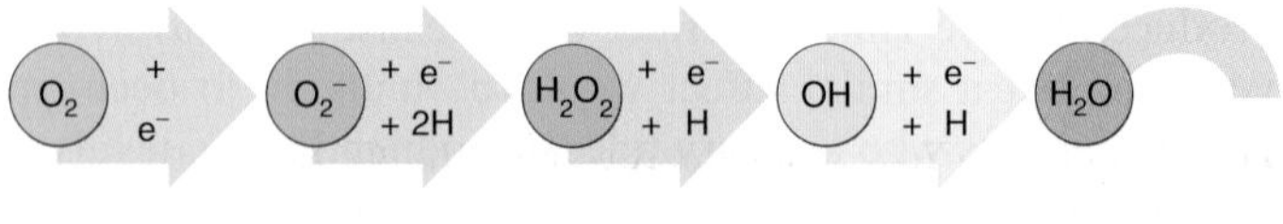
O2
+
e−
O2−
+ e−
+ 2H
H2O2
+ e−
+ H
OH
+ e−
+ H
H2O

FIGURE 10.9. Toxic oxygen radicals.

of their avidity for electrons, the toxic free radicals tend to rob the nearby enzymes, lipids, and DNA of electrons, thereby inactivating them. In particular, the hydroxyl radical and the peroxynitrite anion (the latter is the product of the reaction between H_2O_2 and NO^-) can prove severely damaging (Fig. 10.9).

In general, the higher the concentration of inspired oxygen and the longer that it is inspired, the more the likelihood of alveolar injury (diffuse alveolar damage). No absolute concentration appears to be safe, although it is widely held that FIO_2 at or below 0.5 is unlikely to induce harm even when inhaled for prolonged periods.[17,89] A lung with ongoing alveolitis is more likely to suffer damage than a normal lung. The detrimental effects of oxygen on the lung parenchyma appear to be potentiated by drugs such as bleomycin[6] and amiodarone and by external radiation.

10.4.5 Bronchopulmonary Dysplasia

Described by Northway in 1969, this condition occurs as a result of poorly understood pathologic pathways in premature infants who have received high concentrations of oxygen for several days. Characterized by necrotizing bronchiolitis, squamous metaplasia of the bronchial lining cells, thickening of alveolar walls, and peribronchial and interstitial fibrosis, this entity results in oxygen dependence of the infant for at least a month, but more usually for up to 6 months after birth. Although symptoms generally resolve by the age of 2 years, evidence of pulmonary dysfunction can persist, usually in the form of lung function abnormalities, for several years.

Strategies to minimize oxygen toxicity have been discussed in chapter (section 5.11).

10.4.6 Ventilator-Associated Pneumonia

VAP has been dealt with in the chapter that follows (Chap. 11).

References

1. Adnet F, Jouriles NJ, LeToumelin P, et al Survey of out-of-hospital emergency intubations in the French pre hospital medical system: a milticenter study. *Ann Emerg Med*. 1998;32:454–460
2. Aubier M, Murciano D, Fournier M, et al Central respiratory drive in acute respiratory failure of patients with chronic obstructive pulmonary disease. *Am Rev Respir Dis*. 1980; 122:191
3. Aubier M, Murciano D, Milic-Emili J, et al Effects of the administration of O_2 on ventilation and blood gases in patients with chronic obstructive pulmonary disease during acute respiratory failure. *Am Rev Respir Dis*. 1980;122:747
4. Baleeiro CE, Wilcoxen SE, Morris SB, Standiford TJ, Paine R. Sublethal hyperoxia impairs pulmonary innate immunity. *J Immunol*. 2003;171:955–63
5. Barlettt RH. A procedure for the management of acquired tracheosophageal fistula in ventilator patients. *J Thorac Cardiovasc Surg*. 1976;71:89–95
6. Berend N. Protective effect of hypoxia on bleomycin lung toxicity in the rat. *Am Rev Respir Dis*. 1984;130:307
7. Bernhard WN, Cottrell JE, Sivakumaran C, et al Adjustment of intracuff pressure to prevent aspiration. *Anesthesiology*. 1979;50:363
8. Bernhard WN, Yost L, Joynes D, et al Intracuff pressures in endotracheal and tracheostomy tubes: related cuff physical characteristics. *Chest*. 1985;87:720–25
9. Betbese AJ, Perez M, Bak E, et al A prospective study of unplanned endotracheal extubation in intensive care unit patients. *Crit Care Med*. 1998;26:1108–86
10. Bone RC, Pierce AK, Johnson RL Jr. Controlled oxygen administration in acute respiratory failure in chronic obstructive pulmonary disease. *Am J Med*. 1978;65:896
11. Borrelli E, Roux-Lombard P, Grau GE, et al Plasma concentrations of cytokines, their soluble receptors, and antioxidant vitamins can predict the development of multiple organ failure in patients at risk. *Crit Care Med*. 1996;24:392
12. Boussarsar M, Thierry G, Jaber S, et al Relationship between ventilatory settings and barotrauma in the acute respiratory distress syndrome. *Intensive Care Med*. 2002;28:406
13. Burger EJ, Mead J. Static properties of lungs after oxygen exposure. *J Appl Physiol*. 1969;27:191–7

14. Campbell EJM. Burns Amberson Lecture. The management of acute respiratory failure in chronic bronchitis and emphysema. *Am Rev Respir Dis*. 1967;96:626
15. Chevron V, Menard JF, Richard JC, et al Unplanned extubation: risk factors of development and predictive criteria for reintubation. *Crit Care Med*. 1998;26:1049–53
16. Ching NP, Ayres SM, Paegle RP, et al The contribution of cuff volume and pressure in tracheostomy tube damage. *J Thorac Cardiovasc Surg*. 1971;62:402–408
17. Clark JM, Lambertsen CJ. Pulmonary oxygen toxicity: a review. *Pharmacol Rev*. 1971;23:37–133
18. Comroe JH, Dripps RD, Dumke PR, Deming M. The effect of inhalation of high concentrations of oxygen for 24 hours on normal men at sea level and at a simulated altitude of 18,000. *JAMA*. 1945;128:710
19. Conrady PA, Goodman LR, Laing F, et al Alteration of endotracheal tube position: Flexion and extension of the neck. *Crit Care Med*. 1976;4:8–12
20. Cooper JD, Grillo HC. Experimental production and prevention of injury due to cuffed tracheal tubes. *Surg Gynecol Obstet*. 1969;129:1235–1241
21. Cooper JD. Tracheo-innominate artery fistula: Successful management of 3 consecutive patients. *Ann Thorac Surg*. 1977; 24:439–447
22. Cristiansen J, Douglas CG, Haldane JS. The absorption and dissociation of carbon dioxide by human blood. *J Physiol*. 1914; 48:244
23. Crossley DJ, McGuire GP, Barrow PM, et al Influence of inspired oxygen concentration on deadspace, respiratory drive and $PaCO_2$ in intubated patients with chronic obstructive pulmonary disease. *Crit Care Med*. 1997;25:1522
24. Dane TEB, King EG. A prospective study of complications after tracheostomy for assisted ventilation. *Chest*. 1975;67:398–404
25. Derbyshire DR, Chmielewski A, Fell D, et al Plasma catecholamine responses to tracheal intubation. *Br J Anaesth*. 1983;55:855–860
26. Domino KB, Posner KL, Caplan RA, et al Airway injury during anesthesia. A closed claims analysis. *Anesthesiology*. 1999;91: 1703–1711
27. Dreyfuss D, Saumon G. Barotrauma is volutrauma, but which volume is the one responsible? *Inten Care Med*. 1992;18:139

28. Dreyfuss D, Saumon G. Should the lung be rested or recruited? The Charybdis and Scylla of ventilator management. *Am J Respir Crit Care Med*. 1994;149:1066
29. Dreyfuss D, Saumon G. Barotrauma is volutrauma, but which volume is the one responsible? *Intensive Care Med*. 1992; 18:139
30. Epstein SK. Complications in ventilator-supported patients. In: Tobin MJ, ed. *Principles and Practice of Mechanical Ventilation*. 2nd ed. New York: McGraw-Hill; 2006:877–902
31. Fan C-M, Ko PC-I, Tsai K-C, et al Tracheal rupture complicating emergent endotracheal intubation. *Am J Emerg Med*. 2004;22: 289–93
32. Feller-Kopman DJ, Schwartzstein RM. The use of oxygen in patients with hypercapnia. www.uptodate.com. (800) 998–6374 (781) 237–4788
33. Fox EJ, Sklar GS, Hill CH, et al Complications related to the pressor response to endotracheal intubation. *Anesthesiology*. 1977;47:524–25
34. Fugii Y, Tanaka H, Toyooka H. Circulatory responses to laryngeal mask airway insertion or tracheal intubation in normotensive and hypertensive patients. *Can J Anaesth*. 1995;42: 32–36
35. Gammon RB, Shin MS, Buchalter SE. Pulmonary barotrauma in mechanical ventilation. *Chest*. 1992;102:568
36. Gilbert DL. Oxygen: an overall biological view. In: Gilbert DL, ed. *Oxygen and Living Processes*. New York: Springer; 1981:376
37. Goldberg JS, Rawle PR, Zehnder JL, et al Colorimetric end-tidal carbon dioxide monitoring for tracheal intubation. *Anesth Analg*. 1990;70:191–194
38. Goodman LR, Conrady PA, Laing F, et al Radiographic evaluation of endotracheal tube position. *Am J Roentgenol*. 1976; 127:433–434
39. Grillo HC, Cooper JD, Geffin B, et al A low pressure cuff for tracheostomy tubes to minimize tracheal injury: A comparative clinical trial. *J Thorac Cardiovasc Surg*. 1971;62:898–907
40. Grillo HC. Acquired tracheo-esophageal fistula. In: Grillo HC, Austen WG, et al, eds. *Current Therapy in Cardiothoracic Surgery*. BC Decker: Philadelphia; 1989:54–55
41. Grillo HC. Post-intubation tracheo-esophageal fistula. In: Grillo HC, Eschapasse H, eds. *International Trends of General Thoracic Surgery, Vol 2: Major Challenges*. WB Saunders: Philadelphia; 1987:61–68

42. Guyton DC, Barlow MR, Besselievre TR. Influence of airway pressure on minimum occlusive endotracheal tube cuff pressure. *Crit Care Med*. 1997;25:91–94
43. Hamilton PP, Onayemi A, Smyth JA, et al Comparison of conventional and high-frequency ventilation: Oxygenation and lung pathology. *J Appl Physiol*. 1983;55:131
44. Hanson CW, Marshall B, Frasch HF, Marshall C. Causes of hypercarbia with oxygen therapy in patients with chronic obstructive pulmonary disease. *Crit Care Med*. 1996;24:23
45. Heffner JE, Repine JE. Pulmonary strategies of antioxidant defense. *Am Rev Respir Dis*. 1989;140:531
46. Heffner JE, Miller KS, Saher SA. Tracheostomy in the intensive care unit 2. *Complications chest*. 1986;90:430–436
47. Hickling KG. Ventilatory management of ARDS: can it affect outcome? *Intensive Care Med*. 1990;16:219
48. Hickling, KG. Ventilatory management of ARDS: Can it affect outcome? Intensive Care Med 1990;16:219
49. Hilmi IA, Sullivan E, Quinlan J, et al Esophageal tear: an unusual complication after difficult endotracheal intubation. *Anesth Analg*. 2003;97:911–914
50. American Thoracic Society, The European Society of Intensive Care Medicine, The Societe de Reanimation de Langue Francaise. International consensus conferences in intensive care medicine: Ventilator-Associated Lung Injury in ARDS. *Am J Respir Crit Care Med*. 1999;160:2118
51. Ionescu T. Signs of endotracheal intubation. *Anesthesiol*. 1981;36:422
52. Jones GOM, Hale DE, Wasmuth CE, et al A survey of acute complications associated with endotracheal intubation. *Cleve Clin Q*. 1968;35:23–31
53. Jones JW, Reynolds M, Hewitt RL, et al Tracheoinnominate artery erosion: Successful surgical management of a devastating complication. *Ann Surg*. 1976;184:194–204
54. Kaplan JD, Schuster DP. Physiologic consequences of tracheal intubation. *Clin Chest Med*. 1991;12:425–432
55. Khan F. Reddy NC. *Enlarging intracheal tube cuff diameter: a quantitative roentgenographic study of its value in the early prediction of serious tracheal damage*. 1977;24(1):49–53
56. Lachmann B. Open up the lung and keep the lung open. *Intensive Care Med*. 1992;18:319
57. Lansing AM. Radiological changes in pulmonary atelectasis: Arch. *Surg*. 1965;90:52

58. Law MM, Cryer HG, Abraham E. Elevated levels of soluble ICAM-1 correlate with the development of multiple organ failure in severely injured trauma patients. *J Trauma*. 1994; 37:100
59. Lawson DW, Grillo HC. Closure of persistent tracheal stomas. *Surg Gynecol Obstet*. 1970;130:995–996
60. Levine MS, Scheiner JD, Rubesin SE, et al Diagnosis of pneumoperitoneum on supine abdominal radiographs. *AJR Am J Roentgenol*. 1991;156:731
61. Linko K, Paloheimo M, Tammisto T. Capnography for detection of accidental oesophageal intubation. *Acta Anesthesiol Scand*. 1983;27:199–202
62. Lockhart P, Feldbau EV, Gabel RA, et al Dental complications during and after tracheal intubation. *J Am Dent Assoc*. 1986;112:480–483
63. Lodato RF, Jubran A. Response time, autonomic mediation, and reversibility of hyperoxic bradycardia in conscious dogs. *J Appl Physiol*. 1993;74:634–42
64. Majumdar B, Stevens RW, Obara LG. Retropharyngeal abscess following tracheal intubation. *Anaesthesia*. 1982;37:67–70
65. Malhotra A, Schwartz DR, Schwartzstein RM. www.uptodate.com. (800) 998–6374.(781) 237–4788
66. Manning HL. Peak airway pressure: why the fuss? *Chest*. 1994; 105:242
67. Maunder RJ, Pierson DJ, Hudson LD. Subcutaneous and mediastinal emphysema: pathophysiology, diagnosis and management. *Arch Intern Med*. 1984;144:1447
68. McCulloch TM, Bishop MJ. Complications of translaryngeal intubation. *Clin Chest Med*. 1991;12:507–521
69. Morris WP, Butler BD, Tonnesen AS, et al Continuous venous air embolism in patients receiving positive end-expiratory pressure. *Am Rev Respir Dis*. 1993;147:1034
70. Murry IP, Modell JH. early detection of endotracheal tube accidents by monitoring carbon dioxide concentration in respiratory gas. *Anesthesiology*. 1986;59:344–346
71. Muscedere JG, Mullen JBM, Gan K, Slutsky AS. Tidal ventilation at low airway pressures can augment lung injury. *Am J Respir Crit Care Med*. 1994;149:1327
72. Nahum A, Hoyt J, Schmitz L, et al Effect of mechanical ventilation strategy on dissemination of intratracheally instilled *Escherichia coli* in dogs. *Crit Care Med*. 1997;25:1733

73. Nelems B. Tracheoarterial fistula. In: Grillo HC, Eschapasse H, eds. *International trends in general thoracic surgery, vol 2. Major challenges*. WB Saunders: Pjiladelphia; 1987:69–73
74. Off D, Braun SR, Tompkins B, et al Efficacy of thc minimal lcak technique of cuff inflation in maintaining proper intracuff pressures for patients with cuffed artificial airways. *Respir Care*. 1983;28:1115–1120
75. Orta DA, Cousar JE III, Yergin BM, et al Tracheal laceration with massive subcutaneous emphysema: a rare complication of endotracheal intubation. *Thorax*. 1979;34:665–69
76. Parker JC, Hernandez LA, Longenecker GL, et al Lung edema caused by high peak inspiratory pressures in dogs. Role of increased microvascular filtration pressure and permeability. *Am Rev Respir Dis*. 1990;142:321
77. Parker JC, Hernandez LA, Peevy KJ. Mechanisms of ventilator-induced lung injury. *Crit Care Med*. 1993;21:131–143
78. Payne DK, Anderson WM, Romero MD, et al Tracheo esophageal fistula formation in intubated patients: risk factors and treatment with high frequency jet ventilation. *Chest*. 1990;98:161–164
79. Peppard SB, Dickens JH. Laryngeal injury following short-term intubation. *Ann Otol Rhinol Laryngol*. 1983;92:327–330
80. Pugin J, Dunn I, Jolliet P, et al Activation of human macrophages by mechanical ventilation in vitro. *Am J Physiol*. 1998; 275:L1040
81. Rahn H. The role of N_2 gas in various biological processes with particular reference to the lung. *Harvey Lect*. 1960;55:173
82. Rello J, Sonora R, Jubert P, et al Pneumonia in intubated patients: role of respiratory airways care. *Am J Respir Crit Care Med*. 1996;154:111–115
83. Robinson N, Clancy M. In patients with head injury undergoing rapid sequence intubation, does pretreatment with intravenous lignocaine/lidocaine lead to an improved neurological out-come? A review of the literature. *Emerg Med J*. 2001;18:453–457
84. Robinson TD, Freiberg DB, Regnis JA, Young IH. The role of hypoventilation and ventilation-perfusion redistribution in oxygen-induced hypercapnia during acute exacerbations of chronic obstructive pulmonary disease. *Am J Respir Crit Care Med*. 2000;161:1524
85. Rudolph M, Banks RA, Semple SJG. Hypercapnia during oxygen therapy in acute exacerbations of chronic respiratory failure. *Lancet*. 1977;2:483

86. Sackner MA. LandaJ, Hirsch J, Zapata A. Pulmonary effects of oxygen breathing: A 6-hour study in normal men. *Ann Intern Med*. 1975;82:40–43
87. Sandhar BK, Niblett DJ, Argiras EP, et al Effects of positive end-expiratory pressure on hyaline membrane formation in a rabbit model of the neonatal respiratory distress syndrome. *Intensive Care Med*. 1988;14:538
88. Santos P, Afrassiabi A, Weymuller E. Prospective studies evaluating the standard endotracheal tube and a prototype endotracheal tube. *Am Otol Rhinol Laryngol*. 1989;98:935–940
89. Santos C, Ferrer M, Roca J, et al Pulmonary gas exchange response to oxygen breathing in acute lung injury. *Am J Respir Crit Care Med*. 2000;161:26
90. Schaefer KE. Hyperbaria-O_2 toxicity. In: Loeppky JA, Riedesel ML, eds. *Oxygen transport to human tissues*. New York: ElsevierNorth Holland; 1982:291–304
91. Shennib HF, Barkun AN, Matouk E, Blundell PE. Surgical decompression of a tension pneumomediastinum. A ventilatory complication of status asthmaticus. *Chest*. 1988;93:1301
92. Silen W, Spieker D. Fatal hemorrhage from innominate artery after tracheostomy. *Ann Surg*. 1965;162:1005–1012
93. Singh S, Smith JE. Cardiovascular changes after the three stages of nasotracheal intubation. *Br J Anaesth*. 2003;91:667–671
94. Slutsky AS, Tremblay LN. Multiple system organ failure. Is mechanical ventilation a contributing factor? *Am J Respir Crit Care Med*. 1998;157:1721
95. Slutsky AS. Lung injury caused by mechanical ventilation. Report from the Aspen Lung Conference. *Chest* july 1999 116:1s
96. Stauffer JL, Olson DE, Petty TL. Complications and consequences of endotracheal intubation and tracheotomy: a prospective study of 150 critically ill adults. *Am J Med*. 1981;70:65–76
97. Stauffer JL, Olson DE, Petty TL. Complications and consequences of endotracheal intubation and tracheostomy. *Am J Med*. 1981;70:65–76
98. Stauffer JL, Petty TL. Accidental intubation of the pyriform sinus: a complication of "roadside" resuscitation. *JAMA*. 1977;237:2324–2325
99. Steen JA. Impact of tube design and material on complications of tracheal intubation. *Probl Anesth*. 1988;2:211–224
100. Sternfeld D, Wright S. Tracheal rupture and the creation of a false passage after emergency intubation. *Ann Emerg Med*. 2003;42:88–92

101. Stockley RA. The estimation of the resting reflex hypoxic drive to respiration in normal man. *Respir Physiol.* 1977;31: 217–30
102. Thomas AN. Management of tracheoesophageal fistula caused by cuffed tracheal tubes. *Am J Surg*. 1972;124:181–187
103. Thomas AN. The diagnosis and treatment of tracheoesophageal fistula caused by cuffed tracheal tubes. *J Thorac Cardiovasc Surg*. 1973;65:612–619
104. Thompson DS, Read RC. Rupture of the trachea following endotracheal intubation. *JAMA*. 1968;204:995–997
105. Tremblay L, Valenza F, Ribeiro SP, et al Injurious ventilatory strategies increase cytokines and c-fos m-RNA expression in an isolated rat lung model. *J Clin Invest*. 1997;99:944
106. Tremblay LN, Slutsky AS. Ventilator-induced injury: From barotrauma to biotrauma. *Proc Assoc Am Phys*. 1998;110: 482
107. Utley JR, Dillon ML, Todd EP, et al Giant tracheoesophageal fistula: management by esophageal diversion. *J Thorac Cardiovasc Surg*. 1978;75:373–377
108. Verbrugge SJ, Sorm V, van't V, et al Lung overinflation without positive end-expiratory pressure promotes bacteremia after experimental Klebsiella pneumoniae inoculation. *Intensive Care Med*. 1998;24:172
109. Wagner PD, Laravuso RB, Uhl RR, West JB. Continuous distributions of ventilation-perfusion ratios in normal subjects breathing air and 100 per cent O_2. *J Clin Invest*. 1974;54:54
110. Webb HH, Tierney DF. Experimental pulmonary edema due to intermittent positive pressure ventilation with high inflation pressures. Protection by positive end-expiratory pressure. *Am Rev Respir Dis*. 1974;110:556
111. Williams TJ, Tuxen DV, Scheinkestel CD, et al Risk factors for morbidity in mechanically ventilated patients with acute severe asthma. *Am Rev Respir Dis*. 1992;146(3):607–615
112. Winer-Muram HT, Rumbak MJ, Bain RS Jr. Tension pneumoperitoneum as a complication of barotrauma. *Crit Care Med*. 1993;21:941

Chapter 11
Ventilator-Associated Pneumonia

The area of the alveolar epithelium of the lung is approximately 70 m^2. This area is constantly in contact with the ambient air and is therefore vulnerable to contamination with airborne microbes and particles of respirable size. Due to the configuration of the respiratory tract, airborne particles having diameters in the range of 0.5–2.0 μ can reach and deposit in the terminal part of the tracheobronchial tree – most bacteria are of this size. In reality, very few bacteria cause infections by spreading via the airborne route (e.g., mycobacteria, viruses, and legionella). Most bacteria cause pneumonia by first colonizing the upper respiratory tract and later descending into the tracheobronchial tree.

In contrast to the lower airways, the upper airways are literally teeming with microorganisms, and a multitude of these flourish here even in good health. The majority of them are anaerobes, and these outnumber the aerobes by approximately 3–5 times.

Colonization of the oropharynx begins soon after birth,[58] initially by *E. coli* and other transient contaminants. After a few days, the flora begins to resemble the adult commensal flora, with disappearance of gram-negative rods and appearance of *Streptococcus salivarius*, the lactobacilli, and other anaerobic bacteria. Distinct ecological niches exist within the oral cavity – in areas that are otherwise in anatomical continuity – and in each of these, the dominant organism may differ. A small percentage of normal adults, persistently harbor gram-negative rods in their oropharynxes[116] (see below).

A. Hasan, *Understanding Mechanical Ventilation*,
DOI: 10.1007/978-1-84882-869-8_11,

In healthy adults, the upper respiratory secretions generally contain ten to 100 million organisms per mL of secretion. The number sharply rises in gingivodental disease, when the levels may increase almost 1,000-fold.[90] During sleep, even in healthy individuals, small quantities of upper airway secretions are aspirated into the tracheobronchial tree. About 45% of normal subjects aspirate small quantities during sleep. A much greater proportion of individuals aspirate pharyngeal secretions during sickness. In sick persons, not only is aspiration more frequent but the aspirated flora is different.

Airway mucosa is histologically quite similar, from the nasopharynx through the trachea down to the conducting airways, and is composed of ciliated epithelial cells. Receptors present on epithelial cells allow bacteria to bind to the mucosa via protrusions from bacterial cells called adhesions.[115] In health, the adherence of normal oropharyngeal bacteria to the epithelial cells of the pharynx prevents gram negative aerobes from gaining a foothold on the pharyngeal mucosa, as does the phenomenon of interbacterial inhibition. In less than 1–6% cases, the upper airways of normal subjects are colonized by gram-negative bacteria.

In hospitalized patients, particularly those admitted to intensive care units, proteases eliminate the fibronectins from the epithelial cell surfaces, and a significant change occurs within the oropharyngeal flora. Fibronectins normally prevent bacterial adherence to epithelial surfaces and when the fibronectin film is removed, the adherence of pathogenic bacteria to the oropharyngeal epithelium is facilitated. Increased bacterial adherence leads to colonization of the upper respiratory tract by enteric gram-negative bacteria, and this predisposes to the later development of nosocomial pneumonia (NP). The incidence of colonization with gram-negative rods mounts with the gravity of the illness[75] as well as with the degree of supportive care required by the patient.[159]

Once gram negative aerobes colonize the oropharynx, the stage is set for the aspiration of these noxious organisms into the lower respiratory tract, with the potential peril of NP. The link between NP and oropharyngeal colonization has been established by several studies. In one study, NP occurred in 23%

of patients in whom prior oropharyngeal colonization was documented, but in only 3.3% of noncolonized patients.[75]

11.1 Incidence

Ventilator-associated pneumonia (VAP) is a form of NP, and several mechanisms of pathogenesis are common to the two. NP is the most common infection in the ICU and the most deadly of all nosocomial infections. It is the second most common nosocomial infection overall, second only to urinary tract infection.[64] Although prevalence has been shown to vary between 12 and 29% in different studies,[89] the mortality rate of NP has been uniformly high (20–50%).[1,37] The case fatality ranges between 25 and 33% in most studies,[50] though pneumonia is not necessarily the cause of death in these patients.[35]

Mechanically ventilated patients have extremely high infection rates – the incidence of NP may be 17–23% higher in intubated patients. This means that approximately one of every four mechanically-ventilated patients will get NP at some stage during the course of mechanical ventilation.

The crucial distinction of the ventilated patient is the presence of an endotracheal tube. This by itself (along with certain other factors associated with the care of a mechanically-ventilated patient) predisposes the patient to pneumonia. Ventilated patients may be at 6-20-fold greater risk of contracting pneumonia than are other hospitalized patients.[66] VAP has an even greater mortality rate than NP: the attributable mortality rate of VAP can be as high as 30–50%.[48]

Patients with other comorbidities are prone to NP: smoking, COPD, ARDS, organ failure, major surgery, trauma, burns, and hypoalbuminemia.

11.2 Microbiology

The responsible flora in NP is polymicrobial in many cases, but the dominant organism usually varies from center to center. Aerobic gram-negative bacilli are frequently isolated.

Together with *Staphylococcus aureus*, they may account for as many as 50–70% cases of VAP.[3,95]

The poor outcome in patients with VAP has been strongly linked to the inappropriateness of initial antibiotic therapy. Since initial antibiotic strategy assumes such profound importance, it is essential to realize that initial antibiotic treatment will almost always be empirical – as no test is likely to reveal the etiological agent at a time when initiation of antimicrobials is a medical urgency. It is therefore vital to include under the antibiotic umbrella the most likely etiological agents. Since different organisms prevail in different clinical circumstances – and indeed in different medical units – attempts have been made to formulate guidelines for initial antibiotic therapy depending on the clinical scenario.

Pneumonia developing in less than 5 days from the time of admission (early NP) is likely to be caused by organisms colonizing the patient's upper respiratory tract at the time of intubation[13] – viz., microorganisms that were acquired in the community: this flora is generally drug sensitive – except if antibiotics have been administered recently, or if hospitalization has occurred in the last 90 days. The most common community-acquired pathogens include *Streptococcus pneumoniae*, *Hemophilus influenzae*, and Methicillin-sensitive *Staphylococcus aureus* (MSSA); so antibiotic therapy is directed against these (Fig. 11.1).

Microbiology of early ventilator-associated pneumonia	Microbiology of late ventilator-associated pneumonia
• *Streptococcus pneumoniae* • *Hemophilus influenzae* • Methicillin-sensitive *Staphylococcus aureus* (MSSA)	• *Streptococcus pneumoniae* • *Hemophilus influenzae* • Methicillin-sensitive *Staphylococcus aureus* (MSSA) • *Pseudomonas aeruginosa* • *Acinetobacter* • Methicillin-resistant *Staphylococcus aureus* (MRSA)

FIGURE 11.1. Microbiology of ventilator-associated pneumonia.

The flora in late NP is different: it includes bacteria that are not part of the usual group of community-acquired pathogens – the *Pseudomonas aeruginosa*, Acinetobacter species and Methicillin-resistant *Staphylococcus aureus* (MRSA). , not only is the pattern of antibiotic susceptibility different, but these organisms tend to be multidrug resistant, having thrived on the antibiotic-rich milieu of the intensive care units wherein they proliferate. Predictably, the outcome in this group is palpably worse: not only is this related to the problem of drug resistance, but also to the inadequacy of initial antibiotic prescription which does not always cover these organisms within its ambit.

Different authors have proposed different time-frames for distinguishing between early from late VAPs: a cutoff period of 3 days appears to work just as well as one of 7 days, though a 4 day cutoff (4 days or less, vs. 5 days or more) is the most usually used to set the two apart.

Viral and fungal NPs rarely occur in immunocompetent hosts.

11.3 Risk Factors

Risk factors specific to certain clinical circumstances have been set out in Table 11.1 below.[146]

11.3.1 The Physical Effect of the Endotracheal Tube

As mentioned earlier, the endotracheal tube increases the risk of pneumonia by severalfold. It provides a direct conduit for bacteria to the tracheobronchial tree, bypassing the defenses of the upper respiratory tract. It also interferes with the cough reflex which is an important protective mechanism for the airway. During breathing, the endotracheal tube moves upon the tracheal mucosa (which is especially susceptible to damage in the vicinity of its tip and also in the region

TABLE 11.1. Clinical risk factors specific to pathogens.

Specific risk factor	Pathogen
Aspiration	Anaerobes
Diabetes mellitus	Methicillin-sensitive *Staphylococcus aureus*
Chronic renal failure	Methicillin-sensitive *Staphylococcus aureus*
Steroid therapy	*Legionella, Aspergillus*
Prior antibiotic therapy	*Pseudomonas, Acinetobacter, Enterobacter*
Structural lung disease	*Pseudomonas*
Abdominal surgery	*Anaerobes, Enterococcus*
Coma	Methicillin-sensitive *Staphylococcus aureus*
Prolonged hospitalization	*Pseudomonas, Acinetobacter, Enterobacter*
Intravenous drug abuse	Methicillin-sensitive *Staphylococcus aureus*
COPD	*S. pneumonia, H. influnzae, M. catarrhalis*
Trauma	Methicillin-sensitive *Staphylococcus aureus*

of the cuff).[24] The denudation of the airway epithelium encourages bacterial adherence with subsequent airway colonization.[59] By a foreign-body effect, it also promotes reflex mucus secretion.

11.3.2 Alteration of Mucus Properties

Apart from the overt tracheobronchitis that may be induced by endotracheal or tracheostomy tubes, a chronic low-grade inflammatory state may exist in the intubated patient that may promote the binding of gram-negative bacteria to the airway epithelium; this may be more important in the distal airways than in thc proximal.

One of the important functions of respiratory tract secretions is to trap and neutralize bacteria. To facilitate such an action, airway secretions contain IgA, lactoferrin, and certain bactericidal enzymes. The bacteria and particulate matter trapped in the blanket of mucus that covers the respiratory mucosa are propelled out of the tracheobronchial tree by the coordinated beating of the cilia.

The role of the mucus itself may be quite complex. It is believed that to trap germs, the mucus itself must have receptors for bacteria. If there is reflex mucus hypersecretion as a result of presence of an endotracheal tube, this may mean that more mucus receptors are present for bacterial adherence. The receptors might then serve as a bridge between the bacteria and respiratory epithelium. On the other hand, respiratory mucins may inhibit bacterial binding to the tracheal epithelium by themselves preferentially binding to the bacteria. Either or both the above may be true – the complex interactions between bacteria, mucins and respiratory epithelium are as yet far from clear.[59]

11.3.3 Microaspiration

Pooling of throat secretions frequently occurs above the cuff of the endotracheal tube, and microaspiration between the cuff and the tracheal mucosa is always possible; this could potentially transmit microbes (that have multiplied in the sump created by the pooling of secretions above the endotracheal tube cuff) down into the tracheobronchial tree.[66] The low-pressure high-volume cuff in contemporary use is more effective at preventing aspiration than is the high-pressure low-volume cuff. This is because the low-pressure high-volume cuff lies more closely in apposition with the tracheal wall and assumes the shape of the tracheal lumen with which it is in contact, thereby more reliably preventing aspiration. The possibility of epithelial injury is understandably higher with the low-volume *high-pressure* cuffs,[62] but inadvertent overinflation of a *low-pressure* high-volume cuff may prove just as detrimental.[104]

11.3.4 Biofilms

The luminal surface of the endotracheal tube is invariably contaminated by bacteria-laden secretions coughed out by the patient: it has been shown that within 2 days, the endotracheal tubes of three-fourths of all severely ill patients do get colonized.[138] These bacteria become embedded in a biofilm (glycocalyx) which thinly coats the inner surface of the endotracheal tube. Here, sheltered from the host defenses and antibiotics, these bacteria multiply to enormous numbers.[148] If for some reason, the glycocalyx with its high population of bacteria is dislodged from the wall of the endotracheal tube and enters the tracheobronchial tree, it carries down with it a high burden of infection which can overwhelm host defenses. Such dislodgement is possible when the biofilm is stripped off the tube wall by suction catheters or bronchoscopes, or washed down by liquids deliberately instilled down the endotracheal tube.

Box 11.1 The Endotracheal Tube and Lower Respiratory Tract Infection

Direct conduit for microorganisms by bypassing the upper respiratory tract
Interference with the cough reflex
Denudation of the tracheal mucosa by fricative movement
Alteration of airway mucus properties
Microaspiration of pooled secretions above the cuff
Mucosal injury by overinflated cuff
Biofilm formation

11.3.5 Ventilator Tubings

Like the endotracheal tubes, ventilator tubings can get colonized by bacteria that originate in the patient's secretions. Understandably, colonization is heaviest in the part of the ventilator tubing closest to the patient.[31] The expiratory limb of the ventilator circuit has been found to become colonized approximately after 2–4 days of initiation of mechanical ventilation.[35] Eighty per cent of ventilator condensates are contaminated by bacteria, presumably from the patient's own respiratory tract.[35] The accumulation of pooled condensate in the ventilator tubings provides a haven for bacteria to multiply, sheltered from host defenses and from the effects of antibiotics. When parts of the ventilator tubing are elevated as in the act of raising the bedrail, or when the position of the patient is changed, this condensate may find its way down the endotracheal tube, carrying with it a large "amplified" population of bacteria.[36]

11.3.6 Gastric Feeds

The normally acidic gastric juice discourages the survival of microbiological flora within the stomach, which is therefore sterile. With advancing age and malnutrition, or in achlorhydric states, or indeed with the use of certain drugs that increase the gastric pH,[47] the stomach is liable to get populated with bacteria. Gram-negative bacteria proliferate exponentially with rising in gastric pH: the use of antacids and H_2 blocking agents in the ICU has been shown to be associated with increased gastric colonization.[157]

It appears that the gastric contents can reach the lungs in a number of ways. Recumbency encourages retrograde movement of the gastric contents up the esophagus, facilitating oropharyngeal colonization. Large volume gastric feeds that overwhelm the limited emptying time of the stomach in critically ill patients further encourage reflux. Nasogastric tubes, especially of wide bore interfere with the functioning of the gastroesophageal sphincter, and so promote regurgitation.[159]

The presence of a nasogastric tube can encourage oropharyngeal colonization by various mechanisms. The nasogastric tube may provide a conduit whereby bacteria are transmitted upon its surface in a retrograde fashion from the stomach to the oropharynx, in a manner analogous to the urinary infection that occurs in catheterized patients.[80] Gastric colonization might also be facilitated by the erosion of the oropharyngeal mucosa by the nasogastric tube, in the same manner that endotracheal-induced erosion of tracheal mucosa encourages tracheal colonization with bacteria.[131] Although this sequence of events is certainly plausible, even one study could not prove that nasogastric tubes could indeed predispose to NP.[15]

At this time it is unclear whether initial gastric colonization – with subsequent oropharyngeal colonization, and then aspiration of the contaminated secretions – could be one of the key mechanisms in the genesis of NP. Bacteria isolated from gastric juice have frequently – but not always – been shown to be identical to the bacteria isolated from the lung, and this may imply a causal relationship between the two.[47,77]

11.3.7 Sinusitis

Sinusitis has emerged as an important cause of VAP. As many as 10% of orally intubated patients have been found to have evidence of sinusitis by culture of maxillary sinus secretions,[20] and the incidence may be much higher in nasally intubated patients.[133] The evidence that bacterial sinusitis can lead to VAP is as yet circumstantial, but the flora isolated from the sinuses has been identical to the flora isolated from the lungs in a high proportion of cases of VAP.[133] Indeed, the flora in nosocomial sinus infections tends to be polymicrobial or predominantly gram negative as does the flora in NPs.[147] Anaerobic organisms are also common.[90]

The occurrence of sinusitis in the ICU patient can be related to a variety of mechanisms that are unique to the critically ill patient. Nasogastric[153] and nasotracheal tubes[125] act as foreign bodies, and these elicit a local mucosal reaction. The ensuing mucus hypersecretion and mucosal edema is liable to block sinus ostia, permitting pooling of secretions within the blocked sinuses. Stagnated secretions within the sinuses act as culture media for bacteria; once contaminated, the sinuses act as foci of sepsis, with the potential for dissemination into other areas. It appears that biofilms can form upon plastic nasogastric tubes, much in the same manner as they can within endotracheal tubes.[128]

In the recumbent and immobile ICU patient, the gravitational advantage for natural sinus drainage is lost.[5] Furthermore, in a patient on positive pressure ventilation, the raised intrathoracic pressure diminishes the venous return from the head and neck contributing to nasal mucosal congestion and sinus ostial occlusion.[5] It is also possible that the absence of the normal airflow through the nose in an intubated patient, as also the absence of sneezing and coughing reflexes, may make the patient susceptible to infection.

The paranasal sinuses are the site of production of large quantities of nitric oxide (NO), which is continuously released into the airways through sinus ostia. In quantities as small as 1 part per million, NO can exert substantive antibacterial effects.[100,103] NO is also an important regulating agent for mucociliary activity.[43,102] Ostial blockage can diminish NO production as can sepsis itself.

Box 11.2 Pathologic Mechanisms in Sinusitis

Mucus hypersecretion
Mucosal edema with blockage of sinus ostia
Decreased mucociliary clearance
Biofilm formation
Increased gravitational mucosal congestion
Decreased NO production
Absence of coughing and sneezing

Nosocomial sinusitis usually originates in the maxillary sinuses before spreading to the sphenoid and ethmoid sinuses. Signs of sinusitis in the ICU can be notoriously difficult to appreciate. A high index of suspicion in a febrile patient may unearth sinusitis as the cause of the intercurrent infection. Due to gravitational influences, purulent secretions often trickle down posteriorly, and are aspirated, mimicking symptoms of tracheobronchitis rather than the symptoms of sinusitis.

Box 11.3 Serious Complications of Sinusitis[2,149]

Ventilator-associated pneumonia
Meningitis
Cerebral abscess
Cavernous sinus thrombosis
Orbital infection
Mastoiditis
Bacteremia

The radiographic visualization of sinuses is best achieved with CT scans; sinus opacification and air fluid levels are consistent with sinusitis. Transport of the ventilated patient is itself a risk factor for VAP. Bedside sinus ultrasound, which has a high sensitivity and specificity for maxillary sinusitis[67] – though not for the other sinuses – may obviate the need to transport the patient to the imageology suite.[67]

Attempts should be made at microbiological diagnosis, not merely to identify the organism and its antibiotic sensitivity, but also because the tomographic features of infection are nonspecific and may sometimes be misleading.

11.3.8 Respiratory Therapy Equipment

Respiratory therapy equipment such as mainstream nebulizers can generate contaminated aerosols that can infect the ventilator tubing: contaminated medication nebulizers are capable of inciting infection.[32] Airway interventions like fibreoptic bronchoscopy can also contaminate the airway in much the same way as suction catheters.

11.4 Position

Transportation of the patient out of the ICU appears to be an important risk factor for NP. Positioning the patient supine will not only promote the aspiration of gastric contents or contaminated oropharyngeal secretions, but may cause the condensate in the ventilator tubing to enter the endotracheal tube and so find its way into the lower respiratory tract. In one study, as many as a quarter of all patients transported within the hospital developed NP.[85]

11.5 Diagnosis of VAP

Once introduced into the respiratory tract, the onset of infection and its spread are the factors of the virulence of the organism vis-a-vis the host defenses. The defenses of the critically ill and possibly malnourished host can be further impaired by alveolar hypoxia or neutropenia.

Early and appropriate antibiotic therapy is often crucial to the outcome in NP and VAP. The difficulties of choosing the right regimen are obvious, since it is neither easy to diagnose VAP nor to differentiate it from other confounding conditions that frequently coexist in the ventilated patient. With the insertion of an endotracheal or tracheostomy tube, the normally sterile lower airways become colonized within hours of "tubing" the patient: thus, recovery of at least one bacterial species from the lower airways is frequent, even in the absence of a frank infective process. Also, purulent tracheobronchial secretions are common and do not equate with disease. The occurrence of fever may represent disease elsewhere (e.g., sinusitis, cystitis, or catheter-induced sepsis) and not necessarily infection within the respiratory tract. Pulmonary fibroproliferation occurring later during the course of ARDS may be another noninfectious cause of fever.

Radiological shadows can be cast by a variety of cardiopulmonary conditions in the ventilated patient. Pulmonary infarction, pulmonary edema and areas of atelectasis or alveolar hemorrhage may cause confusion. Importantly, blood cultures, otherwise the *sine qua non* of infection, are frequently positive in ventilated patients even in the absence of pneumonia (Fig. 11.2).

Clinical mimics of VAP	Radiological mimics of VAP	Confounding microbiological issues
• *Fever:* extrapulmonary sepsis (sinusitis, cystitis, catheter induced sepsis) • *Purulent tracheobronchial secretions:* (see text)	• Congestive cardiac failure • Pulmonary infarction • Atelectasis • Alveolar hemorrhage	• The endotracheal tube is colonized within a few hurs of tracheal intubation. • Blood cultures can be positive in ventilated patients in the absence of pneumonia

FIGURE 11.2. Differential diagnosis of ventilator-associated pneumonia (VAP).

When the lower respiratory tract is actually infected, two kinds of infection may occur: infectious tracheobronchitis and pneumonia. When fever and leucocytosis develop along with purulent sputum – but with no new radiological infiltrate – infectious tracheobronchitis is likely.[115] When a new and persistent radiological infiltrate occurs in the setting of leucocytosis and purulent sputum, this indicates that the infection has now involved the pulmonary parenchyma, and a provisional diagnosis of pneumonia should be made.

When purely clinico-radiological criteria are used to identify NP or VAP, over-diagnosis can occur due to the fact that a wide variety of noninfectious clinical conditions can cast radiological shadows (see Fig…). Using bacterial criteria alone to diagnose nosocomial or VAP will result in a large false positive rate, owing to the inadvertent sampling of those organisms causing tracheobronchitis or those merely colonizing the respiratory tract.

Obviously therefore, the diagnosis is more reliable when bacterial criteria are considered in conjunction with clinical criteria. When the patient fulfills all the clinical criteria and the sampling method yields a "representative sample" (see below), pneumonia can be diagnosed with greater assurance.

Since the price to pay for an undiagnosed VAP is heavy, a high index of suspicion must be maintained especially in the situation of a new radiological infiltrate. Although the diagnosis of NP or VAP is untenable without a radiological infiltrate, a new radiological shadow, especially with fresh clinical signs such as fever, increased quantity or purulence of tracheobronchial secretions, or leucocytosis, may be taken to represent VAP unless proven otherwise. Thus, it has proven easier and possibly quite effective to employ a clinical definition for VAP: in epidemiologic studies at least, this has been shown to be quite sensitive – though not quite as specific – for ventilator-induced pulmonary infection.

Once NP or VAP is suspected, every effort should be made to identify the pathogen responsible. Various methods have been developed to sample the proximal and distal airways. Sampling of proximal airways is liable to turn up microbes colonizing the airways rather than true pathogens. Since the trachea may be colonized within a few hours of intubation, sampling by bronchial suction can be expected to yield false positive results.

Interestingly, in the presence of VAP/NP, tracheal suction does frequently yield the pathogen responsible, but will frequently contain as well, bacteria which have merely colonized the respiratory tract and are not responsible for pneumonia. Further confusion is engendered on account of the fact that in a little less than half of all cases, pneumonias may be polymicrobial.

11.5.1 Sampling Methods

Bronchoscopic (protected specimen brushing, bronchoalveolar lavage, protected bronchoalveolar lavage etc.) and nonbronchoscopic methods (telescoping and nontelescoping catheters) of sampling are available and these have varying sensitivities and specificities.[109] The protected bronchoscopic brush is being increasingly favored as the modality least likely to yield contaminated samples and most likely to yield a positive microbiological diagnosis,[24] but much disagreement still remains regarding its sensitivity and specificity.[48] Bronchial washings may be as reliable as protected brush sampling when clinical parameters as suggested above are applied.[150] In difficult situations, open lung biopsy may need to be resorted to.

11.5.2 Interpretation of the Sample

Having isolated a microorganism, it is helpful to ascertain the reliability of the sampling process before treating the microbe as a pathogen – this is because many of the sampling techniques possess less than ideal specificity. To this end, it is desirable to have objective indices wherever possible, but this is easier said than done. Qualitative techniques are generally nonspecific and can lead to unnecessary or inappropriate antibiotic therapy.[52] Quantitative cultures are more representative, but colony counts above the generally accepted levels may not by themselves be diagnostic of pneumonia. Nevertheless, when 1,000 or more colony forming units are grown per milliliter, this means that 1,000–1,000,000 bacteria are present in every mL of the recovered lavage fluid, and this is usually considered significant.[154]

These numbers emerge from the observation that pathogens in distal lung secretions prevail at concentrations of at least 10^5–10^6 colony forming units per milliliter (cfu/mL).[8] Only 1 mL or so of the >100 mL returned is truly representative of one million-odd alveoli sampled during a typical broncho-alveolar lavage (BAL): the number of pathogens in 100 mL of the returning fluid will be about one million cfu. In contrast, colonizing organisms prevail at much lower concentrations (<10^4 cfu/mL). As can be expected, the microbial yield will increase in direct proportion to the quantity of returning lavage fluid.

Box 11.4 Technique of Broncho-Alveolar Lavage (BAL)

1. The bronchoscope is completely wedged into a subsegmental bronchus.
2. Twenty to sixty milliliter aliquots of sterile (buffered or nonbuffered) nonbacteriostatic saline are instilled from a 50 to 60 mL syringe. The saline should ideally be warmed to 37°C, but many centers deviate from this practice.
3. The instilled saline is immediately sucked back into the same syringe using gentle hand suction on the piston: for the next aliquot, a fresh syringe is used. Alternatively the BAL fluid may be collected into a mucus trap using gentle wall suction.
4. At least 120 mL of BAL return should be acheived.[19,107] This usually means the instillation of 3–6 aliqouts.
5. The initial portion of the return represents sampling from the proximal airway, and this is preferably discarded.[9]
6. The lavaged fluid should be stored in a single sterile container of nonadherent plastic or silicon glass: this maximizes the cellular yield.
7. The specimen should be immediately transported to the lab and processed rapidly (usually within half an hour of collection,[18] although cells appear to remain viable for up to 4 h when stored at 25°C.

Processing should be done as per standardized protocols[54]

Bronchoalveolar lavage samples are probably representative if 5% or more lavaged cells show intracellular organisms.[4] In such cases, the likelihood of the sample being representative may be as high as 89–100%,[21] though prior or ongoing antibiotic therapy can substantially reduce the sensitivity of the sampling technique.

When epithelial cells are seen in large numbers, it means that their site of origin is generally the buccal or pharyngeal mucosa. Epithelial cells comprising more than 1% of the total cellular component in bronchoscopic samples imply substantial contamination by oropharyngeal secretions and the samples should not be taken to represent secretions from distal airways or lung parenchyma.[79]

Conversely, the presence of a large number of alveolar macrophages or polymorphs signifies that the sample originated in the terminal air units. When polymorphs are scant, pneumonia is unlikely, or the sample may simply not be adequate. The opposite cannot be said of a high polymorph count, as this may be a nonspecific finding.[108] The presence of elastin fibers in the lavaged fluid may be indicative of gram negative pneumonia.[44]

With both bronchoscopic and nonbronchoscopic techniques, contamination from the upper airways can confound interpretation. For example, Candida colonizing the upper airways can find their way into most samples recovered from the lower respiratory tract: demonstration of the fungus intracellularly within lung biopsy specimens is the only reliable means of confirming the diagnosis.

In spite of the poor sensitivity and specificity of most of these procedures, an attempt should be made to recover a microbiological pathogen, principally because appropriate antimicrobial therapy in the initial stages of NP is so crucial. Recovery of a pathogen may result in retailoring of the antibiotic regimen, with an improvement in outcome.

11.6 Prevention of NP/VAP

11.6.1 Hand-Washing

The old medical adage "prevention is better than cure" holds admirably in the case of NP or VAP, because the outcome of these is often adverse. Vigilance and effective prophylaxis hold the key to successful outcome in a mechanically ventilated patient.

It is surprising to what extent scrupulous hand-washing before and between examining patients can help to reduce the incidence of nosocomially-transmitted infection. Provided it is correctly done, hand-washing remains an extremely important technique for the prevention of nosocomial infection.

11.6.2 Feeding and Nutrition

As discussed earlier, the colonization of the gastrointestinal tract and the subsequent aspiration of its contents may constitute a risk factor for the development of NP/VAP. To reduce the risk of aspiration, the patient must be nursed in a semi-recumbent position wherever possible. Supine head position is an independent risk factor for VAP.[84] Large volume gastric feeds should be avoided.

Adequate nutritional support is important: malnutrition is an independent risk factor for VAP. Septic complications are more frequent with parenteral feeding; carefully regulated enteral feeds are of utmost importance. In the nonintubated patient, all agents which depress the sensorium – and thereby increase the risk of aspiration – must be avoided. Prokinetic agents, by decreasing gastric transit time may reduce the residual gastric volume and prevent aspiration. Large bore feeding tubes by their mechanical effect can promote gastrointestinal sphincter dysfunction and predispose to aspiration; smaller bore feeding tubes may be safer. In theory, enteral placement of the feeding tube could help by introducing the food bolus beyond two valves (gastroesophageal and gastroduodenal), rather than one, but it is uncertain that the risk of pneumonia can be brought down by replacing a gastroduodenal with a gastrojejunal tube.[115]

Before every feed, the gastric residual volumes should be checked: the feed should be delayed or withheld if an excessive volume is aspirated at the time of the scheduled feed. It may be safer to administer enteral nutrition using continuous infusion rather than bolus feeds, using feeding tubes of small bore.

11.6.3 Stress Ulcer Prophylaxis

Mechanical ventilation is intensely stressful for the patient. The risk of stress ulceration in the ICU is extremely high. Stress ulcer prophylaxis is common in ICUs and there may be a tendency to overprescribe these medications. The demerits of pH lowering agents such as H_2 receptor antagonists have been discussed earlier. Sucralfate may offer some advantage over the former in the sense that it does not lower the pH, but rather achieves gastroprotection by acting as a physical barrier between the gastric mucosa and the acidic gastric contents[51]; also, it may have an intrinsic antibacterial activity of its own, theoretically reducing gastric colonization.[155] However, recent studies have, by and large, vindicated the H_2 receptor antagonists,[107] although the last word on the matter has not yet been said.

11.6.4 Topical Antibiotics

Topical antibiotics may be efficacious in treating tracheobronchitis in intubated patients.[83] The rationale behind appears to be that in the absence of florid infection, a topical antibiotic may be able to contain the local tracheobronchial contaminants. Topical antibiotic therapy has been used in the form of drugs delivered to the lower respiratory tract in high concentrations, through a tracheostomy or endotracheal tube.[83] The method of introduction of the antibiotic is usually by nebulization or by direct instillation, but it is not clear which of the two approaches is superior. Aminoglycosides are used in this fashion, usually after pretreatment with a bronchodilator. Although the efficacy of the antibiotics administered by the endotracheal route in preventing VAP has been proven in several studies,[61] their potential for producing bacterial resistance is as yet not ruled out, and as such, the use of topical antibiotics for the prophylaxis of infection is presently discouraged.

Selective digestive decontamination: Application of antibiotic paste to the oropharynx to reduce oropharyngeal colonization, and instillation of antibiotics into the stomach to prevent gastric colonization can possibly prevent bacterial transmission from these sites into the lungs. Used widely in Europe, a mixture of antibiotics like an aminoglycoside or a fluoroquinolone plus a nonabsorbable antibiotic (e.g., polymyxin) and an antifungal agent (either amphotericin B or nystatin) were found to reduce the incidence of pneumonia, but not so much as to favorably alter the outcome.[16] Methodological issues confound the interpretation of a large number of these studies.

In theory, this method of prophylaxis relies on the prevention of colonization of the oropharynx and the stomach for the prevention of the subsequent NP. Therefore it does not prevent the onset of pneumonias that are caused by direct bacterial inoculation into the endotracheal or tracheostomy tubes. Pseudomonas, in particular, has been known to directly colonize the tracheobronchial tree without previously colonizing the gastrointestinal tract or the oropharynx.[115] Again, concerns regarding the emergence of bacterial resistance limit the usage of selective digestive decontamination until more data are available.[160]

Chlorhexidine mouth wash: The use of chlorhexidine – which is an antiseptic – as a mouth wash was found to significantly decrease the incidence of NP in a group of patients undergoing cardiac bypass surgery.[41]

11.7 Interventions Related to the Endotracheal Tube and Ventilator Circuit

Changing of the endotracheal tube with the intent of preventing infection has not been shown to help; indeed, it may actually be harmful, presumably because of the risk of aspiration during such a process, of the pooled pharyngeal secretions collected in the sump above the tube cuff. Also, the act of introducing a new endotracheal tube may itself cause more bacteria to be carried down into the tracheobronchial tree. The answer may lie in the development of new biomaterials for the endotracheal tube that might prevent the development of biofilms. Coating the inside of the endotracheal tube with a silver material appears to reduce biofilm formation and inhibit bacterial colonization, but more trials are necessary.[132] Continuous subglottic suctioning has been shown to be effective: a metaanalysis revealed an almost 50% reduction in the rate of VAP.[42]

Changing the ventilator circuits frequently has also not been shown to have any positive impact in preventing VAP. In fact, one study showed no increase in the rates of VAP if the circuitry was never changed,[46] and patients in whom ventilator circuitry was changed more frequently than every 48 h were shown to actually run a higher risk of VAP.[33] It seems sensible to change tubings only if the circuit appears to be overtly soiled.[152]

Condensate that accumulates in ventilator tubings should be emptied regularly and treated as infectious waste. When airway humidification is required, heat-moisture exchangers (HMEs) are probably safer than heated humidifiers (see section 15.5).

11.8 Treatment of Nosocomial Sinusitis

The treatment of nosocomial sinusitis not only involves the institution of appropriate antibiotic therapy, but also requires the removal of all nasal tubes in order to decrease nasal irritation and mucosal edema. Drainage of stagnant secretions from the sinuses can be aided by opening up the sinus ostia by topical nasal vasoconstrictor drops, and by elevating the head-end of the bed. When maxillary puncture is performed for diagnostic purposes, an antral wash carried out at the same time may prove therapeutic.

11.9 Treatment

In NP, early and aggressive antibiotic therapy strongly correlates with survival. Although attempts to procure respiratory specimens for culture should be swiftly undertaken, antibiotic therapy should never be delayed merely for the purpose of collecting samples.

11.9.1 Antibiotic Resistance

Antibiotic resistance issues have now become the bane of ICUs the world over. Indiscriminate antibiotic usage has resulted in the emergence of resistance, and multidrug resistant bacteria now abound. Indeed, it is true to say that only in the past couple of decades has the gravity of the problem really begun to sink in.

Half of all ICU usage of antibiotics is for lung infections.[11] It is now universally appreciated that indiscriminate antibiotic usage can exert a selective pressure on bacteria, eradicating sensitive organisms and enabling the intrinsically resistant strains to survive and proliferate.[140]

The principles of microbiological resistance (as proposed by Levy) postulate that:

- Given sufficient time and drug use, antibiotic resistance will emerge.
- Antibiotic resistance is progressive, evolving from low levels through intermediate to high levels.
- Organisms that are resistant to one drug are likely to be resistant to other antibiotics.
- Once resistance appears, it is likely to decline slowly, if at all.
- The use of antibiotics by any one person affects others in the extended and immediate environment.

Bacteria can develop antibiotic resistance by several mechanisms: gram-negative bacteria contain a three-layered cell wall. Aqueous porin channels contained within the outer wall allow solutes including antibiotics to diffuse into the bacterial cell.[114] Alteration of porin channels within gram negative bacteria can impede the penetration of the antibiotic into the bacterial cell. The production and concentration of beta-lactamases and other antibiotic-inactivating enzymes within the periplasmic space by gram-negative bacteria has become a cause of troublesome bacterial resistance the world over. In addition, both gram-negative and gram-positive bacteria can have intracellular inactivating enzymes. Bacteria can also alter antibiotic target sites within themselves, or even develop an efflux mechanism to actively pump antibiotics outside the bacterial cell, thereby limiting intracellular antibiotic concentrations. Resistance in gram negative bacteria most frequently is mediated by their production of (beta-lactamase) enzymes that rapidly inactivate the beta-lactam antibiotics. Over 500 beta-lactamases have been identified now; 5 times the number that microbiologists were aware of, 30 years ago.

Beta-lactamase production can result in bacterial resistance to a large spectrum of powerful beta-lactam agents. The enormity of the problem can be appreciated by the fact that it took just 2 years after the introduction of ceftazidime and ceftriaxone for the first extended-spectrum beta-lactamase (ESBL) to be recognized.[140] Since then, there has been a tremendous surge in the frequency with which ESBLs are encountered worldwide. The local prevalence of ESBLs has been shown to vary greatly, and pockets of local dissemination rather than wide-range spread are usual. ESBLs have mostly been encountered in Klebsiella isolates and their incidence worldwide appears to be on the increase. Importantly, once established within the ICU or the hospital, ESBLs can be extremely difficult to eradicate. For the treatment of severe infection by ESBL producing strains, carbapenems like imipenem may be most appropriate.[123]

Certain bacteria, in particular, Pseudomonas and Acinetobacter, are especially adept at developing drug resistance and may do so through several highly specialized and innovative mechanisms. The major mechanism of resistance is chromosomal or plasmid-mediated beta-lactamase production, but Pseudomonas, for instance, can also modify pencillin binding proteins and prevent aminologlycoside binding to ribosomes. Further, Pseudomonas can develop multi-drug resistance (MDR) by decreasing cellular permeability to beta-lactams and four quinolones, in addition to actively pumping these drugs outside the bacterial cell.[25] Resistance to four-quinolones can also develop by mutations at chromosomal loci encoding binding sites on DNA-gyrase.

MDR in gram-negative bacilli has been defined as resistance to at least two – and sometimes as many as eight – key gram-negative antibiotics.[122] When the organisms are resistant to *all* the antibiotics regarded as effective for gram-negative infections (e.g., cefepime, ceftazidime, imipenem, meropenem, piperacillin-tazobactam, ciprofloxacin, and levofloxacin), they are termed panresistant.

Box 11.5 Primary Host-Related Risk Factors for MDR Infection[1]

Antibiotic use in the preceding 90 days

Current hospitalization of 5 days

Admission in a healthcare facility such as a nursing home or a dialysis unit

High incidence of antibiotic resistance in the hospital unit, hospital, or community

Pseudomonas with its advanced mechanisms of developing drug resistance has for some years been recognized as a grave threat, but the recent emergence of multidrug resistant Acinetobacter has been a cause of considerable dismay in certain regions. The revival of the once-redundant colistin is a testament to the desperate need for more antibiotics.

In terms of bacterial resistance, certain gram-positive organisms – such as *S. aureus* – are proving as problematic as aerobic gram-negative bacilli. Pencillin-resistant staphylococci were described shortly after the advent of penicillin, and in just two decades the rates of penicillin resistant strains had spiraled to 90% in some health facilities in England. Currently, nearly all isolates of S. aureus from hospitals, and most community acquired strains are anticipated to be penicillin resistant.[106]

The introduction of methicillin in 1961 did succeed to an extent in overcoming penicillin-resistant strains, but only at the cost of the creation of a new menace, the methicillin-resistant *Staphylococcus aureus* (MRSA). By 1989, MRSA strains comprised 50% of all isolates of *S. aureus* in most major hospitals in the USA. Vancomycin and linezolid are considered the cornerstones for MRSA therapy. Vancomycin-resistant strains of enterococci have now been identified, as have strains of *S. aureus* showing intermediate sensitivity to vancomycin. The vancomycin-intermediate *S. aureus* or glycopeptide-resistant *S. aureus* (VISA, GISA) strains have surfaced under conditions of prolonged exposure to vancomycin, or in situations where dialysis or intravascular device placement was required. Vancomycin-resistant enterococci are capable of spreading vancomycin resistance to other organisms, since the mode of spread is plasmid transmission to other microbes by conjugation.

11.9.2 Pharmacokinetics

An exhaustive discussion on antibiotic pharmacokinetics and pharmacodynamics and indeed of the antibiotic strategy in NP/VAP is beyond the scope of this book.

The efficacy of an antibiotic against a pathogen can be quantified in several ways. These have been summarized in Fig. 11.3.

Choice of antibiotic: The choice of the initial antibiotic for NP is determined not only by the organism likely to be present, the pharmacokinetic profiles of the various antibiotics and their potential toxicity, but also by local resistance issues. As discussed above, organisms that are found in early NP are comparable to those that cause community-acquired pneumonias, and the treatment of the two is generally very

The minimum inhibitory concentration (MIC)

- The smallest concentration of an antibiotic that stops bactetial growth in media containing 10^5 bacteria/mL is called the minimum inhibitory concentration
- Organisms are considered susceptible when their MIC level is below the expected serum level of the antibiotic question
- For effective bacterial killing, antibiotics like the beta-lactams require serum levels to consistently remain above the MIC. Consequently the efficacy of these drugs is on account of time-dependentrather then dose-dependent activity
- These drugs require to be given several times a day in order to maintain their levels constantly above the MICs

AUC/MIC ratio

- The serum level of a given antibiotic increases to a peak and then falls to a trough as the drug is metabolised. The area that falls under the curve representing the serum antibiotic level as a function of time is called the *area under the curve* (AUC)
- For anibiotics such as vancomycin and azithromycin, the AUC/MIC ratio provides a more accurate measure of antibiotic efficacy than does the MIC value taken in isolation

Peak serum level/MIC ratio

- The cure rate of these drugs (e.g.) aminoglycosides and the 4-quinolones) is related to the peak level achived by these drugs in the serum rather than to the time that they remain above the MIC levels
- These antibiotics have a significant postantibiotic effect, which continues to exert an antibacterial effect on microbes even when serum levels have dropped below the MIC´
- Antibiotics such as the aminoglycosides and the 4-quinolones should as a rule, be given in relatively high doses such that a high enough peak serum level is achieved
- A long dosing interval such as a once daily dosing regimen often suffices

FIGURE 11.3. Antibiotic pharmacokinetics.

similar – that is, except, if the patient has been a resident of a nursing home or has other risk factors for antibiotic resistance (see Fig…). For late NP therapeutic decisions are predictably more complex. In general, antibiotic therapy should primarily target gram-negative organisms; in particular the possibility of Pseudomonal infection should be kept in mind. As mentioned above, polymicrobial infections are common and coverage with multiple antibiotics may be needed until microbiological reports are available.

Wherever possible, antibiotic therapy should be guided by microbiology, and the regimen should be restructured in the light of the lab reports. This is essential if the responsible microbe is to be covered with as narrow spectrum antibiotic as possible: the emergence of antibiotic resistance is always a greater concern with broad-spectrum therapy.

Monotherapy may be acceptable in nonbacteremic cases and a carbapenem could be used. A beta-lactam antibiotic with antipseudomonal action plus either an aminoglycoside or ciprofloxacin is a commonly used regimen. Because of resistance issues, dual antibiotic coverage for *Pseudomonas aeruginosa* may be important, especially in bacteremic cases.[70]

Cephalosporins as first-line agents are generally not preferred because of their propensity to select out resistant pseudomonas, and the combination of a broader spectrum penicillin (such as pipercillin with or without tazobactam) along with an aminoglycoside may be more suitable. Indeed, empiric usage of ceftazidime has been incriminated in the emergence of extended spectrum beta-lactamase producing bacteria. It is equally likely that if other antibiotics are used regularly as monotherapy, similar patterns of resistance could emerge. The pharmacokinetics of aminoglycosides preclude their role as *sole* agents for pneumonia. Since the lungs are, in effect, large capillary beds, penetration of most antibiotics into the lungs is adequate; aminoglycosides act poorly in the acidic milieu that is present locally in the pneumonic lung. When the targeted organism is pseudomonas, owing to its sophisticated methods of developing drug resistance, it is necessary to administer at least two antibiotics to which the organism is sensitive.

As regards the specific antibiotics that should be used, there exist no hard and fast rules – except to hit hard (that is, use the antibiotic considered most appropriate up front) – and hit "fast" (that is, to administer the appropriate drug as quickly as possible). It bears emphasis that the choice of an antibiotic for empiric therapy should be based on regional patterns of antibiotic sensitivity, which are generally dynamic and should be continually updated.

Aerosolized antibiotics: The direct delivery of antibiotics into the lungs may provide an alternative to systemic administration.[164] Higher drug concentrations are achievable by nebulizing or instilling antibiotics directly into the lower respiratory tract. Peak drug concentrations in respiratory secretions have been shown to be 200 times those achievable with systemic administration,[121] with sputum trough levels over 20 times those considered adequate.

Reservations about antibiotic resistance have inevitably been voiced,[51] but it may well be that earlier studies relied upon drug delivery systems which did not achieve a satisfactory lung deposition of the aerosolized antibiotic. On the other hand, several investigators have found a much lower incidence of resistance.[12]

At the present time, nebulized antibiotics such as tobramycin[12] may be viewed as being adjunctive treatments to systemic antibiotics in the treatment of VAP[1,65]: most authorities would strenuously discourage their use as prophylactics. There is less clarity as regards their role in the *treatment* of ventilator-associated *tracheobronchitis.*[151] Indeed, if tracheobronchitis be viewed as part of a continuum – of which VAP forms one extreme – aerosolized antibiotics may well have a vital role to play in the future.[121]

All nebulizers do not have similar aerosol outputs in relation to specific drugs: this has been considered in Chap... (Figs. 11.4 and 11.5).

11.9.3 Duration of Therapy

It may be possible to use shorter courses of antibiotics than previously considered necessary. The duration of antibiotic therapy should be individualized to the patient and to the microbe. The speed of resolution of the pneumonia as well as the pathogen incriminated will often help in deciding this. In general, a multilobar or necrotizing pneumonia often presages a delayed response to therapy, as does a poor nutritional status of the host. It is generally possible to eliminate relatively rapidly, the organisms that cause early NP – *H. influenzae* and *S. pneumonia.*[40] On the other hand, the Enterobacteriaceae, *S. aureus* need more prolonged courses of antibiotic.[40] Certain microbes, particularly Pseudomonas or Acinetobacter show high rates of treatment failure and relapse. In such cases antibiotic therapy may be extended to a minimum of 2–3 weeks. Unnecessarily prolonged antibiotic therapy often results in bacterial colonization, and this then presages recurrent VAP.[145]

Pseudomonas aeruginosa	Acinetobacter species	ESBL producing Enterobacteriaceae	MRSA
• Combination therapy has not been shown to alter the rates of resistance[53]; but seem to show a survival benefit[68] • The ATS/IDSA nevertheless recommends combination therapy in proven pseudomonas pneumonia, because the incidence of resistance to monotherapy is so high, and combination therapy is less likely to result in inadequate coverage[1] • A beta lactam antibiotic colud be used with either a quinolone or an aminoglycoside • As a companion antibiotic, an aminoglycoside may result in a trend towards an increased survival than a 4-quinolone[1] • A quinolone as a companion antibiotic is appropriate if local data support its usage: antibiotic resistance is common with overuse[119]Data are scant • Levofloxacin at higher doses (eg 750 mg once daily) may be superior, though at present, there is no evidence to support this presumption[162] • Aerosolized antibiotics may be used as adjuncts[162]	• Combination therapy is generally considered unnecessary[164] • The choice of antibiotics is relatively limited because of the organism's innate resistance to multiple classes of drugs • Appropriate antibiotics: carbapenems, sulbactam (ampicillin-sulbactam), the polymyxins and colistin • When used carbapenems should be used in appropriately high doses to avoid the development of resistance • Aerosolozed antibiotics may be used as adjuncts especially in patients who have shown an unsatisfactory intitial response[65]	• Monotherapy with third generation (Paterson DL, 2001)– and possible also fourth generation– cephalosporins[130] should be avoided • A carbapenem is presently considered effective • Resistance is common to aminoglycosides and 4-quinolones, and so combination therapy is not considered important • The efficacy of piperacillin-tazobactam is uncertain, and the combination should be used with due care when choices are severely limited[77] • Aerosolozed antibiotics may be used as adjuncts especially in patients who have shown an unsatisfactory intitial response[65]	• Both vancomycin or linezolid can be considered effective • Vancomycin drug failures may be related to inadequate dosing[111]– underdosing in renal failure is one example[162] • Vancomycin in combination with rifampin or aminoglycosides has not been shown to be clearly superior to vancomycin as monotherapy[96] • Linezolid penetrates better into the epithelial lining fluid than vancomycin [29]and has been shown to be at least as effective as vancomycin in some clinical trials; it may actually be preferable to vancomycin especially if there are nephrotoxic drugs in the prescription or if there is a coexistent renal faolure[166]

FIGURE 11.4. Empiric choice of antibiotic.

Combination therapy

- Combination therapy is commonly used in antipseudomonas regimens
- The evidence that combination therapy confers clinical advantage is presently scarce
- *Traditional justifications for combination therapy*
  - *To enhance the synergistic activity against Pseudomonas aeruginosa*
  - *To prevent the emergence of resistance against Pseudomonas*
  - *To prevent the emergence of resistance against Enterobacter with third generation cephalosporins* [53,26]
  - *To broaden the coverage of an emperic regimen*
- Antibiotics from different classes should be combined to prevent drug antagonism (e.g., a B-lactam and a 4-quinolone, or a B-lactam and an aminoglycoside)

Monotherapy

- Preferred especially in patients with no risk factors for drug-resistant organisms
- Used for gram positive pneumonias
- May be less succesful in severe NP [145], and should probably not be used unless after an initial course of combination therapy or if LRT secretions are demonstrably sterile[71]
- Acceptable choices: ciprofloxacin, levofloxacin, piperacillin–tazobactam, cefepime, imipenem, and meropenem [53, 72, 162, 17, 143, 120]

FIGURE 11.5. Monotherapy vs. combination therapy.

In responders, an initial course of about 8 days may be as effective as a 14 day course.[23]

11.9.4 Lack of Response to Therapy

An early response – by day 3–5 or so – is a marker of survival.[101] Clinical worsening or a lack of response to what is considered appropriate therapy, often requires a reappraisal of the situation: bacterial causes for the lack of response must of course be considered. The initial pathogens causing NP can persist despite what can be construed as appropriate antibiotic therapy, and such a bacterial persistence has been particularly linked to necrotizing pneumonia and gram-negative bacteremia.[133] The reason for bacterial persistence appears to be drug resistance: the responsible pathogen may have been resistant from the very beginning, or have acquired resistance during the course of therapy. In the case of beta-lactam antibiotics, typically, bacterial isolates show initial susceptibility. However the pathogen at a culture repeated a few days later may be demonstrably resistant to the same antibiotic(s), illustrating the phenomenon of inducible drug resistance.

Clinical lack of response could also mean that the pathogen, by its very generic disposition, is unresponsive to antibiotics as a class: it may be a virus, a fungus or a mycobacterium.

Superinfection pneumonia can emerge when treatment of the dominant organisms allows the other aspirated components of a polymicrobial flora to proliferate,[113] or when reinoculation of infected secretions occurs. The new pathogens generally prove to be much more drug resistant and destructive than their predecessors.[113]

The problem of recurrent pneumonia has been described with regard to Pseudomonas; in practice it may be extremely difficult to differentiate recurrence from superinfection pneumonia.[144] The options in nonresponding patients are not easy and initial broadening of the antibiotic umbrella followed by renewed attempts at directed microbiological sampling may help in clinical problem-solving.

That the pathology is noninfective must also be considered. Congestive cardiac failure, pulmonary infarction, segmental atelectasis, and alveolar hemorrhage are all capable of radiologically mimicking pneumonia. Extrapulmonary sources of infection such as complicated pleural collections may be overlooked, as could catheter induced infection, urinary sepsis, or drug-fever (Fig. 11.6).

11.9.5 Drug Cycling

Drug cycling – in which different antibiotics are deliberately rotated after a period of use – has been proposed as a means to restrict the emergence of antibiotic resistant organisms.

This policy seems to be effective in that resistance to the withdrawn antibiotic can been seen to fall, as reported by some researchers,[56] but the danger inherent in such an approach seems to be that resistance to the antibiotic

Organisms unresponsive to antibacterials by its generic disposition	Antibiotic-resistant bacterium	Noninfective pathology mimicking pneumonia
• Virus (uncommon) • Fungus (uncommon) • Mycobacterium (uncommon)	• Bacterium is innately unresponsive to the chosen class of drug (e.g., a gram-positive organism to a purely gram-negative antibiotic) • Bacterium is resistant from the onset • Bacterium has developed inducible drug resistance on exposure to antibiotic • Treatment of the dominant organisms has allowed other components of a polymicrobial flora to proliferate • Reinfection by reinoculation of infected secretions	• Congestive cardiac failure • Pulmonary infraction • Segmental atelectasis • Alveolar hemorrhage

FIGURE 11.6. Possible causes of a nonresolving pneumonia.

substituted in its place may subsequently rise. John Burke described this phenomenon as "squeezing the balloon of resistance," implying that bacterial resistance may shift its focus to the newly substituted antibiotics when the usage of other antibiotics is restricted. There also remains considerable concern that rotation strategies may expose bacteria sequentially to different classes of antibiotics and thereby lead to a proliferation of multidrug-resistant microbes. Nevertheless, gratifying and sustainable results have been noted by several investigators,[63,86] and in the dynamic scenario that prevails in most ICUs, the subject continues to evoke considerable interest.

References

1. American Thoracic Society/Infectious Diseases Society of America. Guidelines for the management of adults with hospital-acquired, ventilator-associated, and healthcare-associated pneumonia. *Am J Respir Crit Care Med.* 2005;171:388
2. Andrews CP, Coalson JJ, Smith JD, Johanson WG. Diagnosis of nosocomial bacterial pneumonia in acute, diffuse lung injury. *Chest*. 1981;80:254–258
3. Atherton ST, White DJ. Stomach as a source of bacteria colonizing respiratory tract during artificial ventilation. *Lancet*. 1978;2:968–969
4. Aubas S, Aubas P, Capdevila X, et al Bronchoalveolar lavage for diagnosing bacterial pneumonia in mechanically ventilated patients. *Am J Respir Crit Care Med*. 1994;149:860–866
5. Aust R, Drettner B. The patency of maxillary sinusitis in relation to body posture. *Acta Otolaryngol (Stockh)*. 1975;80:443–446
6. Barlett JG, Alexander J, Mayhew J, et al Should fiberoptic bronchoscopy aspirates be cultured? *Am Rev Respir Dis*. 1976;114:73–78
7. Barlett JG, O'Keefee P, Tally FP, et al Bacteriology of hospital acquired pneumonia. *Arch Intern Med*. 1986;146:868–871
8. Bartlett JG, Finegold SM. Bacteriology of expectorated sputum with quantitative culture and wash technique compared to transtracheal aspirates. *Am Rev Respir Dis*. 1978;117:1019–1027
9. Baselski VS, Wunderink RG. Bronchoscopic diagnosis of pneumonia. *Clin Microbiol Rev*. 1994;7:533–558
10. Baughman RP, Thorpe JE, Staneck J, et al Use of the protected specimen brush in patients with endotracheal or tracheostomy tubes. *Chest*. 1987;91:223–235
11. Bergman DC, Bonten MJ, Gaillard CA, et al Indications for antibiotic use in ICU patient: a 1-year prospective surveillance. *J Antimicrob Chemother*. 1997;39:527–535
12. Brown RB, Kruse JA, Counts GW, et al Double-blind study of endotracheal tobramycin in the treatment of gram-negative bacterial pneumonia. The Endotracheal Tobramycin Study Group. *Antimicrob Agents Chemother*. 1990;34:269–272
13. Campbell D, Niederman MS, Brought WA, et al ATS official statement: hospital acquired pneumonia in adults: diagnosis, assessment of severity, initial antimicrobial therapy and

preventive strategies. A consensus statement. *Am J Respir Crit Care Med*. 1996;153:1771–1725

14. CDC: National nosocomial infections study report: annual summary, 1984 MMWR 35:178–29S, 1986
15. Celis R, Torres A, Gatell J, et al Nosocomial pneumonia: a multivariable analysis of risk and prognosis. *Chest*. 1988;93:318–324
16. Chan EY, Ruest A, Meade MO, Cook DJ. Oral decontamination for prevention of pneumonia in mechanically ventilated adults: systematic review and meta-analysis. *BMJ*. 2007; 334:889
17. Chapman TM, Perry CM. Cefepime: a review of its use in the management of hospitalized patients with pneumonia. *Am J Respir Med*. 2003;2:75–107
18. Chastre J, Fagon JY. In: Tobin MJ, ed. *Principles and practice of mechanical ventilation*. McGraw-Hill; 2006;p991–1018
19. Chastre J, Fagon JY. Ventilator- associated pneumonia. *Am J Respir Crit Care Med*. 2002;165:867–903
20. Chastre J, Viau F, Brun P, et al Prospective evaluation of the prected specimen brush for the diagnosis of pulmonary infections in ventilated patients. *Am Rev Respir Dis*. 1984;130: 924–929
21. Chastre J, Fagon JY, Soler P, et al Diagnosis of nosocomial bacterial pneumonia in intubated patients undergoing ventilation: comparison of the usefulness of bronchoalveolar lavage and the protected specimen brush. *Am J Med*. 1988;85:499–506
22. Chastre J, Fagon JY, Bornet-Lesco M, et al Evaluation of bronchoscopic techniques for the diagnosis of nosocomial pneumonia. *Am J Respir Crit Care Med*. 1995;152:231–240
23. Chastre J, Wolff M, Fagon JY, et al Comparison of 8 vs 15 days of antibiotic therapy for ventilator-associated pneumonia in adults: a randomized trial. *JAMA*. 2003;290:2588–2598
24. Chatburn RL. Decontamination of respiratory care equipment: what can be done, what should be done. *Respir Care*. 1989; 34:98–110
25. Chen H, Yan M, Livermore D. Mechanisms to resistance to beta-lactam antibiotics amongst *P.aeruginosa* isolates collected in the UK in 1993. *J Med Microbiol*. 1995;43:300–309
26. Chow JW, Fine MJ, Shlaes DM, et al *Enterobacter* bacteremia: clinical features and emergence of antibiotic resistance during therapy. *Ann Intern Med*. 1991;115:585–590
27. Cometta A, Baumgartner JD, Lew D, et al Prospective randomized comparison of imipenem monotherapy with imipenem plus netilmicin for treatment of severe infections in nonneutropenic patients. *Antimicrob Agents Chemother*. 1994;38: 1309–1313

28. Comhaire A, Lamy M. Contamination of rate of sterilized ventilators in ICU. *Crit Care Med.* 1981;9:546–548
29. Conte JE Jr, Golden JA, Kipps J, Zurlinden E. Intrapulmonary pharmacokinetics of linezolid. *Antimicrob Agents Chemother.* 2002;46:1475–1480
30. Cook DJ, Laine LA, Guyatt GH, et al Nosocomial pneumonia and the role of gastric pH: a meta-analysis. *Chest.* 1991;100:7–13
31. Costerton JW, Irwin RT. The bacterial glycocalyx in nature and disease. *Annu Rev Microbiol.* 1981;35:299–324
32. Craven DE, Driks MR. Nosocomial pneumonia in the intubated patient. *Semin respir Infect.* 1987;2:20–33
33. Craven DE, Steger KA. Nosocomial pneumonia in the intubated patient. *Infect Dis Clin North Am.* 1989;3:843–866
34. Craven DE, Goularte TA, Make BJ. Contaminated condensate in mechanical ventilator circuits: a risk factor for nosocomial pneumonia. *Am Rev Respir Dis.* 1984;129:625–628
35. Craven DE, Kunches LM, Kilinsky V, et al Risk factors for pneumonia and fatality in patients receiving continuous mechanical ventilation. *Am Rev Respir Dis.* 1986;133:792–796
36. Craven DE, Steger KA, Barber TW. Preventing nosocomial pneumonia; state of the art and perspectives for 1990's. *Am J Med.* 1991;91:44S–53S
37. Craven DE, Palladino R, McQuillen DP. Healthcare-associated pneumonia in adults: management principles to improve outcomes. *Infect Dis Clin North Am.* 2004;18:939
38. Cross AS, Roup B. Role of respiratory assistance devices in endemic nosocomial pneumonia. *Am J Med.* 1981;70:681–685
39. de Lassence A, Joly-Guillou ML, Martin-Lefevre L, et al Accuracy of delayed cultures of plugged telescoping catheter samples for diagnosing bacterial pneumonia. *Crit Care Med.* 2001;29:1311–1317
40. Dennesen PJ, Van der Ven AJ, Kessels AG, Ramsay G, Bonten MJ. Resolution of infectious parameters after antimicrobial therapy in patients with ventilator-associated pneumonia. *Am J Respir Crit Care Med.* 2001;163:1371–1375
41. DeRiso AJ II, Ladowski JS, Dillon TA, Justice JW, Peterson AC. Chlorhexidine gluconate 0.12% oral rinse reduces the incidence of total nosocomial respiratory infection and nonprophylactic systemic antibiotic use in patients undergoing heart surgery. *Chest.* 1996;109:1556–1561
42. Dezfulian C, Shojania K, Collard HR, et al Subglottic secretion drainage for preventing ventilator-associated pneumonia: a meta-analysis. *Am J Med.* 2005;118:11

43. Djupesland PG, Chatkin JM, Qian W, Haight JS. Nitric oxide in the nasal airway: a new dimension in otorhinolaryngology. *Am J Otolaryngol.* 2001;22:19–32
44. Downowitz GL, Page MC, Mileur BL, et al Alteration of normal gastric flora in critical care patients receiving antacid and cimetidine therapy. *Infect Control.* 1986;7:23–26
45. Dreyfuss D, Djedaini K, Weber P, et al Prospective study of nosocomial pneumonia and of patient and circuit colonization during mechanical ventilation with circuit changes every 48 hours versus no change. *Am Rev Respir Dis.* 1991;143:738–743
46. Driks MR, Craven DE, Celli BR, et al Nosocomial pneumonia in intubated patients given sucralfate as compared with antacids or histamine type 2 blockers. *N Engl J Med.* 1987;317: 1376–1383
47. El-Ebiary M, Torres A, Gonzalez J, et al Diagnosis of ventilator-associated (VA) pneumonia: diagnostic value of quantitative cultures of endotracheal aspirates (EA). *Am Rev Respir Dis.* 1991;143:A108
48. Fagon JY, Chastre J, Hance AJ, et al Detection of nosocomial lung infection in ventilated patients: use of a protected specimen brush and quantitative culture techniques in 147 patients. *Am Rev Respir Dis.* 1988;138:110–116
49. Fagon JY, Chastre J, Domart Y, et al Nosocomial pneumonia in patients receiving continuous mechanical ventilation: prospective analysis of 52 episodes with use of a protected specimen brush and quantitative culture techniques. *Am Rev Respir Dis.* 1989;139:877–884
50. Fagon JY, Chastre J, Hance AJ, et al Nosocomial pneumonia in ventilated patients: a cohort study evaluating attributable mortality and hospital stay. *Am J Med.* 1993;94:281
51. Feely TW, DuMoulin GC, Hedley-Whyte J, et al Aerosol polymyxin and pneumonia in seriously ill patientsl. *N Engl J Med.* 1975;293:471–475
52. Fiddian-Green RG, Baker S. Nosocomial pneumonia in the critically ill: product of aspiration of translocation? *Crit Care Med.* 1991;19:763–769
53. Fink MP, Snydman DR, Niederman MS, et al Severe Pneumonia Study Group. Treatment of severe pneumonia in hospitalized patients: results of a multicenter, randomized, doubleblind trial comparing intravenous ciprofloxacin with imipenem–cilastatin. *Antimicrob Agents Chemother.* 1994;38:547–557
54. Forceville X, Fiacre A, Faibis F, et al Reproducibility of protected specimen brush and bronchialveolar lavage conserved

at 4 degrees C for 48 hours. *Intensive Care Med.* 2002;28: 857–863

55. Fox RC, Williams GJ, Wunderink RG, et al Follow-up bronchoscopy predicts therapeutic outcome in ventilated patients with nosocomial pneumonia. *Am Rev Respir Dis.* 1991; 143:A109
56. Frdkin SK. Antibiotic cycling: what is the evidence? Program and abstracts of the 41st Interscience Conference on Antimicrobial agents and Chemotherapy; December 16–19. Chicago, Illinois; 2001
57. Garnacho-Montero J, Ortiz-Leyba C, Jimenez-Jimenez FJ, et al Treatment of multidrug-resistant *Acinetobacter baumannii* ventilator-associated pneumonia (VAP) with intravenous colistin: a comparison with imipenem-susceptible VAP. *Clin Infect Dis.* 2003;36:1111–1118
58. Gibbons RJ, van Houte J. Bacterial adherence in oral microbial ecology. *Annu Rev Microbiol.* 1975;29:19–44
59. Grant MM, Poehlman MA, Niederman MS, et al Sputum inhibition of *Pseudomonas aeruginosa* adherence to cells and matrix varies with bacterial strain [abstract]. *Am Rev Respir Dis.* 1990;141:A333
60. Greenfield S, Teres D, Bushnell LS, et al Prevention of gram-negative bacillary pneumonia using aerosol polymyxin as a prophylaxis: effect on colonization pattern of the upper respiratory tract of seriously ill patients. *J Clin Invest.* 1973;52:2935–2940
61. Grey SW, Wunderick RG, Jones CB, et al Correlation of bronchoalveolar lavage neutrophilia with quantitative cultures in the diagnosis of ventilator associated pneumonia. *Am Rev Respir Dis.* 1994;149:970
62. Gross PA, Neu HC, Aswapokee P, et al Deaths from nosocomial infections: experience in a university hospital and community hospital. *Am J Med.* 1980;68:219
63. Gruson D, Hilbert G, Vargas F, et al Strategy of antibiotic rotation: long-term effect on incidence and susceptibilities of gram-negative bacilli responsible for ventilator-associated pneumonia. *Crit Care Med.* 2003;31:1908–1914
64. Haley RW, Hooton TM, Culver DH, et al Nosocomial infections in U.S. hospitals, 1975-1976: estimated frequency by selected characteristics of patients. *Am J Med.* 1981;70:947–959
65. Hamer DH. Treatment of nosocomial pneumonia and tracheobronchitis caused by multidrug-resistant *Pseudomonas aeruginosa*

with aerosolized colistin. *Am J Respir Crit Care Med*. 2000;162:328–330

66. Higuchi JH, Johanson WG Jr. The relationship between adherence of *Pseudomonas aeruginosa* to upper respiratory cells in vitro and susceptibility to colonization in vivo. *J Lab Clin Med*. 1980;95:698–705
67. Hilbert G, Vargas F, Valentino R, et al Comparison of B-mode ultrasound and computed tomography in the diagnosis of maxillary sinusitis in mechanically ventilated patients. *Crit Care Med*. 2001;29:1337–1342
68. Hilf M, Yu V, Sharp J, Zuravleff J, et al Antibiotic therapy for *Pseudomonas aeruginosa* bacteremia: outcome correlations in a prospective study of 200 patients. *Am J Med*. 1989;87:540–546
69. Holzapfel L, Chastang C, Demingeon G, et al A randomized study assessing the systematic search for maxillary sinusitis in nasotracheally mechanically ventilated patients. Influence of nosocomial maxillary sinusitis on the occurrence of ventilator-associated pneumonia. *Am J Respir Crit Care Med*. 1999;159:695–701
70. Huxley EJ, Viroslav J, Gray WR, Pierce AK. Pharyngeal aspiration in normal adults and patients with depressed consciousness. *Am J Med*. 1978;64:564
71. Ibrahim EH, Ward S, Sherman G, Schaiff R, Fraser VJ, Kollef MH. Experience with a clinical guideline for the treatment of ventilator associated pneumonia. *Crit Care Med*. 2001;29:1109–1115
72. Jaccard C, Troillet N, Harbarth S, et al Prospective randomized comparison of imipenem–cilastatin and piperacillin–tazobactam in nosocomial pneumonia or peritonitis. *Antimicrob Agents Chemother*. 1998;42:2966–2972
73. Johanson WG Jr. Ventilator-associated pneumonia: light at the end of the tunnel. *Chest*. 1990;97:1026–1027
74. Johanson WG Jr, Pierce AK, Sanford JP. Changing pharyngeal bacterial flora in hospitalized patients: emergence of gram-negative bacilli. *N Engl J Med*. 1969;281:1137–1140
75. Johanson WG Jr, Pierce AK, Sanford JP, et al Nosocomial respiratory infections with gram-negative bacilli: the significance of colonization of the respiratory tract. *Ann Intern Med*. 1972;77:701–706
76. Joshi JH, Wang KP, DeJongh CA, et al A comparative evaluation of two fiberoptic bronchoscopy catheters: the plugged

telescoping catheter versus the single sheathed nonplugged catheter. *Am Rev Respir Dis*. 1982;126:860–863
77. Joshi N, Localio AR, Hamory BH. A predictive risk index for nosocomial pneumonia in the intensive care unit. *Am J Med*. 1992;93:135–142
78. Joshi M, Bernstein J, Solomkin J, Wester BA, Kuye O, Piperacillin/Tazobactam Nosocomial Pneumonia Study Group. Piperacillin/tazobactam plus tobramycin versus ceftazidime plus tobramycin for the treatment of patients with nosocomial lower respiratory tract infection. *J Antimicrob Chemother.* 1999;43:389–397
79. Kass EH, Schneiderman LJ. Entry of bacteria into the urinary tracts of patients with inlying catheters. *N Engl J Med*. 1957;256:556–557
80. Kerver AJH, Rommes JH, Mevissen-Verhage EAE, et al Prevention of colonization and infection in critically ill patients: a prospective randomized study. *Crit Care Med*. 1988;16: 1087–1093
81. Klainer AS, Turndorf H, Wu WH, et al Surface alterations due to endotracheal intubation. *Am J Med*. 1975;58:674–683
82. Klastersky J, Huysmans E, Weerts D, et al Endotracheally administered gentamicin for the prevention of infections of the respiratory tract in patients with tracheostomy: a double-blind study. *Chest*. 1974;65:650–654
83. Klick JM, DuMoulin GD, Hedley-Whyte J, et al Prevention of gram-negative bacillary pneumonia using polymyxin aerosol as prophylaxis: effect on the incidence of pneumonia in seriously ill patients. *J Clin Invest*. 1975;55:514–519
84. Kollef MH. Ventilator associated pneumonia: a multivariate analysis. *JAMA*. 1993;270:1965–1970
85. Kollef MH, Vlasnik J, Sharpless L, Pasque C, Murphy D, Fraser V. Scheduled change of antibiotic classes: a strategy to decrease the incidence of ventilator-associated pneumonia. *Am J Respir Crit Care Med*. 1997;156:1040–1048
86. Kollef MH, Von Harz B, Prentice D, et al Patient transport from intensive care increases the risk of developing ventilator-associated pneumonia. *Chest*. 1997;112:765–773
87. Lamer C, de Beco V, Soler P, et al Analysis of vancomycin entry into pulmonary lining fluid by bronchoalveolar lavage in critically ill patients. *Antimicrob Agents Chemother*. 1993;37: 281–286
88. Langer M, Cigada M, Mandelli M, et al Early onset pneumonia: a multicenter study in intensive care units. *Inten Care Med*. 1987;13:342–346

89. Langer M, Mosconi P, Cigada M, et al Long term respiratory support and risk of pneumonia in critically ill patients. *Am Rev Respir Dis*. 1989;140:302–305
90. Lassche WJ. *Anerobic bacteria: role in disease*. Springfield, Illinois: Charles C Thomas; 1974
91. Laurenzi GA, Berman L, First M, et al A quantitative study of the deposition and clearance of bacteria in the murine lung. *J clin Invest*. 1964;43:759–768
92. Le Moal G, Lemerre D, Grollier G, et al Nosocomial sinusitis with isolation of anaerobic bacteria in ICU patients. *Intensive Care Med*. 1999;25:1066–1071
93. Leal Noval SR, Alfaro-Rodriquez E, Murillo-Cabeza F, et al Diagnostic value of the blind brush in mechanically ventilated patients with nosocomial pneumonia. *Intensive Care Med*. 1992;18:410–414
94. Ledingham MI, Alcock SR, Eastaway AT, et al Triple regimen of selective decontamination of the digestive tract, systemic cefotaxime and microbiological surveillance for prevention of acquired infection in intensive care. *Lancet*. 1988;1:785–790
95. Leu HS, Kaiser DL, Mori M. Hospital acquired pneumonia. Attributable mortality and morbidity. *Am J Epidemiol*. 1989;129:1258–1267
96. Levine SA, Neiderman MS, Grant MM, et al Regional differences in lower airway epithelial cell bacterial adherence in mechanically ventilated patients. *Chest*. 1990;98:29S
97. Levine DP, Fromm BS, Reddy BR. Slow response to vancomycin or vancomycin plus rifampin in methicillin-resistant *Staphylococcus aureus* endocarditis. *Ann Intern Med*. 1991; 115:674–680
98. Lichtenstein D, Biderman P, Meziere G, Gepner A. The "sinusogram", a real – time ultrasound sign of maxillary sinusitis. *Intensive Care Med*. 1998;24:1057–1061
99. Long R, Light B, Talbot JA. Mycobacteriocidal action of exogenous nitric oxide. *Antimicrob Agents Chemother*. 1999;43: 403–405
100. Lowenstein CJ, Padalko E. iNOS (NOS2) at a glance. *J Cell Sci*. 2004;117:2865–2867
101. Luna CM, Blanzaco D, Niederman MS, et al Resolution of ventilator-associated pneumonia: prospective evaluation of the clinical pulmonary infection score as an early clinical predictor of outcome. *Crit Care Med*. 2003;31:676–682
102. Lundberg JO, Weitzberg E. Nasal nitric oxide in man. *Thorax*. 1999;54:947–952

103. Malawista SE, Montgomery RR, van Blaricom G. Evidence for reactive nitrogen intermediates in killing of staphylococci by human neutrophil cytoplasts. A new microbicidal pathway for polymorphonuclear leukocytes. *J Clin Invest.* 1992;90: 631–636
104. Mangi RJ, Ryan J, Thorton G, et al Cefoperazone vs combination antibiotic therapy of hospital acquired pneumonia. *Am J Med.* 1990;84:68–74
105. Martin LF, Booth FV, Karlstadt RG, et al Continuous intravenous cimetidine decreases stress-related upper gastrointestinal hemorrhage without promoting pneumonia. *Crit Care Med.* 1993;21:19–30
106. Medeiros AA. Evaluation and dissemination of beta-lactamases by generations of beta-lactam antibiotics. *Clin Infect Dis.* 1997;24(Suppl 1):S19–S45
107. Meduri GU, Chastre J. The standardization of bronchoscopic techniques for ventilator-associated pneumonia. *Chest.* 1992;102: 557S–564S
108. Metheny NA, Eisenberg P, Spies M. Aspiration pneumonia in patients fed through nasoenteral tunes. *Heart Lung.* 1986;15: 256–261
109. Middleton RM, Kirkpatrick MB. Comparision of four methods to assess airway bacteriology in the intubated mechanically-ventilated patient. *Am Rev Respir Dis.* 1991;143:A107
110. Middleton RM, Huff W, Kirkpatrick NB. Utility of direct Gram stain from the protected specimen brush in the management of patients with presumed lower respiratory tract infection: a prospective study. *Am Rev Respir Dis.* 1993;147:A651
111. Moise PA, Forrest A, Bhavnani SM, Birmingham MC, Schentag JJ. Area under the inhibitory curve and a pneumonia scoring system for predicting outcomes of vancomycin therapy for respiratory infections by *Staphylococcus aureus*. *Am J Health Syst Pharm.* 2000;57:S4–S9
112. Montecalvo MA, Steger KA, Farber HW, et al Nutritional outcome and pneumonia in critical care patients randomized to gastric versus jejunal tube feedings. *Crit Care Med.* 1992;20: 1377–1387
113. Montravers P, Fagon JY, Chastre J, et al Follow-up protected specimen brushes to asses treatment in nosocomial pneumonia. *Am Rev Respir Dis.* 1993;147:38–44
114. Nakae T. Outer membrane permeability of bacteria. *Crit Rev Microbiol.* 1986;13:1–62
115. Neiderman MS. Bacterial adherence is a mechanism of airway colonization. *Eur J Clin Microbiol Infect Dis.* 1989;8:15–20

116. Neiderman MS, Merrill WW, Polomski L, et al Influence of sputum IgA and elastase on tracheal cell bacterial adherence. *Am Rev Respir Dis*. 1986;133:255–260
117. Neiderman MS, Craven DE, Fein AM, et al Pneumonia in the critically ill hospitalized patients. *Chest*. 1990;97:170–181
118. Neiderman MS, Bass JB, Campbell D, et al ATS Official Statement. Guidelines for the initial management of adults with community-acquired pneumonia: diagnosis, assessment of severity and initial antimicrobial therapy. *Am Rev Respir Dis*. 1993;148:1418–1426
119. Neuhauser MM, Weinstein RA, Rydman R, Danziger LH, Karam G, Quinn JP. Antibiotic resistance among gram-negative bacilli in US intensive care units: implications for fluoroquinolone use. *JAMA*. 2003;289:885–888
120. Nicolau DP, McNabb J, Lacy MK, Quintiliani R, Nightingale CH. Continuous versus intermittent administration of ceftazidime in intensive care unit patients with nosocomial pneumonia. *Int J Antimicrob Agents*. 2001;17:497–504
121. Palmer LB, Smaldone GC, Chen JJ, et al Aerosolized antibiotics and ventilator associated tracheobronchitis in the intensive care unit. *Crit Care Med*. 2008;36(7):2008–2013
122. Paterson DL. The epidemiological profile of infections with multidrug-resistant Pseudomonas aeruginosa and Acinetobacter species. *Clin Infect Dis*. 2006;43(Suppl 2):S432
123. Paterson DL, et al 39th ICAAC, San Fransisco 1999
124. Paterson DL, Ko WC, Von Gottberg A, et al Antibiotic therapy for *Klebsiella neumoniae* bacteremia: implications of production of extended-spectrum B-lactamases. *Clin Infect Dis*. 2004;39:31–37
125. Pedersen J, Schurizek BA, Melsen NC, Juhl B. the effect of nasotracheal intubation on the paransal sinuses. A prospective study of 434 intensive care patients. *Acta Anaesthesiol Scand*. 1991;35:11–13
126. Pham LH, Brun-Buisson C, Legrand P, et al Diagnosis of nosocomial pneumonia in mechanically ventilated patients. Comparison of a plugged telescoping catheter with the protected specimen brush. *Am Rev Respir Dis*. 1991;143:1055–1061
127. Pingleton SK, Fagon JY, Leeper KV Jr. Patient selection for clinical investigation of ventilator-associated pneumonia. Criteria for evaluating diagnostic techniques. *Chest*. 1992;102:553S
128. Poisson DM, Touquet S, Bercault N, Arbeille B. Electron microscopic description of accretions occurring in endotracheal tubes used in adults. *Pathol Biol (Paris)*. 1993;41:537–541

129. Puidupin M, Guiavarch M, Paris A, et al B- mode ultrasound in the diagnosis of maxillary sinusitis in intensive care unit. *Intensive Care Med*. 1997;23:1174–1175
130. Queenan AM, Foleno B, Gownley C, Wira E, Bush K. Effects of inoculum and -lactamase activity in AmpC- and extended-spectrum-lactamase (ESBL)-producing *Escherichia coli* and *Klebsiella pneumoniae* clinical isolates tested by using NCCLS ESBL methodology. *J Clin Microbiol*. 2004;42: 269–275
131. Rello J, Quintana E, Ausina V, et al Risk factors for Staphylococcus aureus pneumonia in critically ill patients. *Am Rev Respir Dis*. 1990;142:1320–1324
132. Rello J, Kollef M, Diaz E, et al Reduced burden of bacterial airway colonization with a novel silver-coated endotracheal tube in a randomized multiple-center feasibility study. *Crit Care Med*. 2006;34:2766
133. Rouby JJ, De Lassale EM, Poete P, et al Nosocomial broncho-pneumonia in the critically ill: histologic and bacteriologic aspects. *Am Rev Respir Dis*. 1992;148:1059–1066
134. Rouby JJ, Laurent P, Gosnach M, et al Risk factors and clinical relevance of nosocomial maxillary sinusitis in the critically ill. *Am J Respir Crit Care Med*. 1994;150:776–783
135. Rubinstein E, Lode H, Grassi C, Antibiotic Study Group. Ceftazidime monotherapy vs. ceftriaxone/tobramycin for serious hospital-acquired gram-negative infections. *Clin Infect Dis.* 1995;20:1217–1228
136. Rubinstein E, Cammarata S, Oliphant T, Wunderink R. Linezolid Nosocomial Pneumonia Study Group. Linezolid (PNU-100766) versus vancomycin in the treatment of hospitalized patients with nosocomial pneumonia: a randomized, double blind, multicenter study. *Clin Infect Dis*. 2001;32: 402 412
137. Rundcrantz H. Postural variations of nasal patency. *Acta Otolryngol*. 1969;68:435–443
138. Safdar N, Crnich CJ, Maki DG. The pathogenesis of ventilator-associated pneumonia: its relevance to developing effective strategies for prevention. *Respir Care*. 2005;50:725
139. Sanchez Garcia M, Cambronero Galache JA, Lopez Diaz J, et al Effectiveness and cost of selective decontamination of the digestive tract in critically ill intubated patients. A randomized, double-blind, placebo-controlled, multicenter trial. *Am J Respir Crit Care Med*. 1998;158:908

140. Sanders CC, Sander WEJ. Beta-lactam resistance in gram-negative bacteria: global trends and clinical impact. *Clin Infect Dis*. 1992;15:824–839
141. Scheld WM. Maintaining fluoroquinolone class efficacy: review of influencing factors. *Emerg Infect Dis*. 2003;9:1–9
142. Sheth NK, Franson TR, Rose HD, et al Colonization of bacteria on polyvinylchloride and Teflon intravascular catheters in hospitalized patients. *J Clin Microbiol*. 1983;18:1061
143. Sieger B, Berman SJ, Geckler RW, Farkas SA. Meropenem Lower Respiratory Infection Group. Empiric treatment of hospital-acquired lower respiratory tract infections with meropenem or ceftazidime with tobramycin: a randomized study. *Crit Care Med*. 1997;25:1663–1670
144. Silver DR, Cohen IL, Weinberg PF. Recurrent *Pseudomonas aeruginosa* pneumonia in an intensive care unit. *Chest*. 1992; 101:194–198
145. Singh N, Rogers P, Atwood CW, Wagener MM, Yu VL. Short-course empiric antibiotic therapy for patients with pulmonary infiltrates in the intensive care unit: a proposed solution for indiscriminate antibiotic prescription. *Am J Respir Crit Care Med*. 2000;162:505–511
146. Sole-Violan J, Rodriguez de Castro F, Rey A, et al Usefulness of microscopic examination of intracellular organisms in lavage fluid in ventilator-associated pneumonia. *Chest*. 1994; 106: 889–894
147. Souweine B, Mom T, Traore O, et al Ventilator- associated sinusitis: microbiological results of sinus aspirates in patients on antibiotics. *Anesthesiology*. 2000;93:1255–1260
148. Stauffer JL, Olson DE, Petty TL. Complications and consequences of endotracheal intubation and tracheostomy. *Am J Med*. 1981;70:65–76
149. Sutherland KR, Steinberg KP, Maunder RJ, et al Pulmonary infection during the acute respiratory distress syndrome. *Am J Respir Crit Care Med*. 1995;152:550–556
150. Timsit JF, Lescale O, Misset B, et al Repeatability of protected specimen brush (PSB) sampling techniques between French centers. *Am Rev Respir Dis*. 1993;147:A654
151. Torres A, Valencia M. Does ventilator-associated tracheo-bronchitis need antibiotic treatment? *Crit Care*. 2005;9: 255–256
152. Torres A, De La Bellacasa JP, Rodriquez-Roisin R, et al Diagnostic value of telescoping plugged catheters in mechanically

ventilated patients with bacterial pneumonia using the Metras catheter. *Am Rev Respir Dis.* 1988;138:117–120
153. Torres A, Aznar R, Gatell JM, et al Incidence, risk, and prognosis factors of nosocomial pneumonia in mechanically ventilated patients. *Am Rev Respir Dis*. 1990;142:523–528
154. Torres A, El-Ebiary M, F'abregas N, et al Value of intracellular bacteria detection in the diagnosis of ventilator-associated pneumonia. *Thorax*. 1996;51:378–384
155. Treloar DM, Stechmiller J. Pulmonary aspiration in tube-fed patients with artificial airways. *Heart Lung*. 1984;13: 667–671
156. Tremblay LN, Slutsky AS. Ventilator-induced injury: from barotrauma to biotrauma. *Proc Assoc Am Phys*. 1998;110:482
157. Tryba M. Risk of acute stress bleeding and nosocomial pneumonia in ventilated intensive care unit patients: Sucralfate versus antacids. *Am J Med*. 1987;83(Suppl 3B): 117–124
158. Tryba M. Sucralfate versus antacids or H2-antagonists for stress ulcer prophylaxis: a meta-analysis on efficacy and pneumonia rate. *Crit Care Med*. 1991;19:942–949
159. Valenti WM, Trudell RG, Bentley DW. Factors predisposing to oropharyngeal colonization with gram-negative bacilli in the aged. *N Engl J Med*. 1978;298:1108–1111
160. Van Saene HFK, Stoutenbeek CC, Stoller JK. Selective decontamionation of digestive tract in the intensive care unit: current Status and future prospects. *Crit Care Med*. 1992;20:691–703
161. Verbrugge SJ, Sorm V, Vant V, et al Lung overinflation without positive end-expiratory pressure promotes bacteremia after experimental Klebsiella pneumoniae inoculation. *Inten Care Med*. 1998;24:172
162. West M, Boulanger BR, Fogarty C, et al Levofloxacin compared with imipenem/cilastatin followed by ciprofloxacin in adult patients with nosocomial pneumonia: a multicenter, prospective, randomized, open-label study. *Clin Ther*. 2003; 25:485–506
163. Westergern V, Berg S, Lundgren J. Ultrasonographic bedside evaluation of maxillary sinus disease in mechanically ventilated patients. *Intensive Care Med*. 1997;23:393–398
164. Wood GC, Swanson JM. Aerosolized antibacterials for the prevention and treatment of hospital acquired pneumonia. *Drugs*. 2007;67:903–917

165. Wood GC, Hanes SD, Croce MA, Fabian TC, Boucher BA. Comparison of ampicillin–sulbactam and imipenem–cilastatin for the treatment of *Acinetobacter* ventilator-associated pneumonia. *Clin Infect Dis*. 2002;34:1425–1430
166. Wunderink RG, Rello J, Cammarata SK, Croos-Dabrera RV, Kollef MH. Linezolid vs vancomycin: analysis of two double-blind studies of patients with methicillin-resistant *Staphylococcus aureus* nosocomial pneumonia. *Chest*. 2003;124: 1789–1797

Chapter 12
Discontinuation of Mechanical Ventilation

Wean (v.t.): induce (when applied to suckling) to feed otherwise than from the breast; cure of, (or) rescue from habit

The Oxford Dictionary

In its truest sense, *weaning* implies a gradual separation of the patient from the ventilator. During this gradual process, the patient is given increasing responsibility for his breathing, culminating in spontaneous unassisted respiration. In actual fact, abrupt separation of the patient from the ventilator is possible, and so the term weaning has been broadened to include rapid separation from the ventilator – as generally occurs in postoperative circumstances – in addition to the more gradual separation as seen, for example, in patients with chronic obstructive lung disease.[37]

The word "separation" has been used to illustrate the process of disengagement from the ventilator; "liberation" means almost the same thing, although it is more evocative of a sense of release and of improvement beyond the need for ventilator support. Some authors have adopted the term "discontinuation" which tacitly implies that the separation is more or less permanent.

Weaning is a crucial milestone for the ventilated patient. The timing of weaning is vital: the price to pay for a premature extubation is reintubation, with all the hazards of a possibly unstable clinical situation – in addition to a significant risk of nosocomial pneumonia. On the other hand, unnecessarily delayed weaning can expose the patient to the risks

A. Hasan, *Understanding Mechanical Ventilation*,
DOI: 10.1007/978-1-84882-869-8_12,

associated with protracted mechanical ventilation. Care must, therefore, be taken to plan for this important event and prepare the patient beforehand.

Weaning should be considered as soon as the patient has recovered sufficiently from his illness to be able to endure the responsibility of sustained spontaneous breathing. The condition for which the patient was ventilated should have improved significantly, although incomplete resolution does not preclude successful weaning. Other prerequisites to weaning include a stable cardiovascular condition and a preserved sensorium. Although it is possible to successfully wean unconscious patients, the ability of these patients to defend their airway is a major concern, and aspiration is always a possibility when the removal of the cuffed endotracheal tube has left the airway unprotected. A reasonable hemoglobin level improves O_2 carriage to the tissues and a normal serum electrolyte level and a well-nourished state further decrease the possibility of respiratory muscle fatigue during the weaning trial.

Certain factors may hamper the weaning process, either by imposing an excessive load upon the respiratory system, or by depressing the neural output from the respiratory center. Metabolic alkalosis depresses the respiratory drive and should be corrected prior to weaning. Gastric distension of any cause offers resistance to the diaphragmatic excursion and so increases the work of breathing. Drugs including sedatives, neuromuscular paralyzing agents, and aminoglycosides should be avoided; while sedatives depress the respiratory center, aminoglycosides and paralyzing agents act on the neuromuscular junctions preventing optimal respiratory muscle contraction.

Weaning is also a stress test – for the left ventricle particularly – and may unmask LV dysfunction (see section 9.1). Sleep deprivation is ubiquitous in a noisy ICU, and can delay weaning through several mechanisms (see Box 12.1).

Box 12.1 The Effect of Sleep Deprivation on the Weaning Process

Decreased ventilatory response to hypercapnia[5]
Decreased ventilatory response to hypoxia[46]
Increased collapsibility of upper airway[35]
Negative nitrogen balance[29]
Decreased respiratory muscle endurance[5]
Increased oxygen consumption[1]
Increased carbon dioxide production[1]

12.1 Weaning Parameters

Since the timing of weaning is so crucial, it is necessary to have reliable information that can help determine the success of the weaning trial. Studies have shown the fallibility of clinical judgment in this regard, and objective predictors have been evolved to assist in the decision-making process.[40]

Often, there is a delay in contemplating weaning. Reliable predictors would obviate unwarranted prolongation of mechanical ventilation by helping to recognize the weanable patient early.[43] Predictors also have the potential for identifying specific physiological derangements responsible for weaning failure. At present, no single predictor, or set of predictors, has the desired reliability.

Weaning parameters can be divided into those that assess the following indices: the oxygenating capabilities of the patient's lungs, the strength and stamina of the respiratory muscles, the respiratory drive, and the work of breathing. Composite indices draw from these categories (see Fig. 12.1).

Weaning criteria are numerically almost identical to those for intubation and ventilation; the major difference lies in that the former are applied in an improving clinical situation, whereas

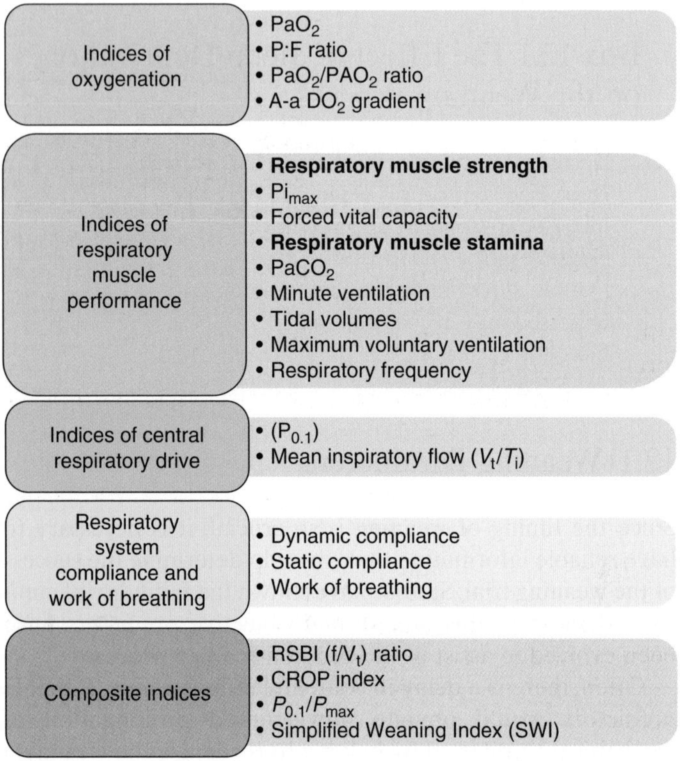
Indices of oxygenation
• PaO_2
• P:F ratio
• PaO_2/PAO_2 ratio
• A-a DO_2 gradient
Indices of respiratory muscle performance
• **Respiratory muscle strength**
• Pi_{max}
• Forced vital capacity
• **Respiratory muscle stamina**
• $PaCO_2$
• Minute ventilation
• Tidal volumes
• Maximum voluntary ventilation
• Respiratory frequency
Indices of central respiratory drive
• ($P_{0.1}$)
• Mean inspiratory flow (V_t/T_i)
Respiratory system compliance and work of breathing
• Dynamic compliance
• Static compliance
• Work of breathing
Composite indices
• RSBI (f/V_t) ratio
• CROP index
• $P_{0.1}/P_{max}$
• Simplified Weaning Index (SWI)

FIGURE 12.1. Weaning indices.

the latter are used under worsening clinical circumstances. Thus, weaning should first be contemplated when the parameters that necessitated ventilation have begun to improve.

12.2 Parameters that Assess Adequacy of Oxygenation

Once off the ventilator, the patient will be capable of being supported reasonably well if he can saturate his hemoglobin with a level of supplementary oxygen that can be delivered by conventional oxygen systems. If on a FIO_2 of 0.4, the arterial oxygen tension is in excess of 55 mmHg, the patient is likely to be operating above the top of the steep part of oxyhemoglobin dissociation curve and his hemoglobin would, thus, be near-saturated. Accordingly, an ability to raise the PaO_2 to 55 mmHg while being given 40% oxygen by the ventilator (with <5cm PEEP) is one of the important indices for discontinuation of mechanical ventilation. In fact, once off the ventilator, the patient is usually given 50–60% oxygen with conventionally available oxygen delivery systems, and this should move him to the top flat part of the oxyhemoglobin dissociation curve and so confer an added measure of safety against hypoxemia.

While operating on the steep part of the oxyhemoglobin dissociation curve, small decrements in PaO_2 produce a steep fall in the hemoglobin saturation, whereas small increments in PaO_2 produce a sharp rise in the hemoglobin saturation. Since the object is to avoid desaturation of hemoglobin with any fluctuations in the PaO_2 that may occur, it is desirable to keep the patient operating on the top *flat* portion of the oxyhemoglobin dissociation curve.

12.2.1 The PaO_2:FIO_2 Ratio

Other indices of oxygenation can also be used in place of PaO_2. Although the P:F ratio (PaO_2/FIO_2 ratio) has been shown to predict weaning successfully in 90% of the patients,[17] it was demonstrably less effective in predicting whether a patient would *fail* a weaning attempt (i.e., its positive predictive value was good, but the negative predictive value poor). The cut-off

TABLE 12.1. Indices of oxygenation.

Parameter of oxygenation	Weaning threshold
PaO_2 (on FIO_2 0.5 and PEEP 5 cm H_2O]	>60 mmHg
PaO_2/FIO_2 ratio ("PF" ratio)	>200
PaO_2/PAO_2 ratio	>0.35
Alveolo-arterial oxygen gradient (A-aDO_2)	<350 mmHg on FIO_2 1.0
Shunt fraction (Qs/Qt ratio)	<0.2 (<20% shunt)

value for the P:F ratio determined in one study to separate weaning success from failure was 238 (roughly equal to a PaO_2 of 50 mmHg while breathing the equivalent of room air).

12.2.2 The A-a DO_2 Gradient

This parameter reflects the ease of oxygen movement from the lungs to the pulmonary capillaries. A high A-a DO_2 indicates that the lungs are poorly capable of oxygenating the blood. Interpreting the A-a DO_2 is easier at the extremes of FIO_2, viz, on 0.21 (room air) and on 100% FIO_2. In normal lungs, the A-a DO_2 is less than 12–15 mmHg on room air and less than 70 mmHg on 100% oxygen. The A-a DO_2 physiologically rises with an increase in FIO_2 and this makes it difficult to interpret on intermediate ranges of FIO_2 (see section 7.1). For a patient on the threshold of weaning, A-a DO_2 of less than 350 on 100% oxygen implies weanability from the oxygenation standpoint.

12.2.3 The PaO_2/PAO_2 Ratio

The PaO_2/PAO_2 ratio is considered a somewhat better index of oxygenation. However, it too has relatively poor positive and negative predictive values for weaning (when a PaO_2/PAO_2 ratio of 0.35 was taken, the positive predictive value was 0.59 and negative predictive value was 0.53).[30,47]

12.3 Parameters that Assess Respiratory Muscle Performance

12.3.1 PI_{max}

One of the time-honored (but possibly not time tested!) measures of respiratory muscle strength is the maximum inspiratory pressure (PI_{max}). PI_{max} is measured when the patient exhales completely to residual volume and then makes a maximum

TABLE 12.2. Indices of respiratory muscle strength and endurance.

Parameter of respiratory muscle performance	Weaning threshold
Respiratory muscle strength	
PI_{max}	<-15 to -30 cm H_2O
Forced VC	>10–15 mL/kg
Respiratory muscle endurance	
$PaCO_2$	<50 mmHg
Minute ventilation (spontaneous)	<10–15 L/min
Tidal volumes	>5 mL/kg
Maximum voluntary ventilation	>20 L/min
Respiratory frequency	<35 breaths/min or >6 breaths/min
f/Vt ratio	<105 breaths/min/L

inspiratory effort against an occluded airway. PI_{max} assesses not only the strength of the diaphragm – which is of course the most important muscle of inspiration – but the collective strength of all the inspiratory muscles. A PI_{max} of less than minus 30 cm H_2O (the ability of the respiratory muscles to generate a negative pressure of at least 30 cm H_2O) is believed to predict successful weaning. Likewise, an inability of respiratory muscles to generate a negative pressure of more than –20 cm H_2O is considered to be predictive of weaning failure (Table 12.2).[30]

Since the maximum inspiratory force is an index of the force the diaphragm can generate, it is essentially an index of strength. Strength does not equate with stamina and the PI_{max} gives no information whatsoever about the diaphragm's ability to *sustain* ventilation. The PI_{max}, therefore, is less effective in assessing the resistance of the diaphragm to fatigue and this is probably the reason the PI_{max} threshold values mentioned earlier (–30 cm H_2O and –20 cm H_2O) are relatively poor in predicting weaning success and failure, respectively.

12.3.2 Vital Capacity

Vital capacity (VC) is a measure of respiratory muscle strength. Measurements of VC have been found to be generally erratic in predicting weaning outcome, and therefore, VC rarely weighs in as a factor for determining weanability. A VC threshold of >10 mL/kg has been proposed as a predictor of successful weaning (the normal VC ranges from 65 to 75 mL/kg).

12.3.3 Minute Ventilation

Another time-honored but perhaps equally unreliable index of weaning is the minute ventilation. Logic dictates that a patient whose cardiopulmonary status has improved and who is therefore weanable, should breathe in a relatively relaxed manner and thus would have a relatively low minute volume. Normal minute ventilation is approximately 6 L/min.[41] A minute ventilation of less than 10 L/min was regarded as an indicator of successful weanability,[11] but again contradictions have surfaced, some studies[47] showing it to be a poor correlate of successful weaning.

12.3.4 Respiratory Rate

The value of physical signs has always been paramount in all aspects of medicine. A thorough physical examination of the spontaneously breathing patient is invaluable. Use of the accessory muscles of respiration is a sign of excessive effort and indicates increased work of breathing. The recruitment of the sternocleidomastoid and ala nasi muscles and the retraction of the intercostal spaces is a sign of excessive effort, whereas paradoxical movement of the diaphragm is a sign that fatigue has set in.

An elevated respiratory rate is perhaps the earliest sign of respiratory muscle fatigue,[34] especially if tidal volumes are falling. A rising heart rate is also a sign that the patient is failing the weaning trial. Respiratory alternans is a late sign of respiratory muscle fatigue and the patient should never be allowed to progress to this stage.

TABLE 12.3. Indices of central respiratory drive.

Parameters that assess central respiratory drive	Weaning threshold
Airway occlusion pressure ($P_{0.1}$)	<2 cm H_2O
Mean inspiratory flow (V_t/T_i)	Low

12.4 Parameters that Assess Central Respiratory Drive

12.4.1 Airway Occlusion Pressure

Airway occlusion pressure ($P_{0.1}$) is determined by making an inspiratory effort against an occluded airway and measuring the airway pressure 0.1 s after the initiation of the inspiratory effort. $P_{0.1}$ is a measure of the intensity of the respiratory drive (normal $P_{0.1}$ values <2 cm H_2O). High values indicate an abnormally high respiratory drive, and therefore, predict weaning failure. It has been shown in some studies that $P_{0.1}$ values above four have a high correlation with weaning failure,[3,11,31] but other studies have yielded conflicting information, and the status of $P_{0.1}$ as a weaning parameter remains uncertain (Table 12.3).

12.4.2 Mean Inspiratory Flow (V_t/T_i)

A drawback of the airway occlusion pressure is that its frequent measurement can modify the respiratory drive.[45] The mean inspiratory flow (V_t/T_i), essentially a ratio of the tidal volume to the inspiratory time, does not suffer from this limitation. Nevertheless, the V_t/T_i is a measure of events taking place much further from the brainstem than is the $P_{0.1}$, and therefore, may considerably underestimate the respiratory drive.[44]

12.5 Respiratory System Compliance and Work of Breathing

12.5.1 Work of Breathing

Unlike the PI_{max}, the work of breathing looks at the ability of the respiratory muscles to endure a *sustained* inspiratory load. At rest, in healthy persons, the work of breathing per liter averages about 0.47 J/L; the average work per minute of ventilation is 4.33 J/min. If the work of breathing is high, the respiratory muscles are clearly making heavy weather of the imposed resistive load, and weaning failure is anticipated. On the other hand, even an excessive work of breathing has been associated with weaning success, and as such, a moderately elevated work of breathing cannot be taken to presage weaning failure (Table 12.4).

Part of the work of breathing in a patient on a spontaneous mode of ventilation is due to the inspiratory resistance imposed by the narrow lumen of the endotracheal tube and by the long ventilator circuits (as discussed in Chap. 3, both the length and luminal diameter of breathing tubes are determinants of airway resistance). It is possible that extubating a patient could take away this component of inspiratory resistance (namely the endotracheal tube and ventilatory circuits) and actually reduce the work of breathing.

On a level of pressure support that is theorically high enough to completely compensate for the inspiratory resistance that is imposed by the ventilator circuitry and the endotracheal tube, increased work of breathing would likely

Table 12.4. Mechanical indices of weaning.

Respiratory system compliance and work of breathing	Weaning threshold
Dynamic compliance	>22 mL/cm H_2O
Static compliance	>33 mL/cm H_2O
Work of breathing	0.47 J/L or 33 J/min

be on account of factors intrinsic to the patient (e.g., high airway resistance or stiff lungs). Under such circumstances, the work of breathing can be expected to be high even after extubation, with the prospect of weaning failure.

12.5.2 Compliance of the Respiratory System

A poorly compliant respiratory system can substantially increase the work of breathing. While operating on the flatter portions of the pressure volume curve, a large inspiratory effort is required to inflate the lungs. A poorly compliant respiratory system may also reflect an unresolved pathologic process within the lung, the pleura, or the chest wall.

The normal static compliance is 60–100 mL/cm H_2O. (Note that these measurements need to be made when the inspiratory muscles are completely at rest: any respiratory muscle activity would bear upon the measured pressures giving fallacious values. Accurate measurement of compliance of the respiratory system would require a well sedated and/or paralyzed patient.) Although C_{dyn} values of >22 mL/cm H_2O and C_{stat} values of >33 mL/cm H_2O are conventionally accepted weaning criteria, one study did find limited predictive values for both weaning success and failure when a respiratory system compliance of 33 mL/cm H_2O was taken as a weaning threshold.[47]

12.6 Integrative Indices

Weaning frequently depends upon the performance of several components of the respiratory system. The simultaneous appraisal of the parameters that reflect these components would be expected to enhance the predictability of its success or failure. As the above discussion may illustrate, many of the solitary indices for the prediction of successful weaning have

TABLE 12.5. Composite indices.

Composite indices	
RSBI (f/Vt) ratio	<105 breaths/min
CROP index	>13 mL/breaths/min
$P_{0.1}/P_{max}$	≤0.9
SWI	<9/min

not been validated with prospective studies. Attempts have been made to combine several of these parameters into integrative indices, so that better predictability of weaning outcome might be possible (Table 12.5).

Respiratory muscle fatigue is associated with falling tidal volumes along with a rise in respiratory frequency, as the patient strives to sustain a minute volume appropriate to his needs. Combining the respiratory rate and tidal volume into an integrative index has been shown to considerably raise the individual predictive power of these two indices. The f/V_t ratio (respiratory frequency divided by the tidal volumes in liters), also called the RSBI (rapid shallow breathing index), has strong positive and negative predictive values of 0.79 and 0.95, respectively,[47] at a cut-off value of 105.

It was, however, found in a separate study[18] that it was not possible to use this index with any degree of certainty in patients whose tidal volumes were boosted with pressure support. It remains a matter for speculation whether this index will validate itself if “just enough” pressure support is used to counter the additional inspiratory resistance imposed by the ventilator circuitry and the endotracheal tube (thereby simulating the inspiratory resistance of the extubated patient as closely as possible). It is also difficult to compute what would constitute “just enough” pressure support as the inspiratory load would vary not only with the caliber of the endotracheal tube, but also with the length of ventilator circuitry and the presence of in-line HMEs. The inspiratory load would also depend upon unquantifiable variables such as secretions within the lumen of the endotracheal tube (since even a minimal compromise in airway diameter can translate into a major increase in airway resistance).[28] At least one study has shown that there is a wide interpatient variability in the level of pressure support that is required to offset the inspiratory load of the endotracheal tube and ventilator circuits.[24]

12.6.1 Simplified Weaning Index (SWI)

The SWI is a measure of the respiratory muscle endurance as well as the efficiency of gas exchange of a patient's lungs.[13] The measurements are made while the patient is receiving full ventilator support.

Box 12.2 Simplified Weaning Index (SWI)

$SWI > [f\,(PIP-PEEP)/MIP] \times [PaCO_2/40]$

f > frequency of respiration

PIP > peak Inspiratory pressure

PEEP > positive end-expiratory pressure

MIP > maximal inspiratory pressure (the maximal negative pressure recorded during a 20-s occlusion of the airway.

An SWI of >9 predicts weaning success 93% of the time; an SWI of >11 is associated with weaning failure.

Box 12.3 The Compliance, Rate, Oxygenation, and Pressure (CROP) Index

The CROP index factors in not only the demands on the respiratory system, but also the ability of the respiratory muscles to handle these demands.

CROP index > $[Cdyn \times MIP \times (PaO_2/PAO_2)]/f$
Cdyn > dynamic compliance
MIP > maximal inspiratory pressure (the maximal negative pressure recorded during a 20-s occlusion of the airway.
PaO_2 > Oxygen tension of the arterial blood
PAO_2 > Oxygen tension of the alveolar air
f > frequency of respiration.
A CROP index of >13 mL/breath per min generally correlates with successful weaning: in one prospective study, its positive and negative predictive values were determined to be 71 and 70%, respectively[47].

Box 12.4 Pressure-Time Product (PTI)

The PTI is another integrative index: it is the time integral of respiratory muscle pressure. Since it quantifies the minute ventilation required to maintain the $PaCO_2$ at 40 mmHg (VE40), it is essentially a measure of respiratory muscle endurance, in addition to being a measure of gas exchange.[13]

12.7 Methods of Weaning

Weaning can either be accomplished by trials of spontaneous breathing on the endotracheal tube for progressively longer periods of time, or by gradually decreasing the level of support on IMV, SIMV+PS, or pressure support ventilation (PSV). As a lead-up to either method, the tidal volumes delivered by the ventilator should be reduced to the tidal volumes the patient is expected to generate when the mechanical ventilatory support is discontinued. Many COPD patients are expected to retain some amount of CO_2 even when they are clinically stable, and their $PaCO_2$ levels should be brought up slowly to their expected "baseline" before commencement of the weaning trial.

12.7.1 Trials of Spontaneous Breathing (T-Piece Weaning)

During a T-piece trial, the patient is disconnected from the ventilator, a T-piece is attached to the endotracheal tube, and an appropriate concentration of O_2 is administered through one limb of the T-piece. The patient is encouraged to breathe on his own through the endotracheal tube, initially for brief intervals of time. These periods of spontaneous breathing are progressively lengthened until the patient is capable of breathing on his own for a reasonable period of time without manifesting any signs of distress.

What constitutes a "reasonable period of time" has not been determined, but clinical experience predicts weanability when the patient is able to comfortably tolerate spontaneous T-piece breathing for 1–24 h. Shorter trials of between 30 and 120 min of spontaneous breathing may be just as effective in predicting weaning success.[7] Neither has it been resolved what intervals of "rest" on the ventilator are optimal between attempts at spontaneous breathing,[6] but again clinical experience points to a range of 1–3 h as sufficient. It is possible that even as few as one trial of spontaneous breathing a day is sufficient.

Trials of spontaneous breathing should be terminated immediately at any stage should any signs of cardiorespiratory distress develop (Fig. 12.2).

Although relatively more labor intensive for the nursing staff and respiratory therapists, the T-piece method serves quite well in patients without significant lung disease. The danger lies in that prolonged trials of spontaneous breathing can deplete

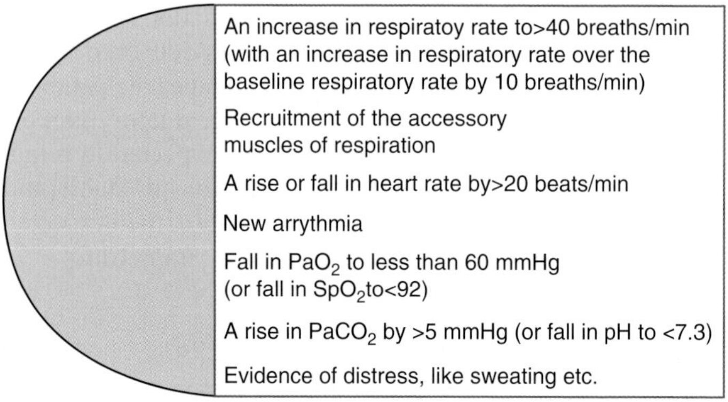
An increase in respiratoy rate to>40 breaths/min (with an increase in respiratory rate over the baseline respiratory rate by 10 breaths/min)
Recruitment of the accessory muscles of respiration
A rise or fall in heart rate by>20 beats/min
New arrythmia
Fall in PaO_2 to less than 60 mmHg (or fall in $SpO_2$to<92)
A rise in $PaCO_2$ by >5 mmHg (or fall in pH to <7.3)
Evidence of distress, like sweating etc.

FIGURE 12.2. Indications for the termination of spontaneous breathing trial.

the tenuous respiratory reserve of a patient with a compromised cardiorespiratory status. Once pushed to the brink of respiratory muscle fatigue, the patient may then require a protracted period of rest; optimization of ventilator strategies is also crucial to the avoidance of excessive work of breathing in order that respiratory muscle strength may be regained.

Not surprisingly, therefore, the emphasis is now shifting to a strategy which applies a limited number of weaning trials a day. Some investigators now regard once a day trials of spontaneous breathing as sufficient to achieve successful weaning without running the risk of exhausting a patient with prolonged periods of spontaneous breathing.

12.7.2 Synchronized IMV

This is one of the methods where the burden of breathing is initially shared between the patient and ventilator; the workload of respiration is gradually transferred to the patient. Enough mandatory breaths are given so that the targeted $PaCO_2$ is achieved without causing the patient any difficulty in breathing. The mandatory breaths are reduced by 1–3 breaths/min at each step. A blood gas sample obtaining after 30 min of reducing the IMV frequency on each occasion enables close monitoring of the $PaCO_2$ and the pH. If the pH continues to remain at a level above 7.35, gradual reduction of the mandatory breaths is continued with blood gas monitoring at each step, until an IMV rate of zero is arrived at. When the patient is able to breathe comfortably at this level for 24 h, extubation is carried out.

The mandatory breaths given in the above protocol are usually synchronized with the patient's inspiratory efforts (SIMV) to avoid any undue work of breathing. The work of breathing can be significant when the patient's attempts to trigger inspiration are not followed by an immediate delivery of a tidal breath.[9,10] In spite of synchronization of the mandatory breaths, a considerable amount of work of breathing can still be done when mandatory breaths are progressively decreased in a stepwise fashion,[22] presumably because of the inability of the respiratory center to cope straightaway with the increased demands imposed upon it.[12] Thus, it appears that intermittent mandatory ventilation – in which the mandatory breaths are perceived to provide supported breaths to the patient and thus reduce the work of breathing – may sometimes actually have the opposite effect and contribute to respiratory muscle fatigue and hamper weaning.[6]

12.7.3 Pressure Support Ventilation (PSV)

In the PSV mode a certain level of pressure support is preset, and this level of pressure is sustained throughout the inspiratory breath till the airflow falls to about 25% of its peak value; at this point, the breath is terminated and exhalation occurs. In weaning, by this mode the physician-preset pressure support level is gradually and progressively reduced and the patient is considered ready for extubation when spontaneous breathing occurs without any sign of distress at a pressure support level of 3–5 cm H_2O, which is the level considered to roughly offset endotracheal tube and ventilator circuit resistance.[2,8] One adapted weaning algorithm is suggested below[15] (Fig. 12.3).

In theory, PSV is an entirely more comfortable mode of ventilation (or of weaning). The patient is afforded much

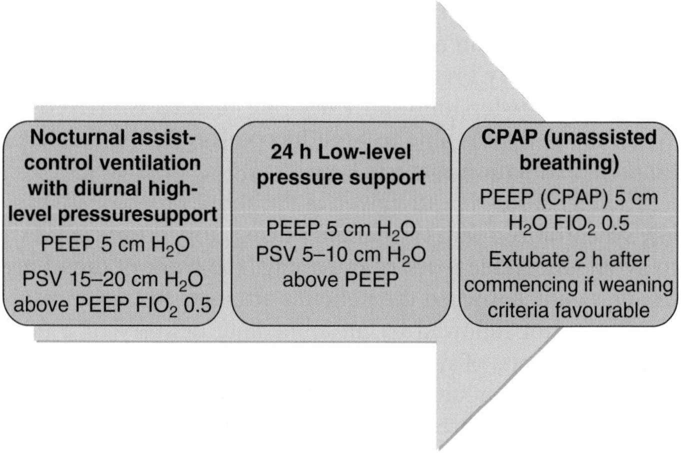
Nocturnal assist-control ventilation with diurnal high-level pressuresupport
PEEP 5 cm H2O
PSV 15–20 cm H2O above PEEP FIO2 0.5
24 h Low-level pressure support
PEEP 5 cm H2O
PSV 5–10 cm H2O above PEEP
CPAP (unassisted breathing)
PEEP (CPAP) 5 cm H2O FIO2 0.5
Extubate 2 h after commencing if weaning criteria favourable

FIGURE 12.3. Weaning with Pressure Support.

more flexibility in the sense that the rate, depth, and flow of the inspired breath can be controlled by the patient according to his or her needs.[21]

Although PSV should offer a near-ideal way to wean, its use is still dogged with controversies and plagued with conflicting results from different studies.[26,39] As discussed in an earlier section, an important step in reducing the work of breathing is to negate the additional inspiratory load imposed by the endotracheal tube and ventilator circuits, by adding an equivalent amount of pressure support. This is easier said than done, because the amount of the inspiratory load contributed by these is extremely difficult to estimate (Fig. 12.3).

Since even a small decrease in endotracheal tube caliber will result in a very large increase in airflow resistance,any internal crusting is enough to create a substantial increase in resistance. Furthermore, different flow rates can also cause airway resistance to vary. Since in PSV the flow rates are largely controlled by the patient, they may differ from breath to breath making even rough estimates of airflow resistance virtually impossible.

Another drawback to weaning by this mode is that due to narrow airways in the obstructed patient, inspiration is frequently prolonged and flow may fail to fall quickly to the level of the peak flow that signals cycling from inspiration to expiration. In such circumstances, the patient may initiate expiration while the ventilator is yet in the process of delivering its breath. Clashing of patient with the ventilator consequently occurs, which considerably interferes with the process of weaning.

12.7.4 Noninvasive Positive Pressure Ventilation (NIPPV)

Not only does NIPPV help decrease the intubation rate in acute type II respiratory failure in COPD patients, but also achieves a high weaning rate.[27] The role of the NIPPV in the weaning of patients with nonhypercapnic respiratory failure is less clear and probably less important. The success of NIPPV can be seriously compromised if leaks are allowed to occur. An ill fitting mask or a large air leak through the mouth while using a nasal mask may severely limit the success of NIPPV as a weaning mode.

12.7.5 Extubation

Weaning is not synonymous with extubation[36]. Extubation should be carried out only after the patient's ability to protect the airway is assured, the prerequisite of which is a satisfactory level of consciousness; a score of >8 on the glasgow coma

Blotter method	Spirometric method
• ETT is disconnected from the ventilator circuit • An index card or a blotting paper is held about 1–2 cm away from the end of the ETT • The patient is instructed to cough forcefully • An ability to moisten the card with three out of four cough attempts correlates 3 times more strongly with successful extubation than does an inability to do so[16]	• A spirometer is introduced into the ventilator circuit • The patient is instructed to cough forcefully • The cough peak flow is measured on the spirometer • A cough peak flow of 60L/min or more correlates 5 times more strongly with successful extubation than does a cough peak flow <60L/min[38]

FIGURE 12.4. Assessment of the strength of cough.

Qualitative assessment for airway patency	Quantitative assessment for airway patency
• The ETT cuff is deflated • The chest piece of the stethoscope is placed on the trachea • A "leak-squeak" during a ventilator delivered positive pressure breath indicates that there is adequate space around the ETT • Lack of a leak-squeak implies the presence of laryngeal edema. And this usually presages extubation failure	• The ETT cuff is deflated • The inpiratory tidal volume and the expiratory tidal volume are both noted for each of six successive breaths • The difference between the inpiratory tidal volume and the expiratory tidal volume is in essence the cuff leak volume • The average of lowest three readings of the cuff leak volume is calculated[23]

FIGURE 12.5. Evaluation of the airway prior to extubation.

scale (GCS) correlates positively with successful extubation.[25] A good cough reflex is also vital; the strength of cough may be assessed by using an index card or a blotting paper, or more formally, by spirometry (see Fig. 12.4).

Box 12.4 Technique of Extubation

The patient is propped up into a sitting position (Fowler's or semi-Fowler's)
Preoxygenation with 100% O_2
The mouth and throat are thoroughly suctioned
The tapes securing the ET tube are loosened
As the cuff is deflated, a fairly large breath is provided
The patient is instructed to cough vigorously as the tube is withdrawn
The ET cuff is completely deflated
The tube is withdrawn in a single swift
The patient is made to cough once more after the withdrawal of the tube
The mouth and throat are suctioned once again
Oxygen is administered through a facemask
The patient's condition, breathing pattern, vitals, ECG, and SpO_2 are closely monitored

Copious airway secretions increase the likelihood of extubation failure.[16] The need for frequent suctioning – e.g., more than once every couple of hours – indicates that extubation is better deferred.

Finally, laryngeal edema or other upper airway problems can compromise the success of extubation, and it is essential to assess the patency of the upper airway before removing the endotracheal tube (Fig. 12.5).

References

1. Bonnet MH, Berry RB, Arand DL. Metabolism during normal, fragmented, and recovery sleep. *J Appl Physiol.* 1991;71:1112–1118
2. Brochard L, Rna F, Lorino H, Lemaire F, Harf A. Inspiratory pressure support compensates for the additional work of breathing caused by the endotracheal tube. *Anesthesiology*. 1991;75:739
3. Capdevila XJ, Perrigault PF, Perey PJ, et al Occlusion pressure and its ratio to maximum inspiratory pressure are useful predictors for successful extubation following T-piece weaning trial. *Chest*. 1995;108:482
4. Chatila W, Ani S, Guaglianone D, et al Cardiac ischemia during weaning from mechanical ventilation. *Chest*. 1996;109:1577–1583.
5. Cooper KR, Phillips BA. Effect of short-term sleep loss on breathing. *J Appl Physiol*. 1982;53:855–858
6. Esteban A, Frutos F, Tobin MJ, et al A comparison of four methods of weaning patients from mechanical ventilation. *N Engl J Med*. 1995;332:345
7. Esteban A, Alia I, Tobin MJ, et al Effect of spontaneous breathing trial duration on outcome of attempts to discontinue mechanical ventilation. *Am J Respir Crit Care Med*. 1999;159:512
8. Fiastro JF, Habib MP, Quan SF. Pressure support compensation for inspiratory work due to endotracheal tubes and demand continuous positive airway pressure. *Chest*. 1988;93:499
9. Gherini S, Peters RM, Virgilio RW. Mechanical work on the lungs and work of breathing with positive end-expiratory pressure and continuous positive airway pressure. *Chest*. 1979;76:251
10. Gibney RTN, Wilson RS, Pontoppidan H. Comparison of work of breathing on high gas flow and demand valve continuous positive airway pressure systems. *Chest*. 1982;82:692

11. Herrera M, Blasco J, Venegas J, et al Mouth occlusion pressure (P0.1) in acute respiratory failure. *Intensive Care Med.* 1985; 11:134
12. Imsand C, Feihl F, Perret C, Fitting JW. Regulation of inspiratory neuromuscular output during synchronised intermittent mechanical ventilation. *Anesthesiol.* 1994;80:13
13. Jabour ER, Rabil DM, Truwit JD, Rochester DF. Evaluation of a new weaning index based on ventilatory endurance and the efficiency of gas exchange. *Am Rev Respir Dis.* 1991;144:531
14. Jubran A, Tobin MJ. Pathophysiologic basis of acute respiratory distress in patients who fail a trial of weaning mechanical ventilation. *Am J Respir Crit Care Med.* 1997;155:906–915
15. Kallet RH, Corral W, Silverman HJ, Luce JM. Implementation of a low tidal volume ventilation protocol for patients with acute lung injury or acute respiratory distress syndrome. *Respir Care.* 2001;46(10):1024–1037
16. Khamiees M, Raju P, DeGirolamo A, et al Predictors of extubation outcome in patients who have successfully completed a spontaneous breathing trial. *Chest.* 2001;120:1262
17. Krieger BP, Ershowsky PF, Becker DA, Gazeroglu HB. Evaluation of conventional criteria for predicting successful weaning from mechanical ventilatory support in elderly patients. *Crit Care Med.* 1989;17:858
18. Lee KH, Hui KP, Chan TB, et al Rapid shallow breathing (frequency-tidal volume ratio) did not predict extubation outcome. *Chest.* 1994;105:540
19. Leiter JC, Knuth SL, Bartlett D Jr. The effect of sleep deprivation on activity of the genioglossus muscle. *Am Rev Respir Dis.* 1985;132:1242–1245
20. Lemaire F, Teboul JL, Cinotti L, et al Acute left ventricular dysfunction during unsuccessful weaning from mechanical ventilation. *Anesthesiology.* 1988;69:171–179
21. MacIntyre NR. Respiratory function during pressure support ventilation. *Chest.* 1986;89:117
22. Marini JJ, Smith TC, Lamb VJ. External work output and force generation during synchronised intermittent mandatory ventilation: effect of machine assistance on breathing effort. *Am Rev Respir Dis.* 1988;138:1169
23. Miller RL, Cole RP. Association between reduced cuff leak volume and postextubation stridor. *Chest.* 1996;110:1035
24. Montgomery AB, Holle RHO, Neagley SR, et al Prediction of successful ventilator weaning using airway occlusion pressure and hypercapnic challenge. *Chest.* 1987;91:496

25. Namen AM, Ely EW, Tatter SB, et al Predictors of successful extubation in neurosurgical patients. *Am J Respir Crit Care Med.* 2001;163:658
26. Nathan SD, Ishaaya AM, Koerner SK, Belman MJ. Prediction of minimal pressure support during weaning from mechanical ventilation. *Chest.* 1993;103:1215
27. Nava S, Ambrosino N, Clini E, et al Non-invasive mechanical ventilation in the weaning of patients with respiratory failure due to chronic obstructive pulmonary disease. A randomised, controlled trial. *Ann Intern Med.* 1998;128:72
28. Proctor HJ, Woolson R. Prediction of respiratory muscle fatigue by measurements of the work of breathing. *Surg Gynecol Obstet.* 1973;136:367
29. Rechtschaffen A, Gilliland MA, Bergmann BM, et al Physiological correlates of prolonged sleep deprivation in rats. *Science.* 1983;221:182–184
30. Sahn SA, Lakshminarayan S. Bedside criteria for discontinuation of mechanical ventilation. *Chest.* 1973;63:1002
31. Sassoon CSH, Mahutte CK. Airway occlusion pressure and breathing pattern as predictors of weaning outcome. *Am Rev Respir Dis.* 1993;148:860
32. Sassoon CSH, Te TT, Mahutte CK, Light RW. Airway occlusion pressure: an important indicator for successful weaning in patients with chronic obstructive pulmonary disease. *Am Rev Respir Dis.* 1987;135:107
33. Scrimshaw NS, Habicht JP, Pellet P, et al Effects of sleep deprivation and reversal of diurnal activity on protein metabolism of young men. *Am J Clin Nutr.* 1919;5:313–319
34. Semmes BJ, Tobin MJ, Snyder JV, Grenvik A. Subjective and objective measurement of tidal volume of critically ill patients. *Chest.* 1985;87:577
35. Series F, Roy N, Marc I. Effect of sleep deprivation and sleep fragmentation on upper airway collapsibility in normal subjects. *Am J Respir Crit Care Med.* 1994;150:481–485
36. Sharar S. Weaning and extubation are not the same. *Respir Care.* 1995;40:239–243
37. Slutsky AS. Mechanical ventilation. American College of Chest Physicians' Consensus Conference. *Chest.* 1993;104:1833
38. Smina M, Salam A, Khamiees M, et al Cough peak flows and extubation outcomes. *Chest.* 2003;124:262
39. Straus C, Louis B, Isabey D, et al Contribution of the endotracheal tube and the upper airway to breathing workload. *Am J Respir Crit Care Med.* 1998;157:23

40. Stroetz RW, Hubmayr RD. Tidal volume maintenance during weaning with pressure support. *Am J Respir Crit Care Med.* 1995;152:1034
41. Tobin MJ. Non invasive monitoring of ventilation. In: Tobin MJ, ed. *Principles and practice of intensive care monitoring*. New York: Mc Graw-Hill; 1998:465–495
42. Tobin MJ, Jubran A. Variable performance of weaning-predictor tests: role of Bayes'theorem and spectrum and test-referral bias. *Intensive Care Med*. 2006;32:2002
43. Tobin MJ, Jubran A. Weaning from mechanical ventilation. In: Jubran A, Tobin MJ, eds. *Principles and Practice of Mechanical Ventilation*. New York: McGraw Hill; 2006:1185
44. Tobin MJ, Jubran A. In: Tobin MJ, ed. *Principles and Practice of Mechanical Ventilation.* McGraw-Hill; 2006 p 1185–1220
45. Tobin MJ, Mador MJ, Guenther SM, Lodato RF, Sackner MA. Variability of resting respiratory drive and timing in healthy subjects. *J Appl Physiol*. 1988;65:309–317
46. White DP, Douglas NJ, Pickett CK, et al Sleep deprivation and the control of ventilation. *Am Rev Respir Dis*. 1983;128:984–986
47. Yang K, Tobin MJ. A prospective study of indexes predicting outcome of trials of weaning from mechanical ventilation. *N Engl J Med*. 1991;324:1445

Chapter 13
Noninvasive Ventilation in Acute Respiratory Failure

Noninvasive ventilation (NIV) entails the administration of positive pressure breaths through the patient's innate airway by means of a close-fitting mask.

13.1 NIV and CPAP

CPAP and NIV are not synonymous. CPAP involves the application of a constant positive pressure to the airway, while the patient spontaneously breathes. Positive pressure breaths are not dispensed and therefore it is not considered a true mode of ventilation. NIV, on the other hand, does provide pressure mechanical breaths, with the objective of boosting tidal volumes and unloading the respiratory muscles; it can therefore be considered a true mode of mechanical ventilation.

13.2 Mechanism of Action

The mechanisms by which NIV improves gas exchange in chronic respiratory failure are not well understood, but can presumed to be more or less similar to those in invasive mechanical ventilation. It is likely that NIV rests the respiratory muscles and reduces pulmonary microatelectasis by the positive pressure it generates. With chronic use, NIV will also

A. Hasan, *Understanding Mechanical Ventilation*,
DOI: 10.1007/978-1-84882-869-8_13,

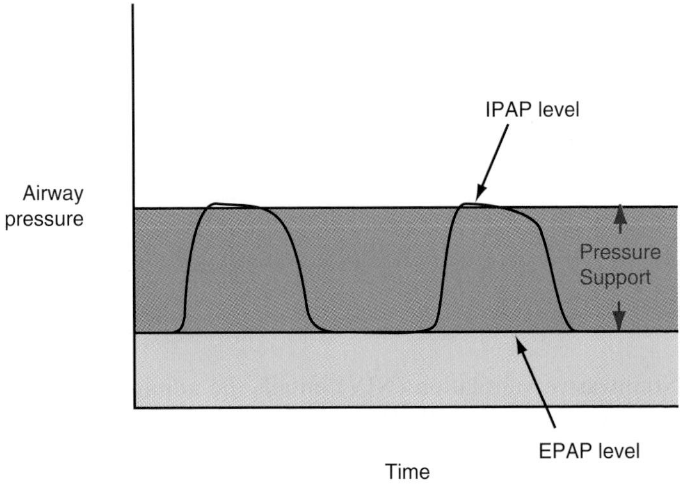
IPAP level
Airway pressure
Pressure Support
EPAP level
Time

FIGURE 13.1. Relationship between PSV, inspiratory positive airway pressure (IPAP), and expiratory positive airway pressure (EPAP).

prevent nocturnal hypoventilation and reset upward the set-point for CO_2. In COPD, NIV likely produces improvements by partly offsetting auto-PEEP and reducing the work of breathing. Any or all of these may contribute to the benefits that accrue (Fig. 13.2).

One of the principal advantages of NIV is in the avoidance of the infections that are associated with the placement of an endotracheal tube. With the innate airway preserved, the patient is able to vocalize, eat, and cough effectively.

Although the use of NIV in several forms of acute respiratory failure (ARF) has been validated, the goals of NIV in many of these situations are disparate. In type I respiratory failure, the aim is to decrease hypoxemia until the process responsible for ARF has resolved. An additional objective in COPD is to unload respiratory muscles and decrease the work of breathing.

In ARF, the role of NIV may be conceptualized as an attempt to avert invasive mechanical ventilation, but recourse

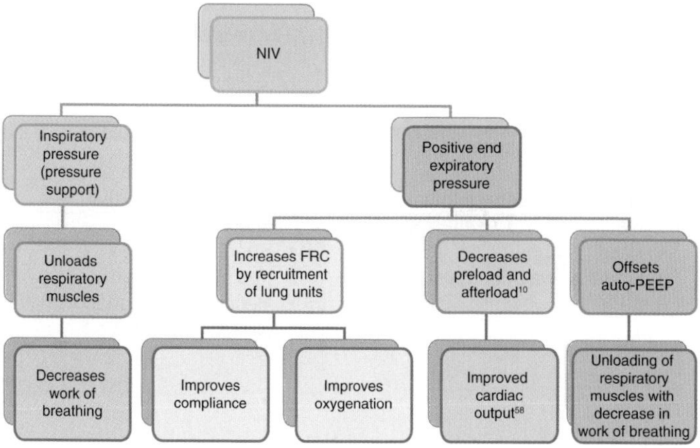
NIV
Inspiratory pressure (pressure support)
Positive end expiratory pressure
Unloads respiratory muscles
Increases FRC by recruitment of lung units
Decreases preload and afterload[10]
Offsets auto-PEEP
Decreases work of breathing
Improves compliance
Improves oxygenation
Improved cardiac output[58]
Unloading of respiratory muscles with decrease in work of breathing

FIGURE 13.2. Mechanisms by which noninvasive ventilation (NIV) improves gas exchange.

to the latter must necessarily be taken in a patient with severe respiratory failure, or in a patient who is failing a trial of NIV. NIV in an unstable patient should always be used within an ICU where personnel and facilities for invasive ventilation are present; invasive mechanical ventilation will eventually be needed in as many as 40% of patients in ARF who are initially treated with NIV.[23]

Nonetheless, the usage of NIV in early respiratory failure has been associated with a gratifying success rate,[20] although, with the currently approved selection criteria, it is presently not possible to predict outcome in a given case. NIV has been shown to be beneficial in acute exacerbations of COPD [15,45,84] and in cardiogenic pulmonary edema.[50,55] NIV has also been widely used as a weaning mode for patients with COPD.[30,59]

It is important to remember that where there is an urgent need for intubation and ventilation, invasive mechanical ventilation must be initiated without delay. Indeed, it has been seen that perseverance with NIV in these situations and

Absolute contraindications

- Need for urgent intubation
- Severe hemodynamic compromise
- Coma, or severe bulbar weakness
- Facial trauma
- Upper airway obstruction

Relative contraindications

- Confusion
- Moderate bulbar weakness
- Unstable angina or evolving myocardial infection
- Poor cough reflex
- Facial deformity
- Recent esophageal or gastric surgery

FIGURE 13.3. Contraindications to NIV.

inordinate delay in the institution of invasive mechanical ventilation have actually been associated with a higher mortality (Fig. 13.3).[82]

The terms CPAP (on the portable ventilator) and PEEP (on a critical care ventilator) are often used interchangeably. On a portable machine, the IPAP is the sum of PSV and PEEP (i.e., the sum of PSV and EPAP). The PSV level (the difference between the IPAP and EPAP) is the real determinant of the inspiratory assistance. Thus, an increase in tidal volume can be accomplished by either increasing the IPAP (without altering the EPAP), or by decreasing the EPAP (without altering the IPAP), both of which will cause the PSV to increase.

13.2.1 *Interface*

Atleast six types of interfaces are now available. In the acute setting, NIV is normally administered by a firmly fitting mask. Cuffs made of soft rubber or plastic help in achieving an effective seal. Six types of masks are now available (Fig. 13.4). In cases where mask fit is problematic, customized masks can be made.

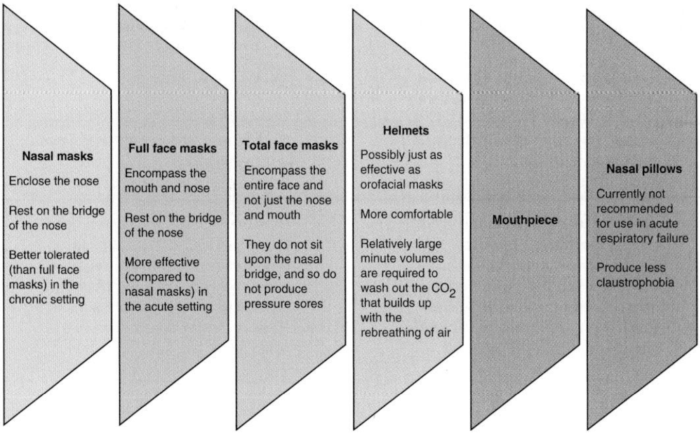
Nasal masks
Enclose the nose
Rest on the bridge of the nose
Better tolerated (than full face masks) in the chronic setting
Full face masks
Encompass the mouth and nose
Rest on the bridge of the nose
More effective (compared to nasal masks) in the acute setting
Total face masks
Encompass the entire face and not just the nose and mouth
They do not sit upon the nasal bridge, and so do not produce pressure sores
Helmets
Possibly just as effective as orofacial masks
More comfortable
Relatively large minute volumes are required to wash out the CO2 that builds up with the rebreathing of air
Mouthpiece
Nasal pillows
Currently not recommended for use in acute respiratory failure
Produce less claustrophobia

FIGURE 13.4. Types of commercially available interfaces.

Either a nasal or a full face mask can be used; each has its special advantages. Total face masks and "helmets" are now available. The nasal plug type "minimasks" are currently not recommended for acute care NIV. Standard nasal masks are available in various sizes and the option of having a choice of size is important to assure a snug, leak-proof, and yet comfortable fit in a given patient. The choice of the right mask size will often prove critical to the success of the NIV. Normally, the selected mask size should be the smallest that fits properly over the nose. A mask that is too large can leak.

Resistance to airflow through the nasal passages can be significant and this may prove to be an important factor at a low level of pressure support (Fig. 13.5).[30]

Being of a much larger volume, the orofacial mask can theoretically increase the dead space; clinically important increases in $PaCO_2$ have, however, rarely been seen to occur.[69,73] In spite of this, arterial blood gases may take longer to normalize with nasal than orofacial masks.[54]

Data on the relative efficacy of nasal and orofacial masks are scant; in acute settings, outcomes appear to be better with the face mask.[60] Therefore, even though patients cannot be as

Nasal mask	Orofacial mask
• Prone to mouth leakages. Leaks may comromise the efficacy of the system	• Mouth covered by the mask
• Less dead space	• More dead space
• Possibly less effective than the orofacial mask in acute situations	• Possibly more effective than nasal mask in acute situations
• Does not work when nasal passages are obstructed	• Not dependent on patency of nasal passages for its efficacy
• Relatively low risk of aspiration since mouth offers egress for vomitus	• Relatively high risk of aspiration since both mouth and nose are covered
• Patient communication more effective	• Patient communication more effective
• Eating, drinking, and expectoration is possible without removal of the mask	• Eating, drinking, and expectoration is possible without removal of the mask
• More comfortable compared to orofacial mask: as a result, better tolerated	• Relatively uncomfortable compared to nasal mask

FIGURE 13.5. A comparison of nasal and orofacial masks.

satisfactorily monitored for aspiration with face masks as they can with nasal masks, the overall superiority of the face mask over the nasal mask may well favor its use, at least at the time of commencement of NIV.[1] On the other hand, in chronic respiratory failure, nasal masks are clearly better tolerated.[60] The preference of the user should be factored into the choice of the mask.

Masks are held in place with head-straps and care must be taken to ensure that these are not secured too tightly in an endeavor to ensure a tight seal between the mask and the face. A too-tight fit can in fact exacerbate air leakage and decrease patient compliance: the head gear should be strapped loosely enough to permit the insertion of a couple of fingers between the strapping and the face (see *air leaks* below).

The patency of the airway within the nose is crucial to the success of a nasal mask, and a topical nasal decongestant may be used as required.

13.2.2 Modes

Most critical care ventilators in current use have capabilities to administer NIV. Either volume-cycled or pressure-cycled ventilation may be utilized.[40] PSV,[15] bilevel positive airway pressure, and CPAP have all been shown to be effective in treating COPD.[45,84]

13.2.3 Devices

Contemporary microprocessor-controlled ventilators of the ICU offer sensitive methods of monitoring the various ventilator parameters, and enable delivery of accurate FIO_2s.[29,44] Large air leaks in the circuit at the patient-mask interface can be reliably detected, and failure rates of NIV thus minimized. In addition, because the inspiratory and expiratory tubings are discrete, these ventilators reduce CO_2 rebreathing. For this reason, it was recommended by several authors that NIV be administered by a standard ventilator in the setting of ARF.[28] Indeed, for the delivery of NIV in acute care units, critical care ventilators have traditionally been favored over the portable bilevel devices.

Dedicated bilevel devices are increasingly becoming sophisticated, and now incorporate better triggering and cycling mechanisms, superior leak compensation, and more alarms. Their performance can now be considered comparable to critical care ventilators.[16] It is probably not important which of the two is used for noninvasive ventilation.

In respect of intubated patients, however, there are clear differences in performance. At low expiratory pressures (around 2–3 cm H_2O), Work of breathing seems to be substantially higher with bilevel ventilators than with critical care ventilators. However, with higher set expiratory pressures (around 5 cm H_2O), there appears to be little difference between the two presumably because $PEEP_i$ is better counterbalanced in the latter circumstance.[63]

With critical care ventilators, internal blenders enable the delivery of an FIO_2 which is more precise.[19] The FIO_2 in bilevel devices depends on the liter-flow of oxygen connected into the circuit from an external source. With the high inspiratory flows that are generated by these machines, an FIO_2 of over 0.5 is seldom possible. The newer bilevel ventilators (such as the Vision™ of Respironics) are fitted with oxygen blenders.

13.2.4 Humidification with NIV (see also Chap. 15)

Whereas portable ventilators use ambient air as the gas-source, critical care ventilators operate on dry air. As a consequence, airway drying is much more common when critical care ventilators are used: this makes airway humidification mandatory.

As far as humidification devices go, HMEs and pass-through humidifiers can considerably increase the work of breathing and may make triggering difficult. Therefore, neither of these ought to be used with NIV: only pass-over humidifiers seem to be suitable at present.

13.3 Air Leaks

Unlike invasive mechanical ventilation, NIV is not a completely closed system and so some air leakage is inevitable. Air leaks from the mouth can compromise the effectiveness of the system, and make it difficult to monitor the delivered tidal volumes. Chin straps are sometimes used to reduce mouth leaks, with variable efficacy.

A full face mask will be effective even if the patient chooses to breathe through the mouth, though air can still leak around the mask apron. Small air leaks at the interface between the mask and the face are in fact common and do not necessarily compromise the effectiveness of ventilation; however, large air leaks can lead to failure of NIV. The full face mask requires a lower amount of patient cooperation, since failure to keep the mouth closed will still result in effective ventilation. Large air leaks will sometimes prevent ventilator cycling, leading to asynchrony between the patient and the machine (see Fig. 13.6). Portable ventilators now have mechanisms for leak compensation, but most critical care machines are less efficient at this.

Unidirectional air leaks through the mouth can produce nasal mucosal drying.[68] The release of local chemokines can then increase nasal airflow resistance, further increasing air

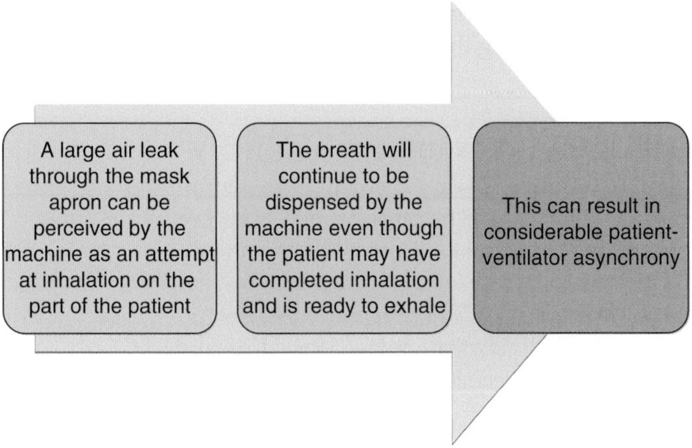
A large air leak through the mask apron can be perceived by the machine as an attempt at inhalation on the part of the patient
The breath will continue to be dispensed by the machine even though the patient may have completed inhalation and is ready to exhale
This can result in considerable patient-ventilator asynchrony

FIGURE 13.6. Patient-ventilator asynchrony with air leaks.

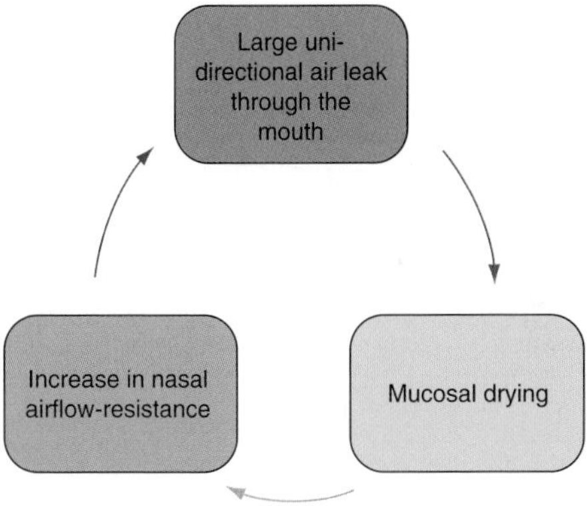
Large uni-directional air leak through the mouth
Mucosal drying
Increase in nasal airflow-resistance

FIGURE 13.7. Unidirectional air leak through the mouth.

leakage through the mouth.[79] The use of heated humidifiers by increasing upper airway humidification may be helpful (Fig. 13.7).[52]

The capacity for leak compensation can vary substantially between ventilators.[56] Pressure-targeted ventilators are superior at compensating for air leaks since they are capable of generating high peak inspiratory flows (120–180 L/min). With volume targeted ventilators, loss of tidal volumes can exceed

50%, but it should be possible to compensate for moderate leaks by increasing the set tidal volumes.[76]

Box 13.1 Advantages of NIPPV

Early support possible, and this may avert need for invasive ventilation with all its attendant complications.
Normal eating, drinking, and communication possible.
Intermittent ventilatory support is possible.
Ventilation in step-down areas (outside ICU) possible.

Box 13.2 Disadvantages of NIPPV

May delay invasive ventilation
Airway protection is suboptimal
Risk of aspiration, especially in obtunded patients
Pressure sores over nasal bridge
Bloating of stomach
Lack of access to the tracheobronchial tree where secretions are troublesome
Claustrophobic patients find mask ventilation distressing
Labor intensive

13.4 Indications for NIV

13.4.1 Hypoxemic Respiratory Failure

The causes of acute hypoxemic respiratory failure (AHRF) are varied, and therefore, the response to NIV in AHRF as a class is not predictable.[6,41,51]

The proportion of patients failing NIV – and subsequently requiring mechanical ventilation – appears to be higher when the respiratory failure is hypoxemic, rather than when it occurs in the setting of COPD (see below). Nevertheless, the use of NIV in ARF has been shown to decrease the length of ICU admission, the incidence of nosocomial pneumonia and sinusitis, and the duration of mechanical ventilation when it was subsequently required.

Significantly, mortality in patients who fail NIV and subsequently require mechanical ventilation tends to be extremely high. This could reflect the severity of disease in patients who progress to endotracheal intubation; equally, it is possible that such patients would have been better off without NIV from the outset, a delay in intubation and the initiation of invasive mechanical ventilation possibly having contributed to the mortality.[82]

Cardiogenic pulmonary edema: outcomes are frequently favorable with NIV in cardiogenic pulmonary edema,[12] and this seems logical considering that positive intrathoracic pressure decreases both preload and afterload. NIV does not appear to hold special advantages over CPAP in this setting, except possibly in patients at risk for intubation,[53] or in whom CPAP has been unsuccessful in reducing the work of breathing.

At least one study has determined that reduced rates of endotracheal intubation in patients treated with NIV do not translate into improved survival.[56] In this study, NIV treated patients had an increased incidence of transmural infarction. It was proposed that methodological limitations may have led to this conclusion and that the results in this study may have been biased by the randomization of a large number of patients with evolving myocardial infarction into the NIV group.[1] On the other hand, it could well be that the rise in intrathoracic pressure could have contributed to myocardial ischemia. Until the issue is clarified, the use of NIV in acute myocardial infarction or active cardiac ischemia should be undertaken with due caution.[14,62]

For patients with pulmonary edema, CPAP should be the noninvasive modality first offered; NIV can be subsequently used if work of breathing remains high or if CO_2 retention is problematic[37]; patients in severe respiratory failure or in whom the respiratory failure cannot be expected to resolve promptly should be intubated forthwith.

13.4.2 Hypercapnic Respitatory Failure

13.4.2.1 COPD Exacerbation

NIV is now an accepted first-line intervention for the hypercapnic respiratory failure of COPD.[21,31,61] The scope of NIV in acute hypercapnic exacerbation of COPD is extensive, and patients have benefited frequently – but not always – with NIV.[13] NIV significantly decreased the rate of intubation, mortality, and length of ICU stay in several trials.[15,45,84] Methodological factors confound the important question as to which subset of patients is likely to benefit from NIV alone, and in what group of patients should endotracheal intubation and invasive mechanical ventilation be directly instituted without a preceding trial of NIV.[42] At the present time it would appear that some patients presenting with exacerbations of COPD are either too ill to require mechanical ventilation straightaway, or not ill enough to require even NIV support; this would leave a group of COPD patients in whom conventional supportive therapy would be likely to fail, and in whom NIV would potentially avert the necessity of invasive mechanical ventilation (Fig. 13.8).[15]

Studies have mostly failed to identify candidates who would be likely to benefit from NIV in COPD exacerbations.[2,35] However, the potential benefits of NIV in COPD exacerbations are great, and unless respiratory failure is advanced, many clinicians feel justified in routinely using NIV in acute hypercapnic COPD exacerbations – provided no contraindications exist – and proceed with the institution of invasive mechanical ventilatory support should patients show a lack of response to the NIV trial.

The most commonly used – and possibly the most effective – mode in COPD exacerbations appears to be PSV (10–15 cm H_2O) with added CPAP (4–8 cm H_2O).[4] The CPAP, by

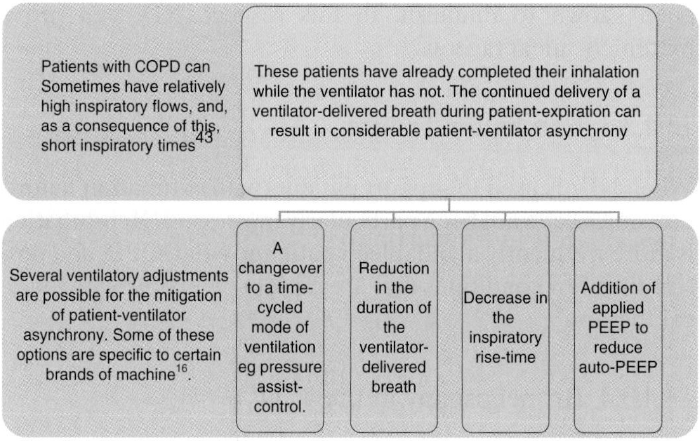
Patients with COPD can Sometimes have relatively high inspiratory flows, and, as a consequence of this, short inspiratory times43
These patients have already completed their inhalation while the ventilator has not. The continued delivery of a ventilator-delivered breath during patient-expiration can result in considerable patient-ventilator asynchrony
Several ventilatory adjustments are possible for the mitigation of patient-ventilator asynchrony. Some of these options are specific to certain brands of machine16.
A changeover to a time-cycled mode of ventilation eg pressure assist-control.
Reduction in the duration of the ventilator-delivered breath
Decrease in the inspiratory rise-time
Addition of applied PEEP to reduce auto-PEEP

FIGURE 13.8. Patient-ventilator asynchrony in COPD patients.

decreasing the inspiratory threshold, enables a greater unloading of the respiratory muscles than does PSV alone.[10]

13.4.2.2 Decompensated Obstructive Sleep Apnea

Lower respiratory tract infections are probably the commonest cause of acute or chronic respiratory failure in patients with OSA. In these patients NIV can be used with benefit.[65]

13.4.3 Miscellaneous Indications

13.4.3.1 Weaning

The role of NIV in weaning has been considered in (Chap. 12.7.4)

13.4.3.2 Acute Respiratory Failure in Immunocompromised Patients

By the very avoidance of endotracheal tube, the risk of nosocomial pneumonia in immunocompromised patients has been shown to diminish. In this respect, NIV can prove extremely advantageous.[3]

13.4.3.3 Extubation Failure

When NIV is used to support patients with extubation failure, outcomes have not been particularly impressive. Reintubation is more frequently avoidable in patients with COPD, and possibly in a few conditions that are rapidly reversible with medical therapy.

13.4.3.4 Bronchoscopy in the ICU

In selected patients with borderline blood gases, NIV can facilitate bronchoscopy[7] and upper GI endoscopy[32] in the intensive care unit; the use of the modern "helmet" has been impressive in increasing patient-comfort and reducing the technical demands on the bronchoscopist.[8]

13.4.4 Steps for the Initiation of NIV

NIV may be initiated either by the incremental (the "high-low") method or the decremental (the "low-high") method (Fig. 13.9) [15,45].

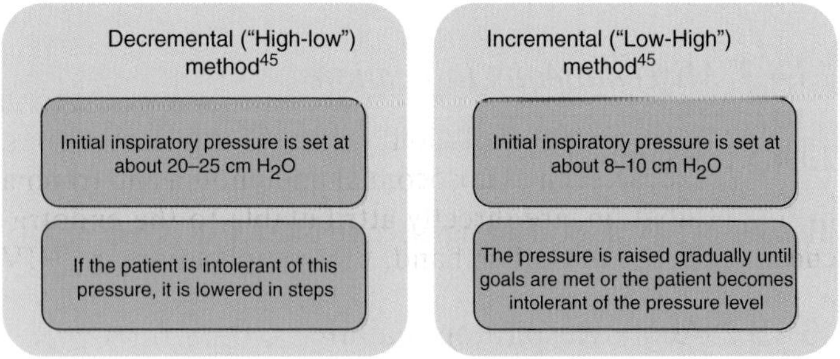
Decremental ("High-low") method[45]
Initial inspiratory pressure is set at about 20–25 cm H_2O
If the patient is intolerant of this pressure, it is lowered in steps
Incremental ("Low-High") method[45]
Initial inspiratory pressure is set at about 8–10 cm H_2O
The pressure is raised gradually until goals are met or the patient becomes intolerant of the pressure level

FIGURE 13.9. The high-low and the low-high methods of initiating NIV.

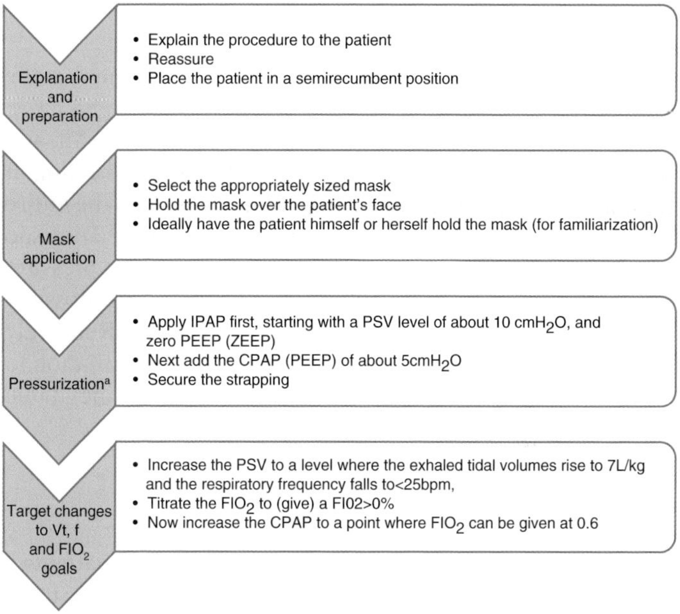
Explanation and preparation
• Explain the procedure to the patient
• Reassure
• Place the patient in a semirecumbent position
Mask application
• Select the appropriately sized mask
• Hold the mask over the patient's face
• Ideally have the patient himself or herself hold the mask (for familiarization)
Pressurization[a]
• Apply IPAP first, starting with a PSV level of about 10 cmH_2O, and zero PEEP (ZEEP)
• Next add the CPAP (PEEP) of about 5cmH_2O
• Secure the strapping
Target changes to Vt, f and FIO_2 goals
• Increase the PSV to a level where the exhaled tidal volumes rise to 7L/kg and the respiratory frequency falls to<25bpm,
• Titrate the FIO_2 to (give) a FI02>0%
• Now increase the CPAP to a point where FIO_2 can be given at 0.6

FIGURE 13.10. Protocol for the initiation of NIV.

One adaptation of the low-high method[38,54] is described in Fig. 13.10.

13.4.5 Complications

Invasive mechanical ventilation is clearly fraught with risks. Several of these, such as nosocomial pneumonia and trauma during intubation, are directly attributable to the endotracheal tube. On the other hand, the complications of NIV are few and infrequent. NIV, at least in theory, can reduce the incidence of nosocomial pneumonia, though the methodology of the studies which suggest this needs critical reappraisal.

13.4.5.1 Skin Ulceration

Pressure necrosis of the skin on the bridge of the nose is the commonest complication of mask-NIV.[36] It can, by and large, be prevented by careful attention to the mask size, its fit, and harness tension. Changing the interface may allow healing of the dermal lesion. Total face masks that encompass the entire face – not just the nose and mouth – are available.[26] These do not sit upon the nasal bridge and so do not produce pressure sores. Compared to orofacial masks, "helmets" are possibly just as effective,[9] and certainly more comfortable.[80] Relatively large minute volumes are required for effective ventilation to prevent the CO_2 retention that occurs with the inevitable rebreathing of air with "helmets."[78]

13.4.5.2 Gastric Distension

Gastric distension can occur in as many as half of all patients.[49] This is more often the case when volume-control NIV is used. Since the resting tone of the esophageal sphincter almost always exceeds 20 mmHg – and is frequently even higher – it will invariably exceed the inspiratory pressures that are usual during NIV.[33] Air insufflation into the stomach is consequently mild, and specific measures to reduce abdominal distension are generally not necessary. When a relatively high insufflation pressure is being used – especially in the presence of a lax esophageal sphincter – discomfort may result.

When thoracic impedance is high, the stomach will be more easily distended by air. Symptoms usually respond to a reduction in mask pressure or to administration of simethicone. In a few cases, changeover from volume-limited to pressure-limited ventilation may be required. Nasogastric tube placement may help, but should not be used "prophylactically."

13.4.5.3 Otalgia

Sinus or ear pain can result from the increased air pressure within the upper airways.

13.4.5.4 Eye Irritation

[49]This can occur due to air leakage from under the apron of the mask. Again excessive strap tension may be causal. Consideration must be given to reducing strap tension, changing mask size, and using emollient eye drops.

13.4.5.5 Hemodynamic Compromise

NIV is known to cause negligible hemodynamic compromise.[23] Certainly, compared with invasive mechanical ventilation, the amount of hemodynamic compromise produced by NIV appears to be minimal.[36] The possibility of hemodynamic depression is greater at higher levels of pressure. The implications of using NIV in patients with evolving myocardial infarction have been mentioned earlier in this chapter.

13.4.5.6 Barotrauma

Barotrauma rarely, if ever, occurs because the insufflation pressures used are relatively low.[27]

13.4.5.7 Asphyxiation with Aspiration

This is another potentially serious complication associated with NIV. Coma or profound bulbar weakness constitutes a contraindication to NIV, and extreme caution is warranted when the patient is confused or has a poor cough reflex. Since orofacial masks allow little egress for vomitus, asphyxiation is much more of a concern with these, than with nasal masks. The presence of an ileus constitutes a relative contraindication to the use of NIV. Gastric decompression with nasogastric tubes is not considered routine with NIV, but may be beneficial when abdominal distension or nausea – which frequently presage emesis and asphyxiation – is present.

Asphyxiation is also possible should ventilator failure occur, and masks these days are designed with straps that can be quickly released; some masks incorporate antiasphyxia valves.

13.4.5.8 Monitoring

One of the crucial factors that determine the success of NIV is patient monitoring. Since it cannot be predetermined whether a given patient on NIV will eventually require invasive mechanical ventilation, early recognition of a failing NIV trial is vitally important if endotracheal intubation is to be carried out in time. Therefore, until it is certain that the patient has clinically stabilized, the patient should be closely observed in an ICU, with meticulous monitoring of vital data, cardiac rhythm, oxygen saturation, and blood gases.

Worsening respiratory failure is obviously one of the prime indications for intubation, and a patient whose $PaCO_2$ worsens over 1–2 h – or indeed fails to improve in about 4 h – must be considered for invasive ventilation.[25] Excessive secretions and a lack of ability to defend the airways are other indications for intubation.

13.4.6 Contraindications

The use of NIV requires the fulfilling of certain preconditions. A normal or a near-normal bulbar function is required. A preserved ability to clear airway secretions and to defend the airway against aspiration, hemodynamic stability, intact gastrointestinal motility, and an ability to cooperate with the treatment are further requirements. Since preservation of the airway reflexes and patient cooperation are essential, it is not possible to heavily sedate (or paralyze) a patient who is synchronizing poorly with the machine. Contraindications to NIV have been summarized in Fig. 13.3.

13.4.7 Outcomes

As mentioned earlier, there are as yet no firm predictors of the outcome of NIV. It has been seen that if an improvement in the respiratory rate and arterial pH is not manifest within 30–120 min of initiation of NIV, the likelihood of success with continued NIV is low (Box 13.3).

When a large air leak exists, there is a significant loss of airway pressure and of tidal volumes. In this situation too, NIV is liable to fail. Excessive airway secretions, a depressed sensorium, inability to coordinate with the NIV breath, high APACHE scores, and a low pH prior to the commencement of NIV have all been linked with significant failure rates.

Box 13.3 Predictors of Failure with NIPPV

Low pH prior to commencement of NIPPV
No improvement in respiratory rates and pH within 30–120 min of applying NIPPV
Significant air leakages
Excessive secretions
Significant neurologic compromise
Inability to coordinate with the NIPPV breath

References

1. Hyzy Robert C. Noninvasive positive pressure ventilation in acute respiratory failure, www.uptodate.com, (800) 998-6374, (781) 237–4788
2. Abou-Shala N, Meduri GU. Non-invasive mechanical ventilation in patients with acute respiratory failure. *Crit Care Med.* 1997;24:705
3. Ambrosino N, Foglio K, Rubini F, et al. Non-invasive mechanical ventilation in acute respiratory failure due to chronic obstructive pulmonary disease: correlates for success. *Thorax.* 1995;50:755–757
4. American Thoracic Society, European Thoracic Society Task Force. *Standards for the diagnosis and management of patients with COPD.* New York: American Thoracic Society; 2004

5. Anton A, Guell R, Gomez J, et al. Predicting the result of noninvasive ventilation in severe acute exacerbations of patients with chronic airflow limitation. *Chest*. 2000;117:828
6. Antonelli M, Conti G, Bufi M, et al. Noninvasive ventilation for treatment of acute respiratory failure in patients undergoing solid organ transplantation: a randomized trial. *JAMA*. 2000;283:235–241
7. Antonelli M, Conti G, Rocco M, et al. Noninvasive positive pressure ventilation vs conventional oxygen supplementation in hypoxemic patients undergoing diagnostic bronchoscopy. *Chest*. 2002;121:1149–1154
8. Antonelli M, Pennisi MA, Conti G, et al. Fiberopticbronchoscopy during noninvasive positive pressure ventilation delivered by helmet. *Intensive Care Med*. 2003;29:126–129
9. Antonelli M, Pennisi MA, Pelosi P, et al. Noninvasive positive pressure ventilation using a helmet in patients with acute exacerbation of chronic obstructive pulmonary disease. *Anesthesiology*. 2004;100:16–24
10. Appendini L, Purro A, Patessio A, et al. Partitioning of inspiratory muscle workload and pressure assistance in ventilator-dependent COPD patients. *Am J Respir Crit Care Med*. 1996;154:1301–1309
11. Bardley TD. Hemodynamic and sympathoinhibitory effect of nasal CPAP in congestive heart failure. *Sleep*. 1996;19:S232–S235
12. Bersten AD, Holt AW, Vedig AE. Treatment of severe cardiogenic pulmonary edema with continuous positive airway pressure delivered by face mask. *N Engl J Med*. 1991;325:1825
13. Bott J, Carroll MP, Conway JH, et al. Randomised controlled trial of nasal ventilation in acute ventilatory failure due to chronic obstructive airways disease. *Lancet*. 1993;341:1555
14. British Thoracic Society Standards of Care Committee. BTS guideline: non-invasive ventilation in acute respiratory failure. *Thorax*. 2002;57:192–211
15. Brochard L, Mancebo J, Wysocki M, et al. Noninvasive ventilation for acute exacerbations of chronic obstructive pulmonary disease. *New Engl J Med*. 1995;333:817–822
16. Bunburaphong T, Imaka H, Nishimura M, et al. Performance characteristics of bilevel pressure ventilators: a lung model study. *Chest*. 1997;111:1050–1060
17. Calderini E, Confalonieri M, Puccio PG, et al. Patient-ventilator asynchrony during noninvasive ventilation: the role of expiratory trigger. *Intensive Care Med*. 1999;25:662–667

18. Capdevila XJ, Perrigault PF, Perey PJ, et al. Occlusion pressure and its ratio to maximum inspiratory pressure are useful predictors for successful extubation following T-piece weaning trial. *Chest*. 1995;108:482
19. Carlucci A, Richard JC, Wysocki M, Lepage E, Brochard L. Noninvasive versus conventional mechanical ventilation. An epidemiologic survey. *Am J Respir Crit Care Med*. 2001;163:874–880
20. Celikel T, Sungur M, Ceyhan B, et al. Comparison of noninvasive positive pressure ventilation with standard medical therapy in hypercapnic respiratory failure. *Chest*. 1998;114:1636
21. Celli BR, MacNee W. ATS/ESR task force: standards for the diagnosis and treatment of patients with COPD: a summary of the ATS/ERS position paper. *Eur Respir J*. 2004;23:932–946
22. Confalonieri M, Gazzaniga P, Gandola L, et al. Haemodynamic response during initiation of non-invasive positive pressure ventilation in COPD patients with acute ventilatory failure. *Respir Med*. 1998;92:331
23. Confalonieri M, Potena A, Carbone G, et al. Acute respiratory failure in patients with severe community-acquired pneumonia: a prospective, randomized evaluation of noninvasive ventilation. *Am J Respir Crit Care Med*. 1999;160:1585–1591
24. Confalonieri M, Potena A, Carbone G, Porta RD, Tolley EA, Umberto Meduri G. Acute respiratory failure in patients with severe community acquired pneumonia. A prospective randomized evaluation of noninvasive ventilation. *Am J Respir Crit Care Med*. 1999;160:1585–1591
25. Confalonieri M, Garuti G, Cattaruzza MS, et al. On behalf of the Italian noninvasive positive pressure ventilation (NPPV) study group. A chart of failure risk for noninvasive ventilation in patients with COPD exacerbation. *Eur Respir J*. 2005;25:348–355
26. Criner GJ, Travaline JM, Brennan KJ, Kreimer DT. Efficacy of a new full face mask for noninvasive positive pressure ventilation. *Chest*. 1994;106:1109–1115
27. Dreyfuss D, Saumon G. Ventilator-induced lung injury: lessons from experimental studies. *Am J Respir Crit Care Med*. 1998;157:294–323
28. Evans TW. International Consensus Conference in Intensive Care Medicine: NIPPV in acute respiratory failure. *Intensive Care Med*. 2001;27:166–178
29. Ferguson GT, Gilmartin M. CO_2 rebreathing during BiPAP ventilatory assistance. *Am J Respir Crit Care Med*. 1995;151:1126

30. Girault C, Daudenthun I, Chevron V, et al. Non-invasive ventilation as a systematic extubation and weaning technique in acute-on-chronic respiratory failure: a prospective, randomised controlled study. *Am J Respir Crit Care Med*. 1999;160:86
31. Global Initiative for Chronic Obstructive Lung Disease (GOLD). Global strategy for the diagnosis, management, and prevention of chronic obstructive pulmonary disease. NHLBI/WHO Workshop report, NIH Publication update 2004
32. Gregory S, Siderowf A, Golaszewski AL, McCluskey L. Gastrostomy insertion in ALS patients with low vital capacity: respiratory support and survival. *Neurology*. 2002;58:485–487
33. Hendrix TR. The motility of the alimentary canal. In: Mountcastle VB, ed. *Medical Physiology*. 14th ed. St. Louis: Mosby; 1980: 1330–1332
34. Herrera M, Blasco J, Venegas J, et al. Mouth occlusion pressure (P0.1) in acute respiratory failure. *Inten Care Med*. 1985;11:134.
35. Hess D. Non-invasive positive pressure ventilation: predictors of success and failure for adult acute care applications. *Respir Care*. 1997;42:424
36. Hill NS. Complications of noninvasive positive pressure ventilation. *Respir Care*. 1997;42:432
37. Hill NS. Noninvasive positive pressure ventilation for non chronic obstructive pulmonary disease causes of acute respiratory failure. In: Hill NS, ed. *Noninvasive positive pressure ventilation: principles and applications*. Futura Publishing Company, Inc Armonk, NY; 2001: 85–104
38. Hill NS, Hess D. Initiation of noninvasive positive pressure ventilation. In: Hill NS, ed. *Noninvasive positive pressure ventilation: principles and applications*. Futura Publishing Company, Inc Armonk, NY; 2001: 85–104
39. Hillberg RE, Johnson DC. Noninvasive ventilation. *N Engl J Med*. 1997;337:1746
40. International Consensus Conferences in Intensive Care Medicine. Noninvasive positive pressure ventilation in acute respiratory failure. Organized jointly by the American Thoracic Society, the European Respiratory Society, the European Society of Intensive Care Medicine, and societé de Réanimation de Langue Francaise and approved by the ATS Board of Directors, December 2000. *Am J Respir Crit Care Med*. 2001;163:283–291
41. Jaber S, Fodil R, Carlucci A, et al. Noninvasive ventilation with heliu-oxygen in acute exacerbations of chronic obstructive pulmonary disease. *Am J Respir Crit Care Med*. 2000;161:1191

42. Jasmer RM, Luce JM, Matthay MA. Non-invasive positive pressure ventilation for acute respiratory failure: underutilised or overrated? *Chest*. 1997;111:1673
43. Jubran A, Van de Graffe WB, Tobin MJ. Variability of patient-ventilator interaction with pressure support ventilation in patients with chronic obstructive pulmonary disease. *Am J Respir Crit Care Med*. 1995;152:129–136
44. Kacmarek RM. Characteristics of pressure-targeted ventilators used for non-invasive positive pressure ventilation. *Respir Care*. 1997;42:380
45. Kramer N, Meyer TJ, Meharg J, Cece RD, Hills NS. Randomized, prospective trial of noninvasive positive pressure ventilation in acute respiratory failure. *Am J Respir Crit Care Med*. 1995;151:1799–1806
46. Krieger BP, Ershowsky PF, Becker DA, Gazeroglu HB. Evaluation of conventional criteria for predicting successful weaning from mechanical ventilatory support in elderly patients. *Crit Care Med*. 1989;17:858
47. L'Her E, Taille S, Deye N, et al. Physiological response of hypoxemic patients to different modes of non-invasive ventilation. *Intensive Care Med*. 2002;28:S49
48. Lee KH, Hui KP, Chan TB, et al. Rapid shallow breathing (frequency-tidal volume ratio) did not predict extubation outcome. *Chest*. 1994;105:540
49. Leger P, Jennequin J, Gerard M, et al. Home positive pressure ventilation via nasal mask for patients with neuromuscular weakness or restrictive lung or chest wall deformities. *Respir Care*. 1989;34:73–77
50. Lin M, Yang Y-F, Chiang H-T, et al. Reappraisal of continuous positive airway pressure therapy in acute cardiogenic pulmonary edema: short-term results and long-term follow-up. *Chest*. 1995;107:1379
51. Martin TJ, Hovis JD, Constantino JP, et al. A randomized, prospective evaluation of noninvasive ventilation for acute respiratory failure. *Am J Respir Crit Care Med*. 2000;161: 807
52. Martins De Araujo MT, Vieira SB, Vasquez EC, Fleury B. Heated humidification or face mask to prevent upper airway dryness during continuous positive airway pressure therapy. *Chest*. 2000;117:142–147
53. Masip J, Paez J, Merino M, et al. Risk factors for intubation as a guide for noninvasive ventilation in patients with severe acute cardiogenic pulmonary disease. *Intensive Care Med*. 2003; 29:1921–1928

54. Meduri GU, Turner RE, Abou-Shala N, Wunderink R, Tolley E. Non-invasive positive pressure ventilation via face mask. First line intervention in patients with acute hypercapnic and hypoxemic respiratory failure. *Chest.* 1996;109:179–193
55. Mehta S, Jay GD, Woolard RH, et al. Randomised, prospective trial of bilevel versus continuous positive airway pressure in acute pulmonary edema. *Crit Care Med.* 1997;25: 620–628
56. Mehta S, McCool FD, Hill NS. Leak compensation in positive pressure ventilators: a lung model study. *Eur Respir J.* 2001; 17:259–267
57. Montgomery AB, Holle RHO, Neagley SR, et al. Prediction of successful ventilator weaning using airway occlusion pressure and hypercapnic challenge. *Chest.* 1987;91:496
58. Naughton MT, Rahman MA, Hara K, et al. Effect of continuous-positive airway pressure on intrathoracic and left ventricular transmural pressures in patients with congestive heart failure. *Circulation.* 1995;91:1725–1731
59. Nava S, Ambrosino N, Clini E, et al. Noninvasive mechanical ventilation in the weaning of patients with respiratory failure due to chronic obstructive pulmonary disease: a randomised, controlled trial. *Ann Intern Med.* 1998;128:721
60. Navalesi P, Fanfulla F, Frigerio P, et al. Physiologic evaluation on noninvasive mechanical ventilation delivered with three types of masks in patients with chronic hypercapnic respiratory failure. *Crit Care Med.* 2000;28:1785
61. NICE (National Institute for Clinical Excellence) guideline on COPD. National clinical guideline on management of chronic obstructive pulmonary disease in adults in primary and secondary care. *Thorax.* 2004;59:1–232
62. Pang D, Keenan SP, Cook DJ, et al. The effect of positive pressure air way support on mortality and the need for intubation in cardiogenic pulmonary edema: a systematic review. *Chest.* 1998;114:1185–1192
63. Patel RG, Petrini MF. Respiratory muscle performance, pulmonary mechanics, and gas exchange between the Bi PAPS/ T-D system and Servo Ventilator 900C with bilevel positive air way pressure ventilation following gradual pressure support weaning. *Chest.* 1998;114:1390–1396
64. Pertusini E, Lellouche F, Catani F, et al. Patient-ventilator asynchronies during NIV does level of pressure support matter? *Intensive Care Med.* 2004;30:S65

65. Piper AJ, Sullivan CE. Effects of short-term NIPPV in the treatment of patients with severe obstructive sleep apnea and hypercapnia. *Chest.* 1994;105:434–444
66. Poponick JM, Renston JP, Bennet RP, Emerman CL. Use of a ventilatory support system (BiPAP) for acute respiratory failure in the emergency department. *Chest.* 1999;116:116–171
67. Proctor HJ, Woolson R. Prediction of respiratory muscle fatigue by measurements of the work of breathing. *Surg Gynecol Obstet.* 1973;136:367
68. Richards GN, Cistulli PA, Ungar RG, Berthon-Jones M, Sullivan CE. Mouth leak with nasal continuous positive airway pressure increases nasal airway resistance. *Am J Respir Crit Care Med.* 1996;154:182–186
69. Saatci E, Miller DM, Sztell IM, et al. Dynamic dead space in face masks used with noninvasive ventilators: a lung model study. *Eur Respir J.* 2004;23:129–135
70. Sahn SA, Lakshminarayan S. Bedside criteria for discontinuation of mechanical ventilation. *Chest.* 1973;63:1002
71. Sassoon CSH, Mahutte CK. Airway occlusion pressure and breathing pattern as predictors of weaning outcome. *Am Rev Respir Dis.* 1993;148:860
72. Sassoon CSH, Te TT, Mahutte CK, Light RW. Airway occlusion pressure: an important indicator for successful weaning in patients with chronic obstructive pulmonary disease. *Am Rev Respir Dis.* 1987;135:107
73. Schettino GPP, Chatmongkolchart S, Hess D, Kacmarek RM. Position of exhalation port and mask design affect CO_2 rebreathing during noninvasive positive pressure ventilation. *Crit Care Med.* 2003;31:2178–2182
74. Semmes BJ, Tobin MJ, Snyder JV, Grenvik A. Subjective and objective measurement of tidal volume of critically ill patients. *Chest.* 1985;87:577
75. Slutsky AS. Mechanical ventilation. American College of Chest Physicians' Consensus Conference. *Chest.* 1993;104:1833
76. Smith IE, Shneerson J. Secondary failure of nasal intermittent positive pressure ventilation using the Monnal D: effects of changing ventilator. *Thorax.* 1997;52:89–91
77. Stroetz RW, Hubmayr RD. Tidal volume maintenance during weaning with pressure support. *Am J Respir Crit Care Med.* 1995;152:1034
78. Taccone P, Hess D, Caironi P, Bigatello LM. Continuous positive airway pressure delivered with a "helmet". Effects on carbon dioxide rebreathing. *Crit Care Med.* 2004;32:2090–2096

79. Togias AG, Naclerio RM, Proud D, et al. Nasal challenge with cold, dry air results in release of inflammatory mediators. Possible mast cell involvement. *J Clin Invest.* 1985;76:1375–1381
80. Tonnelier JM, Prat G, Nowak E, et al. Noninvasive continuous positive airway pressure ventilation using a new helmet interface: a case prospective pilot study. *Intensive Care Med.* 2003;29:2077–2080
81. Vitacca M, Lanini B, Nava S, et al. Inspiratory muscle workload due to dynamic intrinsic PEEP in stable COPD patients: effects of two different settings of non-invasive pressure-support ventilation. *Monaldi Arch Chest Dis.* 2004;61:81–85
82. Wood KA, Lewis L, Von Harz B, Kollef MH. The use of noninvasive positive pressure ventilation in the emergency department: results of a randomized clinical trial. *Chest.* 1998;113:1339–1346
83. Wunderink RG, Hill NS. Continuous and periodic applications of noninvasive ventilation in respiratory failure. *Respir Care.* 1997;42:394
84. Wysocki M, Tric L, Wolff MA, et al. Noninvasive pressure support ventilation in patients with acute respiratory failure: a randomized comparison with conventional therapy. *Chest.* 1995;107:761
85. Yang K, Tobin MJ. A prospective study of indexes predicting outcome of trials of weaning from mechanical ventilation. *N Engl J Med.* 1991;324:1445

Chapter 14
Negative Pressure Ventilation

In essence, the negative pressure ventilator comprises a rigid shell that partly or completely encloses the patient's torso, the pressure within which can be dropped by means of an attached pump.[27] Air enters the lungs as a result of the fall in pleural pressure produced by expansion of the thoracic cage. Expiration is passive. Negative pressure ventilators were introduced in the middle of the nineteenth century and preceded positive pressure devices by nearly a century (see Chap. 1) (Fig. 14.1).

Three types of devices for NPV exist: the iron tank, the cuirass, and the body suit. Since an artificial airway is not

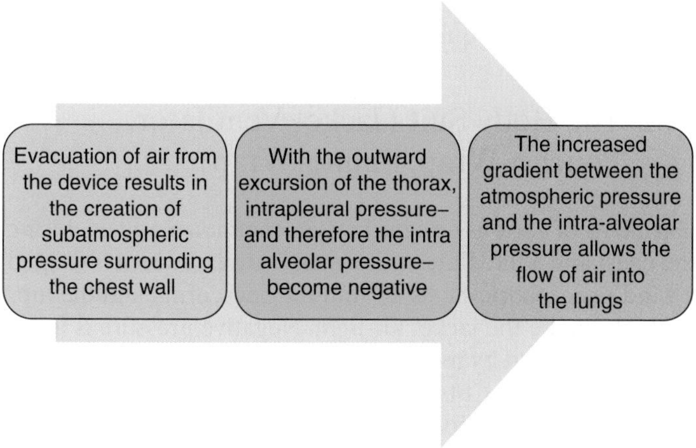
Evacuation of air from the device results in the creation of subatmospheric pressure surrounding the chest wall
With the outward excursion of the thorax, intrapleural pressure– and therefore the intra alveolar pressure– become negative
The increased gradient between the atmospheric pressure and the intra-alveolar pressure allows the flow of air into the lungs

FIGURE 14.1. The principle of Negative Pressure Ventilation (NPV).

A. Hasan, *Understanding Mechanical Ventilation*,
DOI: 10.1007/978-1-84882-869-8_14,

required (unless airway secretions are troublesome), the patient can eat, drink, and talk without hindrance.

14.1 Tank Ventilator (Iron Lung)

Popularly known as iron tanks – though they are now assembled from plastic or aluminum components and are much lighter than the earlier versions – the Porta-Lung of Respironics weighs just 110 pounds (a separate negative pressure unit weighs 45 pounds). These ventilators completely enclose the patient's body from the neck downwards. A padded collar provides an air-tight seal at the neck. Access to the patient for physical examination, nursing, and therapy – necessarily through windows and portholes – is understandably difficult. Moreover, since most of the body lies within the tank, the abdomen is as much subject to the negative pressure generated by the ventilator as is the thorax. Consequently, in some subjects, pooling of blood occurs within the great vessels of the abdomen, reducing the venous return to the heart. The hemodynamic compromise ("tank-shock") can sometimes be severe. Tidal volumes are determined by the magnitude of the negative pressure that is applied, but by and large, there is little scope for finer adjustments to suit the requirements of individual patients.

14.2 The Body Suit (Jacket Ventilator, Poncho-Wrap, Pulmo-Wrap)

Garments of various designs have in common a grid enclosing the chest and a flat plate at the back,[19] around which is draped a wind-proof fabric. Seals around the neck, arms, and the hips or thighs make the jacket air-tight. Negative pressure is intermittently created by means of an external pump connected to a hose. A seal that fits about the pelvis allows access of the patient's perineum for nursing. Leaks (which can produce uncomfortable cooling) are more common with this kind of wrap than with the sort that provides a seal at the thighs or ankles (Pulmobag: Respironics; Pneumobag: Emerson). With the latter type of body suit, an uncomfortable squeezing sensation can be felt about the lower limbs during the negative pressure breath.

With the fabric fashioned into a zippable suit with sleeves and pant legs (Pneumosuit: Emerson; NuMo Suit: Respironics), the movement of the extremities is less restricted. The special fabric (Gore-tex, Gore) is water-permeable, and affords egress for humidity, making for greater patient comfort. The tidal volumes that the device can deliver are lower than those possible with the iron tank.[34]

14.3 Chest: Shell (Cuirass)

The cuirass derives its name from the defensive armor, which consisted of a protective breastplate and a backplate, of the fifteenth century soldier. Mounted soldiers wearing cuirasses were known as Cuirassiers, though this name was later extended to describe any soldier of the heavy cavalry. The cuirass is basically a rigid shell – now made of thermo-molded plastic – enclosing the front of the patient's thorax, the pressure within which is rhythmically lowered by means of a vacuum-creating device linked to it by a hose pipe.

The principle of operation is the same as that of the tank, but since the cuirass encloses only the thorax of the subject, less hemodynamic compromise is encountered. A major advantage is that the patient can be nursed in a seated position, but its smaller surface of apposition also means that as a ventilator, it is rather less efficient than the tank, or even the wrap.[19]

Access for patient care is obviously much better than in the case of iron tank, and unrestricted arm movement is possible. Some models incorporate pressure sensors that detect attempts at inspiration and generate a negative pressure breath in synchrony with it, thus providing an assist mode. Custom-made cuirasses, by and large, eliminate air-leaks that were a problem with earlier models, and the recent incorporation of plastic wrapping around the shell has improved the air-seal.

14.4 Modes of Negative Pressure Ventilation

Several modes of ventilation are possible with NPV, and these have been summarized in Fig.

Negative pressure ventilators still have a role today, especially in the long-term nocturnal ventilation of patients with neuromuscular or chest wall disorders.[20,22] NPV is probably effective in the treatment of acute respiratory failure in COPD[13] and neuromuscular disease[5,26] as well, but currently, positive pressure ventilation is far more popular for this indication (Fig. 14.2).

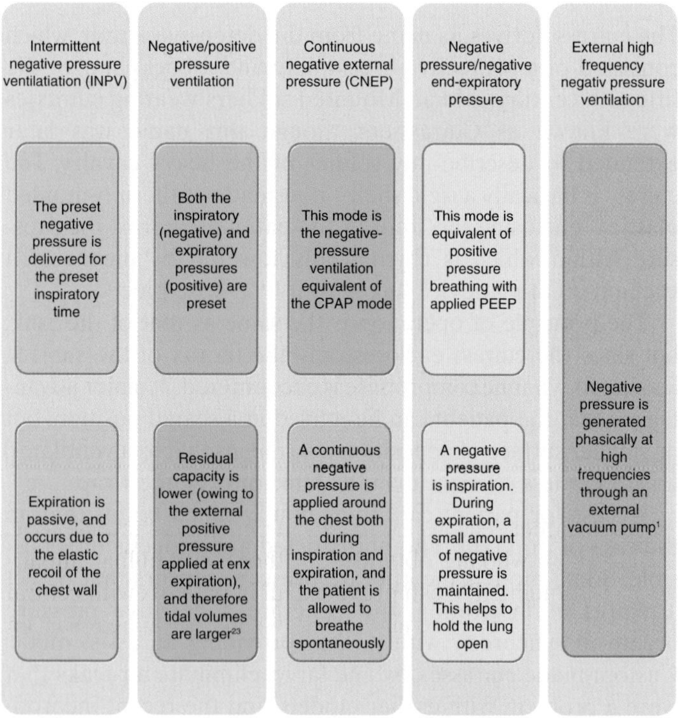
Intermittent negative pressure ventilatiation (INPV)
The preset negative pressure is delivered for the preset inspiratory time
Expiration is passive, and occurs due to the elastic recoil of the chest wall
Negative/positive pressure ventilation
Both the inspiratory (negative) and expiratory pressures (positive) are preset
Residual capacity is lower (owing to the external positive pressure applied at enx expiration), and therefore tidal volumes are larger23
Continuous negative external pressure (CNEP)
This mode is the negative-pressure ventilation equivalent of the CPAP mode
A continuous negative pressure is applied around the chest both during inspiration and expiration, and the patient is allowed to breathe spontaneously
Negative pressure/negative end-expiratory pressure
This mode is equivalent of positive pressure breathing with applied PEEP
A negative pressure is inspiration. During expiration, a small amount of negative pressure is maintained. This helps to hold the lung open
External high frequency negativ pressure ventilation
Negative pressure is generated phasically at high frequencies through an external vacuum pump1

FIGURE 14.2. Modes of Negative Pressure Ventilation.

14.5 Drawbacks of NPV

Unlike positive pressure breathing, intrapleural pressure is negative during inspiration, and airway pressures cycle more or less as they do during physiological respiration. The venous return not being impeded, cardiac output is preserved. Although this is the case with most negative pressure devices, the tank is the exception: since not just the thorax, but the entire body is encompassed by the device, the intrathoracic pressure is actually high relative to the pressure at the body surface.[29] With tank ventilation, therefore, hemodynamic effects may be very similar to those seen during positive pressure ventilation. NIV has on occasion been associated with pneumothorax[39]; rarely rib fractures have been known to occur.[39]

NPV can also be a risk factor for aspiration. NPV is capable of inducing lower esophageal sphincter dysfunction, and its use has sometimes been associated with emesis[10]; prophylaxis with prokinetic agents is desirable.[31] The risk of aspiration is clearly enhanced in patients who are unconscious.

NPV can induce narrowing of the glottis or the supraglottic airway during sleep, provoking apneas and hypopneas.[2,21,24]

Although these effects can as well occur in neuromuscular patients, the overall benefits of NPV in this group outweigh its drawbacks. The mechanism of the upper airway narrowing remains elusive, but it is likely that during sleep with NPV, coordinated respiratory muscle activity may be abolished. With the failure of the pharyngeal muscle tone to increase immediately preceding inspiration, airway walls may be drawn together by the negative inspiratory pressure. The probability of upper airway obstruction appears to be greater in patients who have other reasons for impaired pharyngeal muscle tone, such as those who are obtunded, or those with bulbar impairment. Although NPV can prove useful in patients with central sleep apnea, it is contraindicated when the apnea has an obstructive component to it.[2,21,25]

The supine position that patients with tank or wrap devices are constrained to adopt can produce muscular discomfort and pain.

References

1. Al-Saady NM, Fernando SSD, Petros AJ, Cummin AR, Sidhu VS, Bennett ED. External high frequency oscillation in normal subjects and in patients with acute respiratory failure. *Anesthesia.* 1995;50:1031–1035
2. Bach JR, Penek J. Obstructive sleep apnea complicating negative pressure ventilatory support in patients with chronic paralytic/restrictive ventilatory dysfunction. *Chest.* 1991;99:1386–1393
3. Bailey J, Shapiro MJ. Abdominal compartment syndrome. *Crit Care.* 2000;4:23–29
4. Bloomfield G, Saggi B, Blocher C, et al Physiologic effects of externally applied continuous negative abdominal pressure for intra-abdominal hypertension. *J Trauma.* 1999;46:1009–1014
5. Braun SR, Sufit RL, Giovannoni R. Intermittent negative pressure ventilation in the treatment of respiratory failure in progressive neuromuscular disease. *Neurology.* 1987;37:1874–1875
6. Corrado A, Gorini M. Negative pressure ventilation: is there still a role? *Eur Respir J.* 2002;20:187–197
7. Corrado A, Bruscoli G, Messori A, et al Iron lung treatment of subjects with COPD in acute respiratory failure: evaluation of short and long-term prognosis. *Chest.* 1992;101:692–696
8. Corrado A, De Paola E, Messori A, et al The effect of intermittent negative pressure ventilation and long-term oxygen therapy for patients with COPD: a 4-year study. *Chest.* 1994;105:95–99
9. Corrado A, Gorini M, De Paola E, et al Iron lung treatment of acute on chronic respiratory failure: 16 years of experience. *Monaldi Arch Chest Dis.* 1994;101:692–696
10. Corrado A, Gorini M, Ginanni R, et al Negative pressure ventilation versus conventional mechanical ventilation in the treatment of acute respiratory failure in COPD patients. *Eur Respir J.* 1998;12:519–525
11. Corrado A, Vianello A, Arcaro G, et al Noninvasive mechanical ventilation for the treatment of acute respiratory failure in neuromuscular diseases. *Eur Respir J.* 2000;16:542s
12. Corrado A, Confalonieri M, Marchese S, et al Iron lung versus mask ventilation in the treatment of acute on chronic respiratory failure in COPD patients: a multicenter study. *Chest.* 2002;121:189–195
13. Corrado A, Ginanni R, Villella G, et al Iron lung versus conventional mechanical ventilation in acute exacerbation of COPD. *Eur Respir J.* 2004;23:419–424

14. Del Bufalo C, Fasano L, Quarta CC, et al Use of extrathoracic negative pressure ventilation in weaning COPD and kyphoscopliotic patients from mechanical ventilation. *Respir Care*. 1994;39:21–29
15. Fagon JY, Chastre J, Hance AJ, et al Nosocomial pneumonia in ventilated patients: a cohort study evaluating attributable mortality and hospital stay. *Am J Med*. 1993;94:281–288
16. Garay SM, Turino GM, Goldring RM. Sustained reversal of chronic hypercapnia in patients with alveolar hyperventilation syndrome: long-term maintenance with noninvasive nocturnal mechanical ventilation. *Am J Med*. 1981;70:269–274
17. Gorini M, Ginanni R, Villella G, et al Non-invasive negative and positive pressure ventilation in the treatment of acute on chronic respiratory failure. *Intensive Care Med*. 2004;30:875–881
18. Gunella G. Traitement de'l insuffisance respiratoire aigue des pulmonaires chroniques avec le poumon d'acier: resultat dansune serie de 560 cas. *Ann Med Phys*. 1980;2:317–327
19. Hill NS. Clinical applications of body ventilators. *Chest*. 1986;90:897–905
20. Hill NS. Use of negative pressure ventilation, rocking beds, and pneumobelts. *Respir Care*. 1994;39(5):532
21. Hill NS, Redline S, Carskadon MA, et al Sleep-disordered breathing in patients with Duchenne muscular dystrophy using negative pressure ventilators. *Chest*. 1992;102:1656–1662
22. Holtakers TR, Loosborck LM, Gracey DR. The use of the chest cuirass in respiratory failure of neurological origin. *Respir Care*. 1982;27(3):271
23. Kinnear W, Petch M, Taylor G, Shneerson J. Assisted ventilation using cuirass respirators. *Eur Respir J*. 1988;1:198–203
24. Levy RD, Bradley TD, Newman SL, et al Negative pressure ventilation: effects on ventilation during sleep in normal subjects. *Chest*. 1989;95:95–99
25. Levy RD, Cosio MG, Gibbons L, et al Induction of sleep apnea with negative pressure ventilation in patients with chronic obstructive lung disease. *Thorax*. 1992;47:612–615
26. Libby BM, Briscoe WA, Boyce B, et al Acute respiratory failure in scoliosis or kyphosis. *Am J Med*. 1982;73:532–538
27. Lockhat D, Langleben D, Zidulka A. Hemodynamic differences between continuous positive and two types of negative pressure ventilation. *Am Rev Respir Dis*. 1992;146:677–680
28. Malbrain ML. Abdominal pressure in the critically ill: measurement and clinical relevance. *Intensive Care Med*. 1999;25: 1453–1458

29. Maloney JV, Whittenberger JL. Clinical implication of pressures used in the body respirator. *Am J Med Sci.* 1951;221:425–430
30. Man GCW, Jones RL, McDonald GF, et al Primary alveolar hypoventilation managed by negative pressure ventilators. *Chest.* 1979;76:219
31. Marino WD, Pitchumoni CS. Reversal of negative pressure ventilation induced lower esophageal sphincter dysfunction with metoclopramide. *Am J Gastroenterol.* 1992;87:190–194
32. Mehta S, Hill NS. Noninvasive ventilation. *Am J Respir Crit Care Med.* 2001;163:540–577
33. Pingleton SK. Complications of acute respiratory failure. *Am Rev Respir Dis.* 1988;137:1463–1493
34. Shneerson JM. Non-invasive and domiciliary ventilation: negative pressure techniques. *Thorax.* 1991;46:131–135
35. Sinderby C, Navalesi P, Beck J, et al Neural control of mechanical ventilation in respiratory failure. *Nat Med.* 1999;5:1433–1436
36. Splaingard ML, Frates RC, Jefferson LS, et al Home negative pressure ventilation: report of 20 years of experience in patients with neuromuscular disease. *Arch Phys Med Rehabil.* 1985;66:239
37. Tobin MJ. Mechanical ventilation. *N Engl J Med.* 1994;330: 1056–1061
38. Todisco T, Baglioni S, Eslami A, et al Treatment of acute exacerbations of chronic respiratory failure. *Chest.* 2004;125:2217–2223
39. Zibrack JD, Hill NS, Federman EC, et al Evaluation of intermittent long-term negative pressure ventilation in patients with severe chronic obstructive pulmonary disease. *Am Rev Respir Dis.* 1988;138:1515–1518

Chapter 15
Airway Humidification in the Mechanically Ventilated Patient

15.1 The Role of the Nasal Mucosa

Inhaled air is cold and dry. The highly vascularized nasal mucosa warms and humidifies it, and makes it suitable for breathing.

The surface area of the nasal mucosa is enlarged by the three nasal turbinates. As the air is drawn around these, the laminar airflow becomes turbulent. Eddy currents allow better contact of the inspired air with the mucosa and facilitate the transfer of heat and humidity.

Most of the humidification, by far, occurs in the nose, where the air is warmed to 31–32°C and about 95% saturated with water vapor. By the time inhaled air reaches the middle of the trachea, the temperature would have risen to 34°C and the absolute humidity to 3 mg/L.[39,62] As the airway mucosa gives up its water, it also loses heat – the latent heat of vaporization – which changes the state of the liquid film lining the mucosa to vapor. The heat generated by the bronchial circulation prevents the local airway temperature from falling precipitously.

15.2 The Isothermic Saturation Boundary

Inspired air is eventually warmed to core body temperature, 37°C. It is also completely saturated with water vapor, in which state it carries 44 mg of H_2O per liter. The point at which complete saturation occurs is called the isothermic

A. Hasan, *Understanding Mechanical Ventilation*,
DOI: 10.1007/978-1-84882-869-8_15,

saturation boundary. Proximal to the isothermic saturation boundary, the airway mucosa functions as a heat and moisture exchanger.[20] In this zone, heat and water exchanges vary with the prevailing gradients. Distally, in contrast, the saturation of the air remains constant.

During quiet respiration, the isothermic saturation boundary normally lies within the second order bronchi.[21,38] When cold or dry air is inhaled, the isothermic saturation boundary moves deeper into the lung, and the peripheral airways participate more in the heat and moisture exchange process.[39]

Box 15.1 Water Losses

No more than 20–30% of the water that the mucous membranes add to the inspired air is retrieved by them. During quiet breathing at room temperature (22°C, 50% relative humidity), about 400 gm of water is added daily to the inspired air; only 100–150 gm of this condenses back during exhalation. Thus, 250–300 gm of water – or approximately 150 mL (10 μL per respiratory cycle) – is lost from the respiratory tract each day.[62] Water losses can be much greater when dry air is breathed, or when the minute ventilation high.

Of the 24 mg of water or so lost per liter of air exhaled through the nose, most – about 17 mg/L – comes from the nasal mucosa. A much smaller amount – about 7 mg/L – is lost from the lower respiratory tract. During mouth breathing, overall losses are much higher (29 mg/L), and the amount lost from the lower respiratory tract can increase to 12 mg/L.[44,53,63]

15.3 The Effect of the Endotracheal Tube

The endotracheal tube (ET), by functionally bypassing the nose, delivers relatively unconditioned air directly into the lower respiratory tract. Unlike ambient air, medical gases stored in liquid oxygen and compressed air systems are dry, and water losses from the lower respiratory tract can increase to as much as 32 mg/L.[28,44] Underconditioned inspired air shifts the isothermic saturation boundary well out into the periphery of the bronchial tree, sometimes as much as 15 cm distal to the carina.[20] Dry air can cause irritative bronchospasm by multiple mechanisms: by the direct effect of the cold, by a neural reflex activated by the increased osmolarity of the bronchial fluid, and by the hyperemia of the bronchial circulation it produces.[4]

The ensuing alterations in mucus rheology and surfactant result in microatelectasis, which produces right to left shunting, and worsening of lung compliance. Also, by its physical adjacency and its fricative movement upon the tracheal mucosa, the ETT induces local injury. Repeated suctioning in an attempt to dislodge the thickening secretions compounds the trauma, as also does the high FIO_2 that is often used to control the hypoxemia.[52,60] Disruption of the ciliary structure and function[11,31] and the backwash of infected airway secretions into the distal lung can result in infectious tracheobronchitis and pneumonia.

With dry air, damage to the structural and functional integrity of the airway mucosa can transpire within the hour,[7] and – at least in experimental animals – a near total stagnation of mucous secretions can occur within a few hours.[32,59] Inspissated mucous adheres tenaciously to the walls of the tracheobronchial tree, further disadvantaging the mucociliary escalator.[27]

15.3.1 Overheated Air

The introduction of gas that is warmer than body temperature (for instance, saturated air from a heated humidifier that has been warmed to over 35°C) into the tracheobronchial tree can be equally damaging. The overhydration that overwarmed air induces can flood the mucociliary escalator and severely hinder its performance. Overhydration can also be extremely destructive to surfactant (Box 15.2).[41]

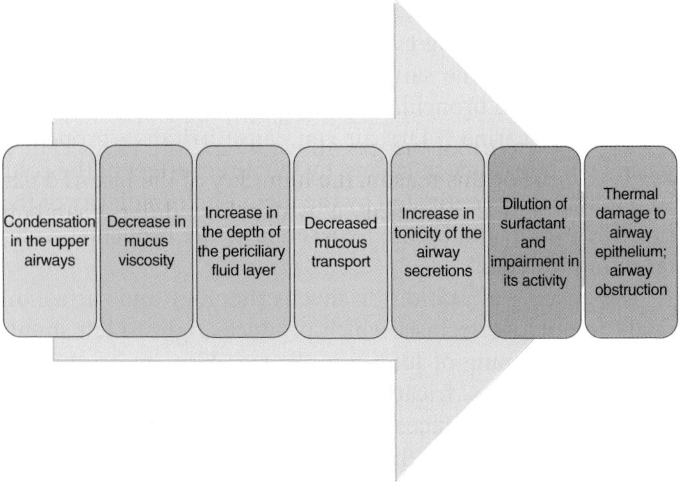
Condensation in the upper airways
Decrease in mucus viscosity
Increase in the depth of the periciliary fluid layer
Decreased mucous transport
Increase in tonicity of the airway secretions
Dilution of surfactant and impairment in its activity
Thermal damage to airway epithelium; airway obstruction

FIGURE 15.1. Sequence of effects of overhumidification.[54,62]

Box 15.2 The Consequences of Overcondensation ("Raining Out")

Interference with airflow sensor readings
Auto-triggering
Increased airway resistance
Nosocomial pneumonia

Hot *dry* air can be more damaging than cold dry air.[38] Overheated-underhumidified air moves the ISB upward: the hot dry gas extracts moisture, drying the airway and inspissating the secretions.

Overwarmed air is capable of causing severe thermal injury, and "hot pot tracheitis" has occasionally been documented.[33]

Two classes of airway humidification devices are employed: heated humidifiers (HHs) and heat-moisture exchangers (HMEs).

15.4 Heated Humidifiers

The evaporation of any liquid within a container is dependent on the surface area that the liquid presents to the gas, the vapor pressure of the gas above it, and the temperature of the liquid. For this reason, the humidity of the inspired gas can be increased by using a wider humidifier chamber, increasing the gas flow rate, or by simply increasing the temperature of the humidifier.

As the conditioned air from the heated humidifier passes through the inspiratory limb of the patient circuit, it cools and condenses upon its walls (heating elements have been used within ventilator circuits to prevent overcondensation, but these circuits are expensive).

Owing to the moisture, HHs frequently get colonized early with potentially pathogenic organisms.[17,48] On these grounds, it has been argued that HHs predispose the patient to nosocomial infection, but this hypothesis remains as yet unproven.[57]

In theory, HHs have superior humidifying ability compared to HMEs.[14] In practice, the difference is not so apparent. Although ET occlusion rates have been demonstrably less with HHs than with the earlier HMEs, modern HMEs do not in any way appear to predispose an excess of this complication.[50] At the customary temperature of 34°C, HHs show no great superiority in performance over HMEs and increasing the temperature to 40°C appears to reduce moisture loss by no more than 7 mg/L over that by the HME.[2]

For overhydration to occur, inhaled gas would require heating to a point considerably above body temperature: therefore, overhydration with HHs is relatively unusual. Similarly, thermal injury due to excessive heating of inspired air is rare.[62] In the vast majority of cases, setting the heated humidifier to 32–34°C and 100% relative humidity appears safe.[54] Higher settings may be required when airway secretions are unusually thick or profuse.

Saturation of the inhaled air to at least 30 mg H_2O/L of absolute humidity is usually acceptable.[3]

15.5 Heat-Moisture Exchangers (HMEs)

Because of the parallel that can be drawn between their mechanism of functioning and that of the nose, HMEs are unofficially referred to as artificial noses.

These light and compact devices are fitted onto the distal end of the endotracheal tube. Since they passively harvest the water that is lost from the lower respiratory tract, the efficacy of HMEs depends on the humidity of the exhaled air, which in turn is dependent on the body temperature. The endotracheal tube and the tracheostomy tube are relatively efficient at preserving heat and moisture of the exhaled air, and so the water content of exhaled air can actually be quite high.[51] Delivered tidal volumes have a substantial bearing upon the performance of the HMEs, the operation declining slightly when large tidal volumes are used.

The functioning of modern HMEs has been greatly improved by a hygroscopic layering of magnesium, calcium, or lithium chloride. A calcium coating is probably just as efficient as a lithium coating – and probably a great deal safer – since the toxic lithium is potentially absorbable by the tracheobronchial mucosa.

After just a few exhalations modern HMEs generally trap enough water within themselves to perform effectively, and a steady state is quickly achieved. Water losses fall to 5–8 mg/L, i.e., to a level below the usual physiological losses.[2]

The proximal retention of moisture results in a relatively dry expiratory circuit, decreasing the potential mechanisms of infection. Some of the currently available HMEs are also coated with bacteriostatic materials.

As can be anticipated, the incorporation of humidification devices into the inspiratory circuit does increase the airways resistance, though the exact significance of this remains presently unclear.

HMEs should be considered potentially harmful in patients having an excess of airway secretions, such as in COPD, infection, pulmonary edema, or pulmonary hemorrhage; here, the obstruction of a HME can prove catastrophic. HMEs should not be used in association with HHs since this can increase the risk of HME occlusion. "Active HMEs" that comprise an integrated heated humidifier have been used in patients requiring large tidal volumes, but these have yet to gain general acceptance.[10] There is a possibility that entrapment of aerosolized medication within HMEs might also increase airflow resistance.

The increase in the airflow resistance that HMEs must undoubtedly produce can prove potentially exhausting for the patient on modes such as CPAP or PSV. This increase in the work of breathing can be offset by increasing the level of pressure support by 5–10 cm H_2O.[35]

The matter of HME-related increase in the work of breathing is also very relevant to patients on noninvasive support, but at the present time the issue awaits clarification.

A theoretical concern with HMEs is the expansion of dead space that they can produce.[29] Available HME devices are capable of increasing dead space by 30–95 mL. Since another 20 mL or so is added by the connecting tube, and 7 mL more by a closed-suction circuit, the cumulative increase in dead space can be expected to impact upon alveolar ventilation. In ARDS or acute severe asthma, where alveolar ventilation is at a premium, HHs may, therefore, prove more advantageous in this respect. When used in ARDS, the HME having the least dead space should normally be chosen.

Because the humidification produced by these devices is dependent on the water content of the expired air, these devices cease to function if expired air is lost, as can happen with a broncho-pleural fistula; for such a patient, a heated humidifier is more appropriate (Fig. 15.2).

Although in most units HMEs are changed on a daily basis, it may be safe to use HMEs for up to a week provided that these devices do not seem visibly clogged or contaminated.[34,58]

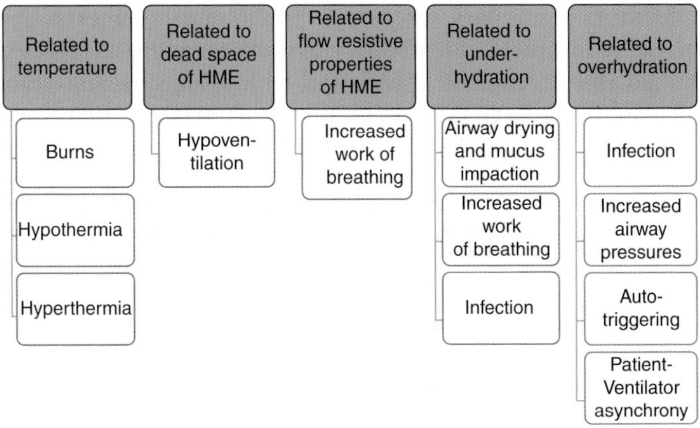
Related to temperature
Burns
Hypothermia
Hyperthermia
Related to dead space of HME
Hypoven-tilation
Related to flow resistive properties of HME
Increased work of breathing
Related to under-hydration
Airway drying and mucus impaction
Increased work of breathing
Infection
Related to overhydration
Infection
Increased airway pressures
Auto-triggering
Patient-Ventilator asynchrony

FIGURE 15.2. Problems associated with the use of humidifiers.

15.6 Airway Humidification During Noninvasive Ventilation

With noninvasive ventilation (NIV), the nasal and oral mucosa can dry very rapidly. During NIV – in contrast to invasive ventilation – the upper airway has not been bypassed by a patient tube, and the humidifying mechanisms of the upper airway are therefore intact. In theory, therefore, there should be no great need for a rigorous humidification exercise. The initial control of inspired air at 28–30°C at 100% relative humidity has been suggested, with further adjustments according to patient comfort.[54] However, with nasal-mask-NIV, mouth leaks are common: such high unidirectional airflows produce a substantial drop in the performance of the nasal mucosa as a heat-moisture exchanger. The consequent increase in the airflow resistance establishes a positive feedback loop.[42]

As discussed earlier, HMEs can increase work of breathing; where humidification is required with NIV, HHs are the devices of choice.

References

1. Markowicz P, Ricard J-D, Dreyfuss D, et al Safety, efficacy and cost effectiveness of mechanical ventilation with humidifying filters changed every 48 hours: a prospective, randomized study. *Crit Care Med* 2000;28(3):665–71
2. Rathgeber J, Henze D, Zuchner K, et al Conditioning of the inspired air with HME's- an effective and cost saving alternative to heated humidifiers in long-term ventilated patients. A prospective randomized clinical study. Anesthetist 1996;45:518–25
3. AARC clinical practice guideline. Humidification during mechanical ventilation. American Association for Respiratory Care. *Respir Care.* 1992;37:887–890
4. Amirav I, Plit M. Temperature and humidity modify airway response to inhaled histamine in normal subjects. *Am Rev Respir Dis*. 1989;140:1416–1420
5. Banner AS, Chausow A, Green J. The tussive effect of hyperpnea with cold air. *Am Rev Respir Dis*. 1985;131:362–367
6. Boisson C, Viviand X, Arnaud S, et al Changing a hydrophobic heat and moisture exchanger after 48 hours rather than 24 hours: a clinical and microbiological evaluation. *Intensive Care Med.* 1999;25:1237–1243
7. Branson RD, Campbell RS, Davis K, et al Anaesthesia circuits, humidity output, and mucociliary structure and function. *Anaesth Intensive Care*. 1998;26:178–183
8. Burton JDK. Effects of dry anesthetic gases on the respiratory mucous membrane. *Lancet*. 1962;1:235–238
9. Caldwell PRB, Gomez DM, Fritts HW. Respiratory heat exchange in normal subjects and in patients with pulmonary disease. *J Appl Physiol*. 1969;26:82–88
10. Campbell RS, Davis K Jr, Johannigman JA, Branson RD. The effects of passive humidifier dead space on respiratory variables in paralyzedand spontaneously breathing patients. *Respir Care*. 2000;45:306–312
11. Chalon J, Loew DAY, Malebranch J. Effects of dry anesthetic gases on tracheobronchial ciliated epithelium. *Anesthesiology*. 1972;37:338–343
12. Chiaranda M, Verona L, Pinamonti O, et al Use of heat and moisture exchanging (HME)filters in mechanically ventilated ICU patients: influence on airway flow-resistance. *Intensive Care Med*. 1993;19:462–466

13. Christopher KL, Saravolatz LD, Bush TL, Conway WA. The potential role of respiratory therapy equipment in cross infection. A study using a canine model for pneumonia. *Am Rev Respir Dis*. 1983;128:271–275
14. Cohen IL, Weinberg PF, Fein IA, Rowinski GS. Endotracheal tube occlusion associated with the use of heat and moisture exchangers in the intensive care unit. *Crit Care Med*. 1988;16: 277–279
15. Cole P. Some aspects of temperature, moisture and heat relationship in the upper respiratory tract. *J Laryngol Otol*. 1953;7:449–456
16. Comhaire A, Lamy M. Contamination rate of sterilized ventilators in an ICU. *Crit Care Med*. 1981;9:546–548
17. Craven DE, Goularte TA, Make BJ. Contaminated condensate in mechanical ventilator circuits. A risk factor for nosocomial pneumonia. *Am Rev Respir Dis*. 1984;129:625–628
18. Davis K Jr, Evans SL, Campbell RS, et al Prolonged use of heat and moisture exchangers does not affect device efficiency or frequency rate of nosocomial pneumonia. *Crit Care Med*. 2000;28:1412–1418
19. Dery R. The evolution of heat and moisture in the respiratory tract during anaesthesia with non-rebreathing system. *Canad Anaesth Soc J*. 1973;20:296–309
20. Dery R. Water balance of the respiratory tract during ventilation with a gas mixture saturated at body temperature. *Can Anaesth Soc J*. 1973;20:719–727
21. Dery R, Pelletier J, Jacques A. Humidity in anaesthesiology III: heat and moisture patterns in the respiratory tract during anaesthesia with the semi-closed system. *Can Anaesth Soc J*. 1967;14: 287–294
22. Déry R, Pelletier J, Jaques A, et al Humidity in anaesthesiology. III. Heat and moisture patterns in the respiratory tract during anaesthesia with the semi-closed system. *Can Anaesth Soc J*. 1967;14:287–298
23. Dhand R, Guntur VP. How best to deliver aerosol medications to mechanically ventilated patients. *Clin Chest Med*. 2008;29(2): 277–296
24. Djedaini K, Billiard M, Mier L, et al Changing heat and moisture exchangers every 48 hours rather than 24 hours does not affect their efficacy and incidence of nosocomial pneumonia. *Am J Respir Crit Care Med*. 1995;152:1562–1569
25. Fonkalsrud EW, Calmes S, Barcliff LT, et al Reduction of operative heat loss and pulmonary secretions in neonates by use of

heated and humidified anesthetic gases. *J Thorac Cardiovasc Surg*. 1980;80:718–723

26. Girault C, Breton L, Richard J, et al Effects of airway humidification devices during difficult weaning from mechanical ventilation. *Am J Respir Crit Care Med*. 2000;161:A560
27. Hirsch JA, Tokayer JL, Robinson MJ, et al Effects of dry air and subsequent humidification on tracheal mucus velocity in dogs. *J Appl Physiol*. 1975;39:242–246
28. Ingelstedt S. Studies of the conditioning of air in the respiratory tract. *Acta Otolaryngol*. 1956;131:1–81
29. Iotti GA, Olivei MC, Palo A, et al Unfavorable mechanical effects of heat and moisture exchangers in ventilated patients. *Intensive Care Med*. 1997;23(4):399–405
30. Kirton O, DeHaven B, Morgan J, Civetta J. A prospective, randomized comparison of an in-line heat and moisture exchange filter and heated wire humidifiers: rates of ventilatior-associated early-onset (community-acquired) or late – onset (hospital-acquired) pneumonia and incidence of endotracheal tube occlusion. *Chest*. 1998;112:1055–1059
31. Kleemann PP. The climatisation of anesthetic gases under conditions of high flow to low flow. *Acta Anaesthesiol Belg*. 1990;41:189–200
32. Kleemann PP. Humidity of anaesthetic gases with respect to low flow anaesthesia. *Anaesth Intensive Care*. 1994;22:396–408
33. Klein EF, Graves SA. "Hot pot" tracheitis. *Chest*. 1974;65:225–226
34. Kollef M, Shapiro S, Boyd V, et al A randomized clinical trial comparing an extended-use hygroscopic condenser humidifier with heated –water humidification in mechanically ventilated patients. *Chest*. 1998;113:759–767
35. Lellouche F, Maggiore SM, Deye N, et al Effect of the humidification device on the work of breathing during noninvasive ventilation. *Intensive Care Med*. 2002;28:1582–1589
36. Lichtiger M, Landa JF, Hirsch JA. Velocity of tracheal mucus in anesthetized women undergoing gynaecologic surgery. *Anesthesiology*. 1975;42:413–419
37. Marfatia S, Donahoe PK, Hendren WH. Effects of dry and humidified gases on the respiratory epithelium in rabbits. *J Paediatr Surg*. 1975;10:583–592
38. McFadden ER. Heat and water exchange in human airways. *Am Rev Respir Dis*. 1992;146:S8-S10
39. McFadden ER, Pichurko BM, Bowman HF, et al Thermal mapping of the airways in humans. *J Appl Physiol*. 1985;58:564–570

40. Misset B, Escudier B, Rivara D, et al Heat and moisture exchanger vs heated humidifier during long-term mechanical ventilation: a prospective randomized study. *Chest*. 1991;100:160–163
41. Modell JH, Giammona ST, Davis JH. Effect of chronic exposure to ultrasonic aerosols in the lung. *Anesthesiology*. 1967;28:680–684
42. Radenrath WJ, Meier J, Genger H, et al Efficiency of cold pass-over and heated humidification under continuous positive airway pressure. *Eur Respir J*. 2002;19:1–4
43. Rashad K, Wilson K, Hurt HH, et al Effect of humidification of anesthetic gases on static compliance. *Anesth Analg Curr Res*. 1967;46:127–133
44. Rathgeber J. Devices used to humidify respired gases. *Respir Care Clin*. 2006;12:165–183
45. Rathgeber J, Zuchner K, Burchardi H. Conditioning of the air in mechanically ventilated patients. In: Vincent JL, ed. *Yearbook of Intensive Care and Emergency Medicine*. Berlin: Springer; 1996:155–164
46. Rathgeber J, Kazmaier S, Penack O, et al Evaluation of heated humidifiers for use on intubated patients. A comparative study of humidifying efficiency, flow resistance and alarm functions using a lung model. *Intensive Care Med*. 2002;28:731–739
47. Ricard J-D, Le Miere E, Markowicz P, et al Efficiency and safety of mechanical ventilation with a heat and moisture exchanger changed only once a week. *Am J Respir Crit Care Med*. 2000;161:104–109
48. Ricard J-D, Hidri N, Blivet A, et al New heated breathing cirtcuits do not prevent condensation and contamination of ventilator circuits with heated humidifiers. *Am J Respir Crit Care Med*. 2003;167:A861
49. Ricard J-D, Boyer A, Dreyfuss D. The effect of humidification on the incidence of ventilator-associated pneumonia. *Respir Care Clin*. 2006;12:263–273
50. Roustan JP, Kienlen J, Aubas P, Aubas S, du Cailar J. Compairson of hydrophobic heat and moistureexchangers with heated humidifier during prolonged mechanical ventilation. *Intensive Care Med*. 1992;18:97–100
51. Ryan SN, Rankin N, Meyer E, et al Energy balance in the intubated human airway is an indicator of optimal gas conditioning. *Crit Care Med*. 2002;30:355–361
52. Sackner MA, Rosen MJ, Wanner A. Estimation of tracheal mucus velocity by bronchofibroscopy. *J Appl Physiol*. 1973;34:495–499
53. Shelley MP. The humidification and filtration functions of the airway. *Respir Care Clin*. 2006;12:139–148

54. Sottiaux TM. Consequences of under- and over-humidification. *Respir Care Clin N Am*. 2006;12(2):233–252
55. Theissen RJ. Filtration of respired gases: theoretical aspects. *Respir Care Clin*. 2006;12:183–201
56. Thiery G, Boyer A, Pigne E, et al Heat and moisture exchangers in mechanical ventilated intensive care unit patients: aplea for an independent assessment of their performance. *Crit Care Med*. 2003;31:699–704
57. Thomachot L, Vialet R, Arnaud S, et al Do the components of heat and moisture exchanger filters affect their humidifying efficacy and the incidence of nosocomial pneumonia ? *Crit Care Med*. 1999;27:923–928
58. Thomachot L, Leone M, Razzouk K, et al Randomized clinical trial of extended use of a hydrophobic condenser humidifier: 1 vs. 7 days. *Crit Care Med*. 2002;30:232–237
59. Todd DA, John E, Osborn RA. Tracheal damage following conventional and high-frequency ventilation at low and high humidity. *Crit Care Med*. 1991;19:1310–1316
60. Wanner A. Clinical aspects of mucociliary clearance. *Am Rev Respir Dis*. 1977;116:73–125
61. Williams RB. The effects of excessive humidity. *Respir Care Clin N Am*. 1998;4:215–226
62. Williams RB, Rankin N, Smith T, et al Relationship between the humidity and temperature of inspired gas and the function of the airway mucosa. *Crit Care Med*. 1996;24:1920–1929
63. Zuchner K. Humidification: measurements and requirements. *Respir Care Clin*. 2006;12:149–163

Chapter 16
Aerosol Therapy in the Mechanically Ventilated Patient

16.1 Terminology

An *aerosol* is defined as a suspension of solid or liquid particles in a gas. Most aerosols in clinical practice are polydisperse, that is to say, the contained particles vary greatly in diameter.

A dust is a suspension of *solid* particles in a gas. Dust particles are irregular.

A spray (or mist) is a suspension of *liquid* particles in a gas. Liquid particles tend to be spherical owing to surface tension forces.

Droplet nuclei are desiccated *complex* suspensions – when the liquid component evaporates, solid particles are left behind (Fig. 16.1).

An aerosol is a suspension of solid or liquid particles in a gas		
Dust	**Spray (mist)**	**Droplet nuclei**
A dust is a suspension of *solid* particles in a gas Dust particles are irregular	A spray (or mist) is a suspension of *liquid* particles in a gas Liquid particles tend to be spherical owing to surface tension forces	Droplet nuclei are dessicated *complex* suspensions When the liquid component evaporates solid particles are left behind

FIGURE 16.1. Aerosols.

A. Hasan, *Understanding Mechanical Ventilation*,
DOI: 10.1007/978-1-84882-869-8_16,

16.2 The Behavior of Particles

In the absence of air currents, the rate of sedimentation of particles is finite. Initially, a given particle falls with increasing velocity, and in doing so, encounters increasing airway resistance. At a certain point, the airway resistance does not permit it to fall any faster and a *settling velocity* is reached. Particles of differing densities – even though their sizes may be the same – do not settle with the same velocity. Depending upon the settling velocity of a particle, its aerodynamic diameter is computed; this may differ from its actual diameter. The aerodynamic diameter is measured by devices such as the Cascade sampler or Anderson's sampler. The average particle "size" determined by the aerodynamic method is termed its mass median aerosol diameter (MMAD).

Droplet nuclei remain airborne for relatively long periods of time. Evaporation shrinks particle size rapidly and makes it lighter and slower to settle. A particle less than 3 μ in size may remain airborne indefinitely.

The size of a particle determines its behavior within the airways (see Fig. 16.2). Not all particles can be inhaled; not all particles inhaled can be respired; and not all respirable particles are retained within the lower airways.

Typically, the particle diameter in an exhaled breath ranges from 0.3 to 2,000 μ.[20,54]

16.3 Devices for Aerosol Delivery

Three classes of device for aerosol delivery are available: nebulizers, metered-dose inhalers, and dry powder (inhalers). The last class is unsuitable for mechanically ventilated patients.

Nebulizers break up liquids into aerosols. Three types of nebulizers – jet, ultrasonic, and vibrating mesh nebulizers (VMNs) – are in use for patients on mechanical ventilation.

16.3.1 Jet Nebulizers (Syn: Pneumatic Nebulizers)

Gas is pumped under pressure through a Venturi system, which is essentially a very narrow orifice. Distally, there is a sharp

Inhalable fraction (0.1–185μ)	Thoracic fraction (<10–30μ)	Respirable fraction(<5μ)	Fine particles
• All particles that can be inhaled into the upper respiratory tract constitute the inhalable fraction • The larger of these particles will deposit on the walls of the upper airways, mostly by inertial impaction	• All particles that can enter the thorax after traversing the larynx constitute the thoracic fraction • The thoracic fraction consists predominantly of particles les then 10–30μ in diameter • Particles bigger than this are lost by impaction upon the walls of the upper aiway	• These are the particles that have the potential to reach the respiratory zone of the lung • Most such particles are around 1μ in size • Yet, only about 20% of the particles less than 1μ (and 14% of particles < 0.3μ) do eventually deposit here[39,44] • Humidity can expand the size of these particles, promoting their deposition[44,63]	• Very fine particles below 0.5μ in diameter frequently fail to deposit in the airway lumen, and are exhaled

FIGURE 16.2. Size related behavior of particles in the innate airway.

drop in pressure, and this causes the gas velocity to increase sharply. The nebulizer solution that is fed into the system through a separate conduit is first drawn into fine ligaments, which then, with the forces of surface tension, shatter into tiny droplets.[49] The smaller of these – the respirable droplets – enter the proximal part of the nebulizer circuit and are inhaled; the largest droplets collide with plates – called baffles – and are returned to the solution within the reservoir.

Since well over 90% of the particle load impacts upon the baffles, the fraction of the drug output is necessarily low.[49] Of the drug that is aerosolized, a large proportion dissipates into the surrounding air especially during exhalation, and a considerable amount is deposited upon upper airway (in the nonintubated patient): thus, at least half of the aerosol is eventually lost. Intermittent nebulizers, which nebulize the drug only during inhalation, are more efficient. Also, at the end of nebulization, sometimes as much as two thirds of the drug may remain behind in the nebulization chamber.

Nebulizers typically produce a polydispersed aerosol. Although particles less than 5 μ in diameter are widely regarded as respirable, it is not by any means certain that all such particles reach the lower respiratory tract. Often, the amount of useful drug that reaches the lungs is no more than about 10%, the greatest portion of the drug never reaching its intended destination.[4,67] With jet nebulizers, the nebulization time is prolonged compared to ultrasonic nebulizers (see below).

All jet nebulizers are not alike with regard to the size of the orifice of air-jet, the diameter of the capillary tube, and in the baffle design. These differences translate into different output characteristics, which may in fact differ considerably between brands.[36,45] This may have greater relevance for those medications that require their doses to be tightly controlled – such as pentamidine, ribavirin, rhDNAase, and tobramycin – than for inhaled bronchodilators (Figs. 16.3 and 16.4).

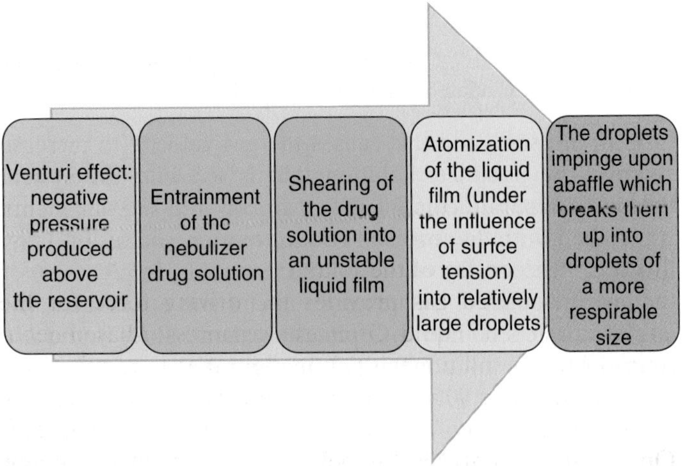
Venturi effect: negative pressure produced above the reservoir
Entrainment of the nebulizer drug solution
Shearing of the drug solution into an unstable liquid film
Atomization of the liquid film (under the influence of surfce tension) into relatively large droplets
The droplets impinge upon abaffle which breaks them up into droplets of a more respirable size

FIGURE 16.3. Aerosolization of nebulized particles.

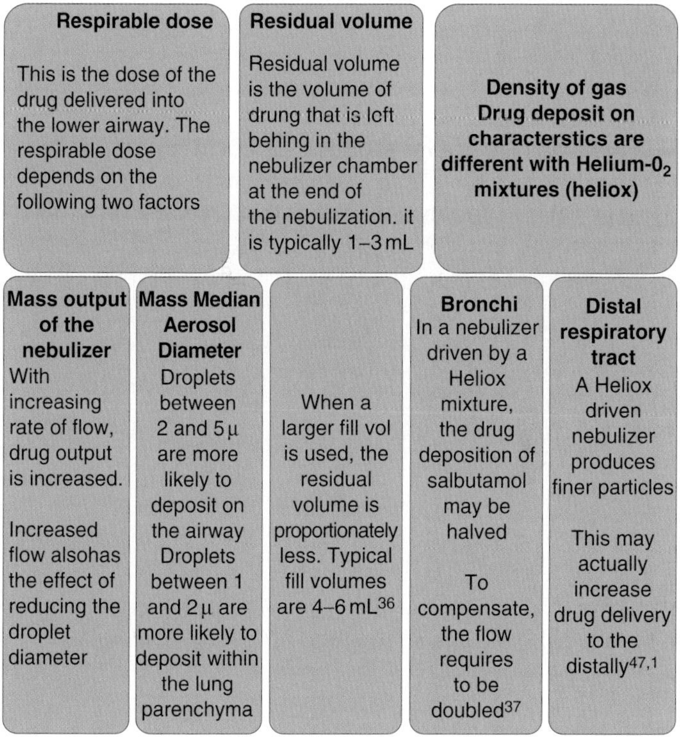
Respirable dose
This is the dose of the drug delivered into the lower airway. The respirable dose depends on the following two factors
Residual volume
Residual volume is the volume of drung that is left behing in the nebulizer chamber at the end of the nebulization. it is typically 1–3 mL
Density of gas
Drug deposit on characterstics are different with Helium-0_2 mixtures (heliox)
Mass output of the nebulizer
With increasing rate of flow, drug output is increased.
Increased flow alsohas the effect of reducing the droplet diameter
Mass Median Aerosol Diameter
Droplets between 2 and 5 μ are more likely to deposit on the airway Droplets between 1 and 2 μ are more likely to deposit within the lung parenchyma
When a larger fill vol is used, the residual volume is proportionately less. Typical fill volumes are 4–6 mL[36]
Bronchi
In a nebulizer driven by a Heliox mixture, the drug deposition of salbutamol may be halved
To compensate, the flow requires to be doubled[37]
Distal respiratory tract
A Heliox driven nebulizer produces finer particles
This may actually increase drug delivery to the distally[47,1]

FIGURE 16.4. Factors affecting aerosol delivery during nebulization.

Since proportionately more water than drug evaporates, the solution within the chamber becomes increasingly concentrated during the course of nebulization. Evaporation also results in the cooling of the solution.

The pressurized gas provides the driving force for the atomization of the liquid. Often, the compressor-based nebulizers do not generate the 8 L/m flow that is required for optimum nebulization.[57,60] With a higher rate of flow, the drug output is increased, and the droplet diameter attenuated.[37] One of the techniques for nebulizer use is set out below (Fig. 16.5).[22]

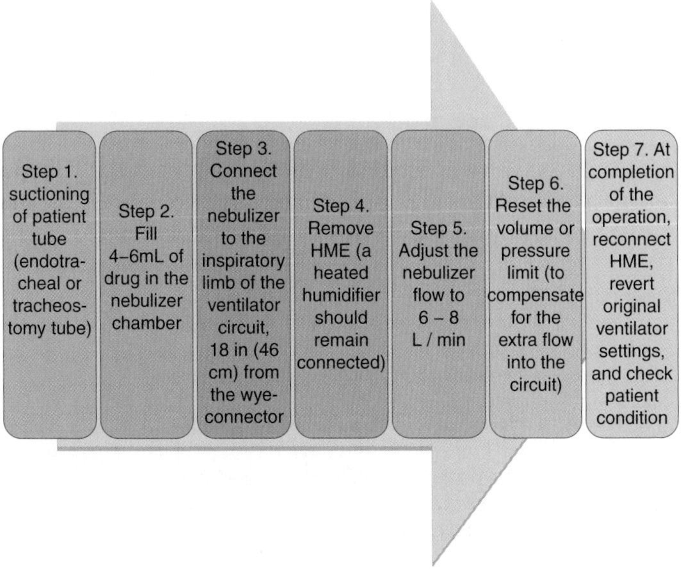
Step 1. suctioning of patient tube (endotracheal or tracheostomy tube)
Step 2. Fill 4–6mL of drug in the nebulizer chamber
Step 3. Connect the nebulizer to the inspiratory limb of the ventilator circuit, 18 in (46 cm) from the wye-connector
Step 4. Remove HME (a heated humidifier should remain connected)
Step 5. Adjust the nebulizer flow to 6 – 8 L / min
Step 6. Reset the volume or pressure limit (to compensate for the extra flow into the circuit)
Step 7. At completion of the operation, reconnect HME, revert original ventilator settings, and check patient condition

FIGURE 16.5. Technique for drug delivery by jet nebulizer. *Flow-by (or continuous flow) should be turned off during nebulization.*

16.3.2 Ultrasonic Nebulizers

Ultrasonic nebulizers incorporate a piezo-electric crystal which vibrates at a high frequency. The acoustic vibrations generate standing waves in the solution contained above the crystal. The crests of these waves fracture into droplets, and aerosolization of the solution occurs. The size of the aerosol droplet is inversely proportional to the frequency of vibration of the piezo-electric crystal; therefore, it is the frequency that determines the drug output.[29,56]

In general, the droplet size tends to be larger than that produced by the jet, and this increases drug wastage through deposition into ventilator tubings and the proximal respiratory tract. Again, the larger droplets are removed from the nebulisate when they impact upon baffles. Earlier versions of the ultrasonic nebulizers were superior in terms of drug delivery and nebulization time compared to earlier jet nebulizers, but the modern versions of the latter are more efficient and have come to be preferred. With most ultrasonic nebulizers, nebulization time is shorter.[33] Newer ultrasonic nebs are more efficient and relatively portable.[55]

For the delivery of inhaled bronchodilators, small volume ultrasonic nebulizers are appropriate; large volume ultrasonic nebulizers are used mostly for sputum induction. Concerns that ultrasonic waves can inactivate certain formulations have not been substantiated.

16.3.3 Vibrating Mesh Nebulizers (VMNs)

These novel devices incorporate a mesh which by its vibrations generates an aerosol.[8] VMNs are relatively efficient and can synchronize aerosol delivery with inspiration.[14] VMNs, by design, have no baffle. They have a low residual volume[66] and an excellent drug output – at least twice that of jet nebulizers.[8] Although the size of the aerosol particle that VMNs generate can vary, the particle size in general is quite small (a greater proportion of droplets of less than 3.3 μ are produced) and drug delivery into the target zone is therefore much better.[66]

The lower frequency of vibration of VMNs means that low-powered electrical units can be used, for which reason their operation is much quieter. They can be operated on battery pack in addition to wall current.[25]

16.3.4 Nebulization in the Ventilated Patient

Under the best of conditions, the delivery of aerosols into the peripheral airways is low. In intubated patients, the presence of an artificial airway will severely curtail deposition.[46] This is true for both aerosols released by pressurized metered-dose inhalers (MDIs) and nebulizers.[26] Lately, with the availability of better aerosol generators and improved techniques, results have significantly improved.[14]

Several factors can affect the deposition of aerosol in the peripheral airways: the size of the aerosol particle, the characteristics of the artificial airway and ventilator circuit, ventilator settings, and even the positioning of the patient.

Airway conditions: Large quantities of aerosol can be lost on the walls of the endotracheal tube[29]; a comparatively small amount will deposit upon the walls of the tracheostomy tube.[52] The narrow endotracheal tube in infants can significantly decrease aerosol penetration; in adults, differences in endotracheal tube size do not seem to compromise delivery as much.[6]

Severe airflow limitation will substantially impair drug deposition.[16] Increasing humidity will encourage the deposition of aerosol into the ventilator circuit and will substantially increase aerosol losses as well.[24] Drug losses – both from MDIs and nebulizers – are to the order of about 40% in a humidified system, compared to when dry gas is breathed.[43] Although a dry circuit is sometimes used when drug delivery is critical – as with antibiotics and prostaglandins – deliberately reducing the circuit humidity cannot be recommended for bronchodilator therapy. When employed, “dry circuit” nebulization time should be minimized to less than 10 min or so, in order to prevent airway dehydration.

Ventilator circuit: Jet nebulizers are best hooked into the circuit at a distance of a foot and a half from the endotracheal tube than between the patient Y-piece and endotracheal tube.[40,50] In contrast, the performance of ultrasonic nebulizers does not appear to depend as much upon the site of placement.[50]

Ventilator modes and settings: Modern ventilators are capable of coordinating the delivery of the aerosol to the inspiration, and compensating for the flow such that the tidal volumes and minute ventilation remains unaffected during the nebulization period.[11,15] Recent ventilators incorporating in-built nebulizers appear to be more efficient in this respect.[9,47] In spite of this, the drop in the driving pressure can decrease the drug output.[40,47]

Drug delivery with nebulizers appears to be lower when the pressure-controlled mode is used, compared to volume-control ventilation[38] (in contrast, drug delivery with MDIs seems not to be influenced by the mode of ventilation). For nebulizers (as well as for MDIs), aerosol delivery is greater with larger tidal volumes, a slower inspiratory flow rate and a longer inspiratory time.[18] However, these effects are probably not clinically significant in patients with COPD.[48] In theory, the use of flow triggering could reduce nebulizer (but not MDI) efficiency by increasing drug wastage during the expiratory cycle.[23] PEEP seems to have a variable effect on aerosol delivery.[30,65]

Position of the patient: In the supine patient, drug delivery is reduced,[16] and propping the patient to about 20–30° will improve the efficiency of nebulization.

Compared to invasive mechanical ventilation, aerosol delivery during noninvasive positive-pressure ventilation is consistently lower (see Chap. 13).

16.3.5 Nebulization of Other Drugs

The aerosol output of nebulizers is especially important with regard to critical drugs like antibiotics.

Jet nebulizers that are operated by a continuous external gas flow will promote drug deposition on ventilator circuitry during expiration; on the other hand when operated intermittently, their drug output suffers. Their chambers have relatively small reservoirs, and large residual volume result in further drug wastage. They are therefore less than ideal as far as drug nebulization goes.

Ultrasonic nebulizers are superior in the sense that they have larger reservoirs and generate finer particles ($<5\,\mu$).

While jet nebulizers will cool the nebulized solution, ultrasonic nebulizers will warm it by 10–15°C. This will generally not affect the viability of antibiotics such as aminoglycosides and colistin,[44] though it can denature peptides and proteins.[61] With VMNs, the temperature of the solution does not change, and so VMNs appear especially suited to protein and peptide drug nebulization.[8,14]

16.3.6 Pressurized Metered-Dose Inhalers (MDIs)

Contrary to the prevailing impression, MDIs are just as effective as nebulizers in ventilated patients.[10,19] Because of their

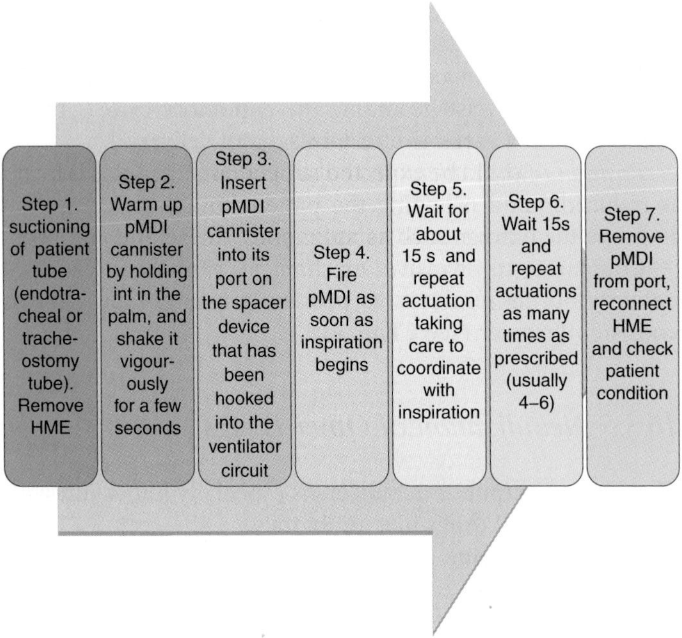
Step 1. suctioning of patient tube (endotracheal or tracheostomy tube). Remove HME
Step 2. Warm up pMDI cannister by holding int in the palm, and shake it vigourously for a few seconds
Step 3. Insert pMDI cannister into its port on the spacer device that has been hooked into the ventilator circuit
Step 4. Fire pMDI as soon as inspiration begins
Step 5. Wait for about 15 s and repeat actuation taking care to coordinate with inspiration
Step 6. Wait 15s and repeat actuations as many times as prescribed (usually 4–6)
Step 7. Remove pMDI from port, reconnect HME and check patient condition

FIGURE 16.6. Metered-dose inhaler (MDI) technique in ventilated patients.

uniform particle size, MDIs are excellent at bronchodilator drug delivery, and being much less intrusive, they are far less likely to contaminate the patient circuit.[5,32] For these reasons, there has been a definite increase in MDI usage in ICUs.[2] One technique of using MDIs in ventilated patients has been suggested in Fig. 16.6.[13]

Spacers: Several kinds of spacers/adapters are available for use with MDIs. The kind of adapter fitted to the MDI can have a profound effect on aerosol delivery.[10,58] A large volume spacer will generally deliver 4–6 times as much drug as will an elbow adapter or a unidirectional inline spacer.[3,27] When the MDI device is inserted into the circuit immediately adjoining the endotracheal tube, drug wastage can be very high[7]: the MDI-spacer assembly is ideally inserted into the circuit around 15 cm from the endotracheal tube.[17]

The newer environment-friendly hydrofluoroalkane (HFA) MDIs produce weaker plumes than the chlorofluorocarbon (CFC) MDIs. Wasteful drug deposition upon the walls of spacing chambers would be expected to decrease,[28] but this is by no means certain.[24]

At present, drugs such as antibiotics, surfactant, and prostaglandins are not available in MDIs[12]; for these reasons, nebulizers are still required.

References

1. Anderson M, Svartengren M, Philipson K, et al Deposition in man of particles suspended in air or in helium-oxygen mixture at different flow rates. *J Aerosol Med*. 1990;3:209
2. Ballard J, Lugo RA, Salyer JW. A survey of albuterol administration practices in intubated patients in the neonatal intensive care unit. *Respir Care*. 2002;47:31–38
3. Bishop MJ, Larson RP, Buschman DL. Metered dose inhaler aerosol characteristics are affected by the endotracheal tube actuator/adapter used. *Anesthesiology*. 1990;73:1263–1265
4. Clay MM, Clarke SW. Wastage of drug from nebulizers: a review. *J R Soc Med*. 1987;80:38–39
5. Craven DE, Lichtenberg DA, Goularte TA, et al Contaminated medication nebulizers in mechanical ventilator circuits. Source of bacterial aerosols. *Am J Med*. 1984;77:824–838
6. Crogan SJ, Bishop MJ. Delivery efficiency of metered dose aerosols given via endotracheal tubes. *Anesthesiology*. 1989;70:1008–1010
7. Dhand R. Special problems in aerosol delivery: artificial airways. *Respir Care*. 2000;45:636–645
8. Dhand R. Nebulizers that use a vibrating mesh or plate with multiple apertures to generate aerosol. *Respir Care*. 2002;47:1406–1416
9. Dhand R. Aerosol therapy during mechanical ventilation: getting ready for prime time. *Am J Respir Crit Care Med*. 2003;168(10): 1148–1149
10. Dhand R. Inhalation therapy with metered-dose inhalers and dry powder inhalers in mechanically-ventilated patients. *Respir Care*. 2005;50(10):1331–1344

11. Dhand R. Bronchodilator therapy. In: Tobin M, ed. *Principles and Practice of Mechanical Ventilation*. 2nd ed. New York: McGraw Hill; 2006:1277–1310
12. Dhand R. Inhalation therapy in invasive and noninvasive mechanical ventilation. *Curr Opin Crit Care*. 2007;13(1):27–38
13. Dhand R, Guntur VP. How best to deliver aerosol medications to mechanically ventilated patients. *Clin Chest Med*. 2008;29(2): 277–296
14. Dhand R, Sohal H. Pulmonary drug delivery system for inhalation therapy in mechanically ventilated patients. *Expert Rev Med Devices*. 2008;5(1):9–18
15. Dhand R, Tobin MJ. Inhaled drug therapy in mechanically-ventilated patients (pulmonary perspective). *Am J Respir Crit Care Med*. 1997;156:3–10
16. Dhand R, Jubran A, Tobin MJ. Bronchodilator delivery by metered-dose inhaler in ventilator-supported patients. *Am J Respir Crit Care Med*. 1995;151(6):1827–1833
17. Dhand R, Duarte AG, Jubran A, et al Dose-response to bronchodilator delivered by metered-dose inhaler in ventilator-supported patients. *Am J Respir Crit Care Med*. 1996;154:388–393
18. Dolovich MA. Influence of inspiratory flow rate, particle size, and airway caliber on aerosolized drug delivery to the lung. *Respir Care*. 2000;45:597–608
19. Duarte AG, Momii K, Bidani A. Bronchodilator therapy with metered-dose inhaler and spacer versus nebulizer in mechanically ventilated patients: comparison of magnitude and duration of response. *Respir Care*. 2000;45(7):817–823
20. Duguid JP. The size and the duration of air carriage of respiratory droplets and droplet nuclei. *J Hyg (Lond)*. 1946;44:471–479
21. Fink JB. Aerosol device selection: evidence to practice. *Respir Care*. 2000;45:874
22. Fink JB. Aerosol drug therapy. In: Wilkins RL, Stoller JK, Scanlan CL, eds. *Egan's Fundamentals of Respiratory Care*. 8th ed. St. Louis (MO): Mosby; 2003:761–800
23. Fink JB, Dhand R, Duarte AG, et al Aerosol delivery from a metered-dose inhaler during mechanical ventilation. An in vitro model. *Am J Respir Crit Care Med*. 1996;154:382–387
24. Fink JB, Dhand R, Grychowski J, et al Reconciling in-vitro and in-vivo measurements of aerosol delivery from a metered-dose inhaler during mechanical ventilation, and defining efficiency enhancing factors. *Am J Respir Crit Care Med*. 1999;159:63–68

25. Fink JB, Barraza P, Bisgaard J. Aerosol delivery during mechanical ventilation with high frequency oscillation: an in vitro evaluation (abstract). *Chest*. 2001;120:S277
26. Fuller HD, Dolovich MB, Posmituck G, et al Pressurized aerosol versus jet aerosol delivery to mechanically ventilated patients. Comparison of dose to the lungs. *Am Rev Respir Dis*. 1990;141: 440–444
27. Fuller HD, Dolovich MB, Turpie FH, et al Efficiency of bronchodilator aerosol delivery to the lungs from the metered dose inhaler in mechanically ventilated patients. A study comparing four different actuator devices. *Chest*. 1994;105:214–218
28. Gabrio BJ, Stein SW, Velasquez DJ. A new method to evaluate plume characteristics of hydrofluoroalkane and chlorofluorocarbon metered dose inhalers. *Int J Pharm*. 1999;186:3–12
29. Greenspan BJ. Ultrasonic and Electrohydrodynamic Methods for Aerosol Generation. In: Hickey AJ, ed. *Inhalation aerosols: physical and biologic basis for therapy. Lung biology in health and disease. vol. 94*. New York: Marcel Dekker; 1996
30. Guerin C, Durand PG, Pereira C, et al Effects of inhaled fenoterol and positive end-expiratory pressure on the respiratory mechanics of patients with chronic obstructive pulmonary disease. *Can Respir J*. 2005;12(6):329–335
31. Habib DM, Garner SS, Brandeburg S. Effect of helium-oxygen on delivery of albuterol in a pediatric, volume-cycled, ventilated lung model. *Pharmacotherapy*. 1999;19:143
32. Hamill RJ, Houston ED, Georghiou PR, et al An outbreak of Burkholderia (formerly Pseudomonas) cepacia respiratory tract colonization and infection associated with nebulized albuterol therapy. *Ann Intern Med*. 1995;122:762–766
33. Harvey CJ, O'Doherty MJ, Page CJ, et al Comparison of jet and ultrasonic nebulizer pulmonary aerosol deposition during mechanical ventilation. *Eur Respir J*. 1997;10:905–909
34. Henry RR, Mudaliar SR, Howland WC III, et al Inhaled insulin using the AERx insulin diabetes management system in healthy and asthmatic subjects. *Diabetes Care*. 2003;26:764
35. Hess D, Daugherty A, Simmons M. The volume of gas emitted from five metered dose inhalers at three levels of fullness. *Respir Care*. 1992;37:444
36. Hess D, Fisher D, Williams P, et al Medication nebulizer performance. Effects of diluent volume, nebulizer flow, and nebulizer brand. *Chest*. 1996;110:498

37. Hess DR, Acosta FL, Ritz RH, et al The effect of heliox on nebulizer function using a beta-agonist bronchodilator. *Chest.* 1999;115:184
38. Hess DR, Dillman C, Kacmarek RM. In vitro evaluation of aerosol bronchodilator delivery during mechanical ventilation: pressure control vs. volume control ventilation. *Intensive Care Med.* 2003;29(7):1145–1150
39. Hinds WC. *Aerosol Technology: Properties, Behaviour, and Measurement of Airborne Particles*. 2nd ed. New York: Wiley; 1999:42–74
40. Hughes JM, Saez J. Effect of nebulizer mode and position in a mechanical ventilator circuit on dose efficiency. *Respir Care.* 1987;32:1131–1135
41. Kacmarek RM, Hess D. The interface between patient and aerosol generator. *Respir Care*. 1991;36:952
42. Kress JP, North I, Gelbach BK, et al The utility of albuterol nebulized with heliox during acute asthma exacerbations. *Am J Respir Crit Care Med*. 2002;165:1317
43. Lange CF, Finlay WH. Overcoming the adverse effect of humidity in aerosol delivery via pressurized metered-dose in halers during mechanical ventilation. *Am J Respir Crit Care Med*. 2000;161: 1614–1618
44. Le Conte P, Potel G, Peltier P, et al Lung distribution and pharmacokinetics of aerosolized tobramycin. *Am Rev Respir Dis*. 1993;147:1279–1282
45. Leung K, Louca E, Coates AL. Comparison of breath-enhanced to breath-actuated nebulizers for rate, consistency, and efficiency. *Chest*. 2004;126:1619
46. Maclntyre NR, Silver RM, Miller CW, et al Aerosol delivery in intubated, mechanically ventilated patients. *Crit Care Med*. 1985; 13:81–84
47. Miller DD, Amin MM, Palmer LB, et al Aerosol delivery and modern mechanical: in vitro/in vivo evaluation. *Am J Respir Crit Care Med*. 2003;168:1205–1209
48. Mouloudi E, Prinianakis G, Kondili E, et al Bronchodilator delivery by metered-dose inhaler in mechanically ventilated COPD patients: influence of flow pattern. *Eur Respir J*. 2000;16:263–268
49. Nerbrink O, Dahlback M, Hansson HC. Why do medical nebulisers differ in their output and particle size characteristics? *J Aerosol Med*. 1994;7:259–276
50. O'Doherty MJ, Thomas SH, Page CJ, et al Delivery of a nebulized aerosol to a lung model during mechanical ventilation.

Effect of ventilator settings and nebulizer type, position, and volume of fill. *Am Rev Respir Dis*. 1992;146:383–388

51. O'Riordan TG, Greco MJ, Perry RJ, et al Nebulizer function during mechanical ventilation. *Am Rev Respir Dis*. 1992;145(5): 1117–1122
52. O'Riordan TG, Palmer LB, Smaldone GC. Aerosol deposition in mechanically ventilated patents. Optimizing nebulizer delivery. *Am J Respir Crit Care Med*. 1994;149:214–219
53. Olschewski H, Simonneau G, Galie N, et al Inhaled iloprost for severe pulmonary hypertension. *N Engl J Med*. 2002;347:322
54. Papineni RS, Rosenthal FS. The size distribution of droplets in the exhaled breath of healthy human subjects. *J Aerosol Med*. 1997;10(2):105–116
55. Phipps PR, Gonda I. Droplets produced by mechanical nebulizers. Some factors affecting their size and solute concentration. *Chest*. 1990;97:1327–1332
56. Rau JL. Design principles of liquid nebulization devices currently in use. *Respir Care*. 2002;47:1257–1275
57. Reisner C, Katial RK, Bartelson BB, et al Characterization of aerosol output from various nebulizer/compressor combinations. *Ann Allergy Asthma Immunol*. 2001;86:566
58. Rubin BK, Fink JB. Optimizing aerosol delivery by pressurized metered-dose inhalers. *Respir Care*. 2005;50:1191–1197
59. Standaert TA, Vandevanter D, Ramsey BW, et al The choice of compressor effects the aerosol parameters and the delivery of tobramycin from a single model nebulizer. *J Aerosol Med*. 2000;13:147
60. Standaert TA, Bohn SE, Aitken ML, Ramsey B. The equivalence of compressor pressure-flow relationships with respect to jet nebulizer aerosolization characteristics. *J Aerosol Med*. 2001;14:31
61. Steckel H, Eskandar F. Factors affecting aerosol performance during nebulization with jet and ultrasonic nebulizers. *Eur J Pharm Sci*. 2003;19:443–455
62. Svartengern M, Anderson M, Philison K, et al Human lung deposition of particles suspended in air or in helium-oxygen mixture. *Exp Lung Res*. 1989;15:575
63. Theissen RJ. Filtration of respired gases: theoretical aspects. *Resp Care Clin*. 2002;12:183–201
64. Thomas SH, O'Doherty MJ, Page CJ, et al Delivery of ultrasonic nebulized aerosols to a lung model during mechanical ventilation. *Am Rev Respir Dis*. 1993;148:872–877
65. Tzoufi M, Mentzelopoulos SD, Roussos C, et al The effects of nebulized salbutamol, external positive end-expiratory pressure,

and their combination on respiratory mechanics, hemodynamics, and gas exchange in mechanically ventilated chronic obstructive pulmonary disease patients. *Anesth Analg*. 2005;101(3):843–850

66. Waldrep JC, Berlinski A, Dhand R. Comparative analysis of methods to measure aerosol generated by vibrating mesh nebulizer. *J Aerosol Med*. 2007;20(3):310–319
67. Zainudin BMZ, Biddiscombe M, Tolfree SEJ, Short M, Spiro SG. Comparison of bronchodilator responses and deposition patterns of salbutamol inhaled from a pressurized, metered dose inhaler, as a dry powder, and as a nebulized solution. *Thorax*. 1990;45:469–473

Chapter 17 Nonconventional Modes and Adjunctive Therapies for Mechanical Ventilation

The science of mechanical ventilation is as yet imperfect. As newer innovations further the frontiers of artificial life support, it is clear that this area will continue to burgeon in the foreseeable future. Several innovations have fallen by the wayside despite showing early promise, but other exciting options have appeared on the horizon. What follows is a brief discussion of the (as yet) unconventional modes of ventilation, some of which have already gained a measure of acceptance.

Box 17.1 Inverse Ratio Ventilation

The basis of using a longer inspiratory time for the purposes of improving oxygenation is based upon the physiological assumption that diseased alveoli have different lung constants compared to healthy air units and therefore require a longer time to fill and to empty. These alveoli can be recruited to provide useful ventilation if the inspiratory time is increased. Indeed, inverse ratio ventilation, which is defined by the deliberate prolongation of the inspiratory time to equal or exceed the expiratory time, has been shown to improve oxygenation; it is less clear, however, whether the increase in oxygenation translates to an increase in survival.

A. Hasan, *Understanding Mechanical Ventilation*,
DOI: 10.1007/978-1-84882-869-8_17,

Poor patient tolerance of the "inverted" pattern of breathing often requires heavy sedation and possibly pharmacological paralysis, and the shortened expiratory time increases the likelihood of air-trapping, resulting in a high incidence of hemodynamic instability and barotrauma.

Inverse ratio ventilation has been discussed in sections 5.12.3 and 9.4.3.9 ...and ....

Box 17.1.1 Prone ventilation

Like inverse ratio ventilation, ventilating the patient in the prone position does improve oxygenation, though its ability to improve the outcome is less certain. The mechanisms by which the improvement in oxygenation occurs are uncertain and several hypotheses exist. These theories do not satisfactorily elucidate the underlying mechanisms and it is clear that other as yet undefined pathways must be operative. Nevertheless, it does appear that improvements once obtained are sustained, though the maintenance of the partial pressure of oxygen at the improved level may be on account of the other therapeutic strategies already in place.

Prone ventilation has been discussed in section 9.4.3.12

17.1 High-Frequency Ventilation

HFV was first described in 1969.

In HFV breaths are delivered at extremely high respiratory frequencies – 150–3,000 cycles/min[11]; the tidal volumes are therefore less than the anatomical dead space, but effective gas exchange does occur in spite of this. The delivered gas presumably reaches the alveoli by augmented gas diffusion and Taylor dispersion; but this is by no means certain.

It has also been proposed that lateral dispersion of gas molecules and CO_2 washout from the central airways (streaming) facilitate gas exchange, as does a degree of cross-ventilation between alveoli having different time constants (pendelluft).

Compared to low-frequency ventilation, where most of the tidal breath is directed to the lower lobes, HFV leads to better homogeneity of ventilation. Four forms of HFV – namely high-frequency positive pressure ventilation (HFPPV), high-frequency jet ventilation (HFJV), high-frequency oscillation (HFO), and high-frequency percussive ventilation (HFPV) – have evolved in response to the need for safe ventilation of those patients likely to have unacceptably high airway pressures with the conventional modes of ventilation. A fifth, High-Frequency Flow Interruption, is currently used for investigational purposes. These modes are classified according to the frequencies at which the pulsatile airflow is delivered, and by the manner in which the breaths are delivered. The use of the various HFV modes is more common in neonatal and pediatric ICUs: only high-frequency oscillatory ventilation (HFOV) (see below), and occasionally, percussive ventilation is used to any extent to ventilate selected adults who present difficulties in oxygenation.[26]

Even today, the specific applications of HFV remain nebulous.[56] HFV has been used with varying results in ventilating patients with bronchopleural fistula (BPF),[5] inhalational injury, and head injury,[22] but it is its potential role in ALI/ARDS that has evoked the most interest. Low tidal volumes are of proven value in the management of acute lung injury, and the small tidal volumes that are possible with HFV theoretically make HFV an attractive option under these circumstances; indeed, its use has been justified by clinicians when hypoxemia has worsened despite conventional mechanical ventilation – especially early in the course of ARDS.[16,44]

While ALI and ARDS are important potential indications for HFV, airway obstruction is not; air-trapping and barotrauma can very quickly occur (see below).

17.2 High-Frequency Positive Pressure Ventilation (HFPPV)

HFPPV is delivered through conventional ventilators at frequencies ranging between 60 and 150 breaths/min (1–2.5 Hz).[11] The USFDA defines HFV as any mode that uses a breath rate of 150/min and above, and so HFPPV technically does not qualify as a high-frequency mode. Its use has now been more or less supplanted by the other HFV modes discussed below.

17.3 High-Frequency Jet Ventilation (HFJV)

HFJV can either be used alone, or in conjunction with conventional mechanical ventilation. A special adapter attached to a conventional endotracheal tube has been used, but special triple lumen endotracheal tubes are now in vogue. The large central lumen is used for conventional positive pressure breaths or for the application of CPAP. The peripheral conduits are used for jet ventilation – with gas pulsed at frequencies of 240–660 breaths/min[11] – and for monitoring peripheral airway pressure. Expiration is passive. The air exits through a port a third of the distance from the distal end of the endotracheal tube.

Respiratory frequency and driving pressure are adjusted according to patient requirements. High respiratory rates are poorly tolerated, and excessive movement can interfere with gas exchange, so sedation is invariably – and paralysis frequently – required. Usual initial settings are a respiratory rate of between 100 and 150 breaths/min, an inspiratory fraction (which is the inspiratory time divided by the respiratory cycle time) of 40% or less, and a driving pressure of approximately 35 pounds per square inch (psi). With progressively increasing support, an effective "capture" is signaled by an abrupt improvement in gas exchange.

Applied PEEP is generally quite high in HFJV, but the lower tidal volumes keep the airway pressures within the limits considered safe.[60,70]

Concomitantly, CMV breaths can be given, and are usually required at relatively low frequencies – 10 breaths/min or

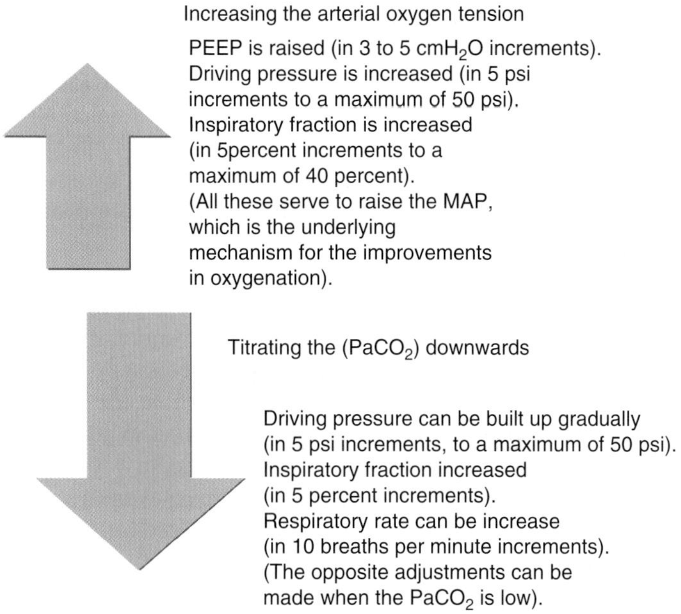
Increasing the arterial oxygen tension
PEEP is raised (in 3 to 5 cmH_2O increments).
Driving pressure is increased (in 5 psi increments to a maximum of 50 psi).
Inspiratory fraction is increased (in 5percent increments to a maximum of 40 percent).
(All these serve to raise the MAP, which is the underlying mechanism for the improvements in oxygenation).
Titrating the ($PaCO_2$) downwards
Driving pressure can be built up gradually (in 5 psi increments, to a maximum of 50 psi).
Inspiratory fraction increased (in 5 percent increments).
Respiratory rate can be increase (in 10 breaths per minute increments).
(The opposite adjustments can be made when the $PaCO_2$ is low).

FIGURE 17.1. HFJV: adjustment in ventilator settings.

less. When the lung has been well recruited by the PEEP, HFJV ventilation may by itself suffice and CMV breaths can be discontinued.[60]

In adults, HFJV has also been used in selected patients in the setting of BPF, although the rationale of ventilation is very different to that in ARDS. It is believed that the lower airway pressure manageable through the use of HFJV decreases air leakage through the fistula, improving its chances of closure.

Obviously, in this setting, no attempt to generate intrinsic PEEP is made, and the emphasis is on minimizing airway pressures to the bare minimum required for effective ventilation. Although HFJV has been used with a measure of success in patients with large BPFs, generally, its use in BPFs that occur in the setting of ARDS can actually worsen gas exchange.[5] In fact, there is as yet no convincing evidence that HFJV can actually help BPF to heal.[5]

Although the lower tidal volumes possible with HFJV may achieve a lower peak airway pressure, dynamic hyperinflation can still occur on account of the high respiratory rate. For this reason, the use of HFJV is relatively contraindicated in obstructive airway disease. In fact, the mean airway pressure developed may be no lower than that seen with conventional ventilation and the incidence of hemodynamic compromise and barotrauma may be just as high.[30]

The side effects with HFJV may be no less common than with conventional ventilation; because of the high flow rates used, they may actually exceed those of conventional ventilation. The large drop in pressure across the injection system will cause the injected gas to expand upon reaching the trachea, and this can result in substantial airway cooling. When HFJV is used for longer than 8 h, dehydration of the airway mucosa can predispose to several problems including severe necrotising tracheobronchitis; special devices are required for adequate airway humidification. It is now being realized that the collision of high pressure gas "bullets" with the mucosa may be the main cause for the necrotizing tracheobronchitis.[46]

17.4 High-Frequency Oscillatory Ventilation (HFOV)

HFOV is now the commonest used form of HFV for infants and young children. In HFOV even higher respiratory frequencies (480–1,800 breaths/min) are made possible by a device that incorporates a reciprocating pump, piston, or diaphragm. Unlike in HFPPV and HFJV, exhalation in HFO is active: the negative stroke of the piston assists evacuation of gas which exits the circuit directly opposite its entry point. The exit valve offers higher impedance to oscillating gas than it does to the more slowly flowing "exhaled" air, and this enables venting of expired air to the exterior. The rapid oscillations of gas cause the airway pressure to oscillate around a steady mean airway pressure. The mean airway pressure can be dialed in directly on some devices; on others, it is controlled by regulating the inspiratory flow rate and expiratory back pressure.[24]

With HFOV, mean airway pressures are higher than with most other modes: derecruitment is prevented, while excessive peak airway pressures are avoided.

When a smaller endotracheal tube is used or a higher respiratory frequency applied, a smaller tidal volume – also termed amplitude – results.[32] Control of oxygenation is achieved by manipulating the mean airway pressure or the FIO_2. $PaCO_2$ is controlled by regulating the tidal volume or respiratory rate. The "right" respiratory rate is determined by a "wiggling" of the patient's trunk.

Among the high-frequency modes, HFOV has been the subject of the most scrutiny, at least among adult patients with ALI and ARDS.[45] In these patients HFOV, by elevating mean airway pressure, has produced significant improvements in oxygenation. The improvements were, however, not sustained beyond 24 h.[45] Nevertheless, based upon these studies, the role of HFO cannot be dismissed since the trials were performed with tidal volumes later recognized as being clearly excessive.

The benefits of HFOV, in terms of oxygenation though not in terms of outcomes, can be complemented with inhaled nitric oxide and by recruitment maneuvers.[23,43] To an extent, the gains in oxygenation can be sustained when a proned patient is put back into the supine position.[18]

17.5 High-Frequency Percussive Ventilation (HFPV)

HFPV makes use of a phasitron, an inspiratory–expiratory valve through which gas at high pressure is driven phasically.

In HFPV, HFV breaths are superimposed upon conventional pressure-controlled, time-cycled machine breaths. HFV breaths are pulsed at about 200–900 breaths/min, over "background" PCV breaths cycled at about 10–15 times a minute. In other words, HFOV breaths are given at alternating – inspiratory and expiratory – pressure levels.[56] Ventilation at relatively low airway pressures is made possible. Thus, HFPV is capable of improving both oxygenation and ventilation without exposing the patient to the effects of high intrathoracic pressure. As a consequence, it has less of a propensity to produce hypotension, barotrauma, or intracranial hypertension in blunt head injury than do other modes.[56]

HFPV appears to be superior at mobilizing secretions than are other modes of HFV.[56] Pharmacologic paralysis is not generally required.

17.6 Extracorporeal Life Support (ECLS)

ECLS is a method of life support that enables gas exchange to occur outside the body, and thus allows the native lungs to rest.

17.6.1 Extracorporeal Membrane Oxygenation (ECMO)

Although ECMO has been used in some pediatric units in the past, its use in adults has only recently increased. ECMO can be administered either through a veno-arterial bypass (VA-ECMO) or a veno-venous bypass (VV-ECMO). VA-ECMO is used when hemodynamic shock complicates respiratory failure; VV-ECMO is the method of choice when cardiac function is preserved.

17.6.1.1 VA-ECMO (Veno-Arterial Bypass)

Venous access is secured by cannulating the right atrium through the internal jugular vein. The oxygenated blood is perfused back into the aorta usually through the right common carotid – alternatively, the femoral artery can be used for arterial access – in which case blood is retrogradely perfused back up the aorta. If the heart stops pumping – which it frequently does – this can predispose it to thrombosis; since the left side of the motionless heart will continue to receive the blood from the bronchial and thesbesian veins, its overdistension can cause back-pressures in the pulmonary circulation to rise sharply, leading to pulmonary edema.

17.6.1.2 VV-ECMO (Veno-Venous Bypass)

Blood is drawn out from the right atrium through a cannula introduced into the internal jugular vein; after oxygenation, blood is reintroduced into the right atrium through the cannulated femoral vein. Since all the blood continues to pass through the pulmonary vascular bed, there is now a much smaller danger of thrombosis within the left-sided cardiac chambers.

17.6.2 Extracorporeal CO_2 Removal

With extracorporeal CO_2 removal ($ECCO_2R$) systems, a VV-ECMO is created and gas exchange occurs extracorporeally; the patient's native lungs (which are kept apneic) are made use of to augment oxygenation.[27] In this case, it is the patient's own cardiac output that determines systemic perfusion. Extracorporeal CO_2 removal may be combined with low-frequency positive pressure ventilation (LFPPV–$ECCO_2R$) and the rested lung is inflated with just 2–3 breaths/min to preserve FRC and lung compliance.[9,28]

ECMO requires anticoagulation; consequently, patients run a substantial risk for bleeding. On the other hand, the heparinized membrane lung used for $ECCO_2R$ eliminates the need for systemic anticoagulation and the risk of bleeding is commensurately low.

17.6.3 Indications for ECLS

ECLS may be considered when severe, yet potentially reversible respiratory failure does not respond to conventional methods of ventilation.[3] Patients in severe ARDS, pneumonia, or pulmonary embolism would at present seem reasonable candidates for ECLS, as would patients with severe but potentially reversible myocardial dysfunction[40] and patients with impending organ replacement.

17.6.4 Contraindications to ECLS

Contraindications to ECLS include a bleeding diathesis, recent surgery within the preceding 3 days, severe systemic sepsis, and indeed any condition (such as severe brain injury) that could make long-term survival meaningless. Clearly, patients having incurable or potentially irreversible conditions (such as an untreatable systemic condition, malignancy, or an ARDS that is considered irremediable) cannot be considered for ECLS. Although the results of ECLS in earlier studies were uniformly discouraging,[70] more recent clinical data have shown a much more improved survival.[33] This possibly reflects the ventilation of patients at lower mean airway pressures compared to those before and earlier recourse to ECMO under worsening circumstances. It is also possible that better supportive care of patients may have played an important role in the increased survival noted in the above studies. This dramatic increase in survival rates should probably be viewed with circumspection, though it is likely that with improving technology, ECLS may well assume a key role in the not too distant future.[48]

17.7 Nitric Oxide

Before nitric oxide (NO) was recognized as one of the major players in pulmonary pathophysiology, it was largely considered an air pollutant. The behavior of nitric oxide within the human body is ill understood as yet and there is reason to believe that it may play a complex part in the regulation of numerous cellular processes (see Fig. 17.2).

Normally, NO produced within the nasopharynx and the paranasal sinuses – within the maxillary sinuses in particular – is drawn into the well-ventilated regions of the lung, producing selective vasodilatation. By so redistributing perfusion from ill-ventilated to well-ventilated units, it improves V/Q

Constitutive neuronal NOS (nNOS)	Constitutive endothelial Nos (eNOS)	Inducible NOS (iNOS)
• Expressed by peripheral nerves • Regulates bronchial smooth muscle relaxation	• Expressed by vascular endothelial cells • Regulates vascular tone in systemic and pulmonary arteries	• Expressed by inflammatory cells • Regulates anti inflammatory effects

FIGURE 17.2. Isoforms of nitric oxide synthetase.

matching. In intubated patients, tracheal NO concentrations are palpably lower; this may have consequences for the mechanically ventilated patient.

Nitric oxide may be inducible or constitutive; there are several isoforms of nitric oxide synthetase, the enzyme that produces nitric oxide from arginine (Fig. 17.2).

That the effects of nitric acid are local and not manifest at sites distant to its origin is principally on account of its propensity to rapidly combine with the heme portion of hemoglobin to form methemoglobin, and in doing so, to inactivate itself (In spite of this, it has recently been demonstrated that a small proportion of NO can in fact spill over into the systemic circulation and decrease the systemic vascular resistance).[51] The diffusibility of nitric oxide across biological membranes is on account of its lipophilicity. Its biological effects seem to occur as a result of the reactivity conferred upon it by its unpaired electron. Diffusion of nitric oxide from the site of its production – the vasculature – to the subjacent smooth muscle cells where it activates guanylate cyclase appears to be central to its role as a vascular smooth muscle relaxant, and therefore, as a modulant of blood flow. The benefits of inhaled nitric oxide may go beyond the V/Q matching it promotes and the lowering of the pulmonary arterial pressures that it facilitates. Nitric oxide may have intrinsic anti-inflammatory properties and may modulate platelet adhesiveness and endothelial permeability.

Inhaled nitric oxide has been shown to produce remarkable improvement in oxygenation when administered to ARDS patients and these effects were most apparent in prone patients.[53] Because inhaled NO can only access the pulmonary circulation through well-ventilated air units, it is likely that recruitment manoeuvers may enhance its effects.[49,50] In ARDS, the pulmonary arterial pressures exhibit a dose-dependent effect with inhaled NO. In contrast, it takes miniscule concentrations of inhaled NO – 10 parts/billion – to significantly decrease hypoxemia. It is helpful to construct dose-response curves to determine the precise dosage requirements in individual cases.[29] In any case, the improvements in oxygenation appear to be transient and seem not to translate into improved survival. Not all patients respond to the administration of NO, and no predictive indices that could identify potential responders are as yet known. Furthermore, it is possible that a rebound worsening may occur in the pulmonary hypertension[14] or oxygenation[55] if inhaled nitric oxide were to be suddenly withdrawn. It is also possible that NO – especially when administered in high concentrations – may engender toxic radicals such as dinitrogen trioxide and peroxynitrite; whether these are less or more harmful than the toxic oxygen radicals to which the patient breathing high fractions of oxygen is exposed is not presently known.

Box 17.2 Functions of Endogenous Nitric Oxide

Pulmonary vasodilation
Microbicidal effect
Increased ciliary motility and mucous clearance
Increased mucus production
Bronchodilation by regulation of the basal bronchomotor tone
Regulation of platelet adhesion
Modulation of endothelial permeability

Box 17.3 Side Effects of Inhaled Nitric Oxide[31]

Met-hemoglobinemia
Pulmonary edema
Alveolar hemorrhage
Rebound pulmonary vasoconstriction
Rebound hypoxemia
Type II pneumocyte hyperplasia
Increase in alveolar inflammatory cells
Formation of toxic radicals
Impairment of surfactant action
Decreased platelet aggregation
Breakages in chromatin

17.8 Surfactant Therapy

In a completely fluid-filled lung, no air–liquid interface exists, and therefore, no forces of surface tension exist. In the normal airway lumen, liquid–air interfaces generate forces of surface tension, which tend to collapse the airways. Healthy alveoli would collapse entirely at end expiration, were it not for the surface tension lowering properties of the surfactant that lines them.[55] Surfactant-depleted alveoli do collapse at end expiration, producing right to left shunting, decreased pulmonary compliance, and predisposing the lung to atelectrauma.

Pulmonary surfactant, produced by the type II pneumocytes, is composed of two principal components: four known surfactant-specific proteins (SP-A, SP-B, SP-C, SP-D) and lipids.[4] The bulk (approximately 90%) of surfactant is composed of lipids, of which the principal ones are the two phospholipids – phosphatidylcholine and phosphatidylglycerol.[63,64]

The varied and complex role of surfactant is being increasingly recognized. Surfactant defends the air spaces against flooding by preventing fluid transudation across the alveolo–capillary membrane,[39] and against infection by the lectins contained within its SP-A and SP-D moieties.[66] It also facilitates the clearance of mucus and the debris of apoptotic cells from the air spaces. The role of surfactant in scavenging reactive O_2 species also appears important in the limitation of inflammation.

The functional form of surfactant is gathered into large aggregated (LA). The LA form can decline into a vesicular form comprising small aggregates (SA).[49,50]

When large phasic changes in the surface area of air units occur – as they do the application of excessive tidal volumes – the LAs become altered into the relatively ineffective SAs.[64] In ARDS, the seepage of a protein and fibrin rich exudate into the alveoli can seriously impair surfactant function.[57]

In theory, surfactant replacement therapy in ARDS is a rational therapeutic intervention, given the role of surfactant in the genesis of this condition. Surfactant can be aerosolized into the bronchial tree by nebulization,[65] but this method has

Box 17.4 LaPlace's Law

$$\Delta P > 2\delta / r$$

Where
P > pressure
δ > surface tension
R > radius

LaPlace's Law states that the change in pressure within an air bubble is inversely proportional to its radius. Applied to the air unit, during exhalation, as the denominator in the equation (the radius of the alveolus) decreases, the change in pressure within will tend to collapse it – unless the numerator (the surface tension) shows a parallel decrease. In other words, an air unit will remain stable only when a reduction in its radius is paralleled by a reduction in the surface tension. Surface tension forces within the alveolus are dynamic and match the alveolar diameter: they can range from 40 dynes/cm at end inspiration to 10 dynes/cm at end expiration.

the inherent drawback that surfactant does not precisely aerosolize to its targeted site – the surfactant-depleted atelectatic alveoli. It may, therefore, be more effectual to directly instill surfactant boluses into the endotracheal tube[62] or lavage the bronchopulmonary segments with surfactant through the bronchoscope.[65] Postinstillation, adequate PEEP and tidal volumes must be applied to ensure the success of the treatment.[38] Unfortunately, surfactant replacement therapy has not yet fulfilled the promise it initially showed, though with the advent of superior formulations not only ARDS but other diseases such as alveolar proteinosis,[21] interstitial lung disease,[42] asthma, and cystic fibrosis[19] could be targeted as well.

17.9 Helium–Oxygen Mixtures

As described in Chap. 3, airflow is turbulent in the larger airways and more laminar in the smaller.

The flow of gases through straight and rigid tubes is governed by physical laws. At low velocities, particles travel in a streamlined manner, parallel to the sides of the tube: this is termed laminar flow. The gas front is parabolic, since the particles in the center of the tube move faster than those at the periphery. At high velocities, particles move in an unpredictable chaotic manner; this is termed turbulent flow. The critical mathematical parameter that determines that the flow is laminar or turbulent is a dimensionless number – the Reynold number. Reynold number is itself a function of the diameter of the tube as well as the density, velocity, and the viscosity of the gas. The last of these is relevant to the discussion that follows.

Looking at the equation (Box 17.5) it is evident that in a given tube – or airway – when flow is constant, it is the density of the gas which determines whether the airflow is laminar or turbulent. In a straight, rigid, smooth nonbranching tube, a Reynold number below 2,000 results in laminar flow; a number above 4,000 determines turbulent flow. Unfortunately the airway is none of these, and as a result of considerable turbulence, the above equation, applied to the human airway, lacks precision. It, nevertheless, follows that if gas with a lower density than air is breathed, turbulence can be reduced.

Helium is such a gas, with a density of 0.8 g/L (that of air is 1.29 g/L). The addition of helium (in place of nitrogen) to oxygen lowers the Reynolds number of the gas mixture, and so reduces turbulence. Mixtures of helium and oxygen (heliox) in the proportion 80:20 or 70:30 are used in clinical practice to try to overcome the high airway pressure in refractory asthma and respiratory distress syndrome in children.[8,37]

The flow of gas through an orifice being inversely proportional to the square root of its density (Graham's Law), Heliox will flow almost twice as fast than an oxygen flow-meter indicates.[20] Unless the lower density of this gas mixture is factored in, errors can occur during the calculation of flows while ventilating patients with heliox. Similarly, since the set FIO_2 may not reflect the fraction of oxygen actually delivered to the patient who is breathing heliox, oxygen analyzers must be relied upon while programming oxygen delivery on the ventilator.

Box 17.5 Determinants of the Reynold Number

$$R > pdv/u$$

where,
R > Reynolds number
p > density
d > airway diameter
v > velocity of gas
u > viscosity of the gas

17.10 Liquid Ventilation

Liquid ventilation involves the insufflation of lungs by perfluorochemicals rather than air for the purpose of gas exchange. Attempts to improve oxygen diffusion through diseased lungs using hyperbaric saline ventilation[41] led to the development of perfluorocarbons as media for facilitating gas exchange.[12]

When the hydrogen atoms of hydrocarbons are replaced by the halogen fluorine, biologically inert perfluorocarbons are formed. Perfluorocarbons are colorless but radio-opaque fluids. O_2 and CO_2 have a high solubility into these chemicals, which as a result, provide a large reservoir for these gases. The solubility of oxygen within perfluorocarbons exceeds by approximately 15-fold that within plasma.[59]

Perfluorocarbons have certain properties which make them well suited for their purpose as media for liquid ventilation. Unlike saline, they do not remove surfactant from alveoli.[17] By abolishing the air–liquid interface at the surface of the alveolar epithelium, they substantially diminish surface tension especially in surfactant-depleted air units. By filling up alveoli, they prevent alveolar closure, recruit alveoli, and improve functional residual capacity. It is possible that the reason for improvement in oxygenation is alveolar recruitment. The gravitational descent of the dense liquid into the nether regions of the lung may also be responsible for the redistribution of perfusion to the relatively well-ventilated nondependent areas.

By assuring alveolar patency even at relatively low airway pressures, perfluorocarbons can lower the risk for barotrauma. Inappropriately large boluses of perfluorocarbons can in fact distend the lung in a similar manner to PEEP, and are similarly capable of compromising the cardiac output. Since they are denser than water, perfluorocarbons gravitate to the dependent air units where the lung pathology is often most severe; mucus and inflammatory debris being lighter than perfluorocarbons float upward and can so be removed. The rinsing of the lung of inflammatory mediators may possibly modify neutrophil function and help limit lung inflammation and injury.[61] Owing to their higher heat capacity, perfluorocarbons can be utilized to regulate core body temperature.[25,58] Perfluorocarbons are immiscible with body fluids and negligible quantities diffuse into pulmonary capillary blood.[67]

17.10.1 Total Liquid Ventilation

During total liquid lung ventilation (TLV), the lungs are completely filled up with oxygenated perfluorocarbons and tidal boluses of perfluorocarbons are periodically pumped in and out of the lungs. This involves the use of complex equipment for the transportation of these dense fluids to and from the lungs and for the extracorporeal oxygenation and CO_2 removal from the fluid. The repeated instillation into and removal of perfluorocarbons from the lungs also serves to rinse the alveoli.[54]

17.10.2 Partial Liquid Ventilation

Technically less demanding, partial liquid ventilation involves the instillation of perfluorocarbons that are quantitatively equivalent to the functional residual capacity of the lungs. In this way, the partially filled lungs can be ventilated by a conventional mechanical ventilator rather than the complex equipment used for TLV. Experimentally, partial liquid lung ventilation has been convincingly shown to improve lung compliance, reduce the shunt fraction, and improve gas exchange.[1,47] As in the case of TLV, inflammatory debris from the distal parts of the lung is mobilized proximally; unlike in TLV, since fluid exchanges are not carried out, exudates have to be suctioned out of the proximal airways.[34,36]

Indications: Potential applications for liquid ventilation include neonatal hyaline membrane disease,[54] meconium aspiration,[35] and persistent primary pulmonary hypertension of the newborn.[13]

Although the role of liquid ventilation in adults appears to be most relevant in ARDS, its use has also been proposed in pneumonia where the lavaging of infected lungs with perfluorocarbons enables purging of bacteria and exudates,[35] and even facilitates the delivery of antibiotics suspended within the perfluorocarbon directly to the infected alveoli.[15] Perfluorocarbons have also been utilized for the prevention of lung injury during cardiopulmonary bypass,[10] and for conservation donor lungs before transplantation.[68]

The potential side effects – including bleeding, mucous plug formation, and pneumothorax – are inseparable from those of the inciting pathology.[34] Because they are radio-opaque, perfluorocarbons dramatically opacify the lungs; needless to say, their use negates the diagnostic value of the chest radiograph.

Uncontrolled trials in humans have certainly shown reason for optimism, though the specific role of liquid ventilation yet remains to be defined.

17.11 NAVA

Neurally adjusted ventilatory assist (NAVA)[60] is a novel closed-loop mode of ventilation that was specifically designed to counteract patient-ventilator asynchrony.

The delay between the neural trigger and the ventilator response time is an important cause of patient-ventilator asynchrony. At the present time, the diaphragm is the most proximal level at which a neural trigger signal can be electrically sensed. In NAVA, an array of nasogastric tube-mounted electrodes placed at the level of the diaphragm detects the intensity of the patient's neural output, and the strength of this signal, integrated to the ventilator output, determines support provided by the ventilator. The ventilator cycles on at the onset of neural inspiration and cycles off when neural expiration begins. Since the patient interacts intimately with the machine, in theory at least, synchronization is better.

17.12 Conclusion

As in any other field in clinical medicine, mechanical ventilation is not an exact science. Much conceptual change has occurred during the past three decades and many of the strategies of ventilation will continue to change. It is almost certain that the near future will see a major revolution in this field, which should fill up the deficiencies that exist in current practice.

References

1. Al-Rahmani A, Awad K, Miller TF, Wolfson MR, Shaffer TH. Effects of partial liquid ventilation with perfluorodecalin in the juvenile rabbit lung after saline injury. *Crit Care Med.* 2000;28:1459–1464
2. Anderson HL, Steimle C, Shapiro M, et al Extracorporeal life support for adult cardiorespiratory failure. *Surgery.* 1993;114:161
3. Bartlett RH. Extracorporeal life support for cardiopulmonary failure. *Curr Probl Surg.* 1990;27:621
4. Bernhard W, Haslam PL, Floros J. From birds to humans: new concepts on airways relative to alveolar surfactant. *Am J Respir Cell Mol Biol.* 2004;30:6–11
5. Bishop MJ, Benson MS, Sato P, et al Comparison of high frequency ventilation with conventional mechanical ventilation for bronchopleural fistula. *Anesth Analg.* 1987;66:833
6. Bollen CW, van Well GT, Sherry T, et al High frequency oscillatory ventilation compared with conventional mechanical ventilation in adult respiratory distress syndrome: a randomized controlled trial. *Crit Care.* 2005;9:R430
7. Bone RC, Slotman G, Maunder R, et al Randomised double-blind, multicenter study of prostaglandin E1 in patients with the adult respiratory distress syndrome. Prostaglandin E1 Study Group. *Chest.* 1989;96:114
8. Boorstein JM, Boorstein SM, Humphries GN, Johnston CC. Using helium-oxygen mixtures in the emergency management of acute upper airway obstruction. *Ann Emerg Med.* 1989;18:688
9. Brunet F, Belghith M, Mira JP, et al Extracorporeal carbon dioxide removal and low-frequency positive-pressure ventilation. Improvement in arterial oxygenation with reduction of risk of pulmonary barotrauma in patients with adult respiratory distress syndrome. *Chest.* 1993;104:889
10. Cannon ML, Cheifetz IM, Craig DM, et al Optimizing liquid ventilation as a lung protection strategy for neonatal cardiopulmonary bypass: full functional residual capacity dosing is more effective than half functional residual capacity dosing. *Crit Care Med.* 1999;27:1140
11. Whittaker KB. Neonatal mechanical ventilation In: Chang DW. Clinical Applications of Mechanical Ventilation. 3rd ed. Delmar learning; 2006;541–549
12. Clark JC Jr, Gollan F. Survival of mammals breathing organic liquids equilibrated with oxygen at atmospheric pressure. *Science.* 1966;152:1755

13. Cox CA, Wolfson MR, Shaffer TH. Liquid ventilation: a comprehensive overview. *Neonatal Netw*. 1996;15(3):31–43
14. Cueto E, Lopez-Herce J, Sanchez A, et al Life-threatening effects of discountinuing inhaled nitric oxide in children. *Acta Paediatr*. 1997;86:1337–1339
15. Cullen AB, Cox CA, Hip SJ, et al Intra-tracheal delivery strategy of gentamicin with partial liquid ventilation. *Respir Med*. 1999; 93:770
16. David M, Weiler N, Heinrichs W, et al High-frequency oscillatory ventilation in adult acute respiratory distress syndrome. *Intensive Care Med*. 2003;29:1656
17. Degraeuwe PLJ, Vos GD, Blanco CE. Perfluorochemical liquid ventilation: from the animal laboratory to the intensive care unit. *Int J Artif Organs*. 1995;18:674
18. Demory D, Michelet P, Arnal JM, et al High-frequency oscillatory ventilation following prone positioning prevents a further impairment in oxygenation. *Crit Care Med*. 2007;35:106
19. DeSanctis GT, Tomkiewicz RP, Rubin BK, et al Exogenous surfactant enhances mucociliary clearance in the anesthetized dog. *Eur Respir J*. 1994;7:1616–1621
20. Devabhaktuni VG, Torres A Jr, Wilson S, Yeh MP. Effect of nitric oxide, perfluorocarbon, and heliox on minute volume measurement and ventilator volumes delivered. *Crit Care Med*. 1999;27:1603
21. Doyle IR, Davidson KG, Barr HA, et al Quantity and structure of surfactant proteins vary among patients with alveolar proteinosis. *Am J Respir Crit Care Med*. 1998;157:658–664
22. Eastman A, Holland D, Higgins J, et al High-frequency percussive ventilation improves oxygenation in trauma patients with acute respiratory distress syndrome: a retrospective review. *Am J Surg*. 2006;192:191
23. Ferguson ND, Chiche JD, Kacmarek RM, et al Combining high-frequency oscillatory ventilation and recruitment maneuvers in adults with early acute respiratory distress syndrome: the treatment with oscillation and an open lung strategy (TOOLS) Trial pilot study. *Crit Care Med*. 2005;33:479
24. Fessler HE, Derdak S, Ferguson ND, et al A protocol for high-frequency oscillatory ventilation in adults: results from a roundtable discussion. *Crit Care Med*. 2007;35:1649
25. Forman DL, et al A new approach to induced hypothermia. *J Surg Res*. 1986;40:36
26. Froese AB. Unconventional methods of ventilator support: high frequency ventilation. In: Tobin MJ, ed. *Principles and Practice of Mechanical Ventilation*. McGraw-Hill; 2006

27. Frumin MJ, Epstein RM, Cohen G. Apneic oxygenation in man. *Anesthesiology*. 1959;20:789–798
28. Gattinoni L, Kolobow T, Tomlinson T, et al Low-frequency positive pressure ventilation with extracorporeal carbon dioxide removal (LFPPV-ECCO2R): an experimental study. *Anesth Analg*. 1978;57:470–477
29. Gerlach H, Rossaint R, Pappert D, et al Time-course and dose-response of nitric oxide inhalation for systemic oxygenation and pulmonary hypertension in patients with adult respiratory distress syndrome. *Eur J Clin Invest*. 1993;23:499–502
30. Gluck E, Heard S, Patel C, et al Use of ultrahigh frequency ventilation in patients with ARDS: a preliminary report. *Chest*. 1993;103:1413
31. Greenbaum R, Bay J, Hargreaves MD, et al Effects of higher oxides of nitrogen on the anaesthetized dog. *Br J Anaesth*. 1967;39:393–404
32. Hager DN, Fessler HE, Kaczka DW, et al Tidal volume delivery during high-frequency oscillatory ventilation in adults with acute respiratory distress syndrome. *Crit Care Med*. 2007;35:1522
33. Hemmila MR, Rowe SA, Boules TN, et al Extracorporeal life support for sever acute respiratory distress syndrome in adults. *Ann Surg*. 2004;240:595
34. Hirschl RB. Advances in the management of respiratory failure. Liquid ventilation in the setting of respiratory failure. *ASAIO J*. 1996;42:20
35. Hirschl RB, Pranikoff T, Gauger P, et al Liquid ventilation in adults, children and full-term neonates. *Lancet*. 1995;346:1201
36. Hirschl RB, Pranikoff T, Wise C, et al Initial experience with partial liquid ventilation in adult patients with the acute respiratory distress syndrome. *JAMA*. 1996;275:383
37. Hohlfeld J, Fabel H, Hamm H. The role of pulmonary surfactant in obstructive airway disease. *Eur Respir J*. 1997;10:482–491
38. Ito Y, Manwell SEE, Kerr CL, et al Effect of ventilation strategies on the efficacy of exogenous surfactant therapy in a rabbit model of acute lung injury. *Am J Respir Crit Care Med*. 1998;157:149–155
39. Kobayashi T, Nitta K, Ganzuka M, et al Inactivation of exogenous surfactant by pulmonary edema fluid. *Pediatr Res*. 1991;29:353–356
40. Kolla S, Lee WA, Hirschl RB, Bartlett RH. Extracorporeal life support for cardiovascular support in adults. *ASAIO J*. 1996;42:M809
41. Kylstra JA, Tissing MO, Van der Maen A. Of mice as fish. *ASAIO Trans*. 1962;8:378

42. McCormack FX, King TEJ, Voelker DR, et al Idiopathic pulmonary fibrosis. Abnormalities in the bronchoalveolar lavage content of surfactant protein A. *Am Rev Respir Dis*. 1991;144:160–166
43. Mehta S, MacDonald R, Hallett DC, et al Acute oxygenation response to inhaled nitric oxide when combined with high-frequency oscillatory ventilation in adults with acute respiratory distress syndrome. *Crit Care Med*. 2003;31:383
44. Mehta S, Granton J, MacDonald RJ, et al High-frequency oscillatory ventilation in adults: the Toronto experience. *Chest*. 2004;126:518
45. Mentzelopoulos SD, Roussos C, Koutsoukou A, et al Acute effects of combined high-frequency oscillation and tracheal gas insufflation in severe acute respiratory distress syndrome. *Crit Care Med*. 2007;35:1500
46. Milner AD, Hoskins EW. High frequency positive pressure ventilation in neonates. *Arch Dis Child*. 1989;64(1):1–3; [Fetal Neonatal ed]
47. Papo MC, Paczan PR, Fuhrman BP, et al Perfluorocarbon associated gas exchange improves oxygenation, lung mechanics, and survival in a model of adult respiratory distress syndrome. *Crit Care Med*. 1996;24:466–474
48. Peek GJ, Clemens F, Elbourne D, et al CESAR: conventional ventilatory support vs extracorporeal membrane oxygenation for severe adult respiratory failure. *BMC Health Serv Res*. 2006; 6:163
49. Putensen C, Rasanen J, Lopez FA, et al Continuous positive air way pressure modulates effect of inhaled nitric oxide on the ventilation- perfusion distributions in canine lung injury. *Chest*. 1994;106:1563–1569
50. Puybasset L, Rouby JJ, Mourgeon E, et al Factors influencing cardiopulmonary effects of inhaled nitric oxide in acute respiratory failure. *Am J Respir Crit Care Med*. 1995;152:318–328
51. Quezado ZM, Natanson C, Karzai W, et al Cardiopulmonary effects of inhaled nitric oxide in normal dogs and during E. coli pneumonia and sepsis. *J Appl Physiol*. 1998;84:107–115
52. Reper P, Wibaux O, Van Laeke P, et al High frequency percussive ventilation and conventional ventilation after smoke inhalation: a randomised study. *Burns*. 2002;28:503
53. Rialp G, Betbese AJ, Peres-Marquez M, et al Short-term effects of inhaled nitric oxide and prone position in pulmonary and extrapulmonary acute respiratory distress syndrome. *Am J Respir Crit Care Med*. 2001;164:243–249

54. Richman PS, Wolfson MR, Shaffer TH. Lung lavage with oxygenated perfluorochemical liquid in acute lung injury. *Crit Care Med.* 1993;21:768
55. Rossaint R, Falke KJ, Lopez F, et al Inhaled nitric oxide for the adult respiratory distress syndrome. *N Engl J Med.* 1993;328: 399–405
56. Salim A, Martin M. High-frequency percussive ventilation. *Crit Care Med.* 2005;33:S241
57. Seeger W, Grube C, Gunther A, Schmidt R. Surfactant inhibition by plasma proteins: differential sensitivity of various surfactant preparations. *Eur Respir J.* 1993;6:971–977
58. Shaffer TH, Forman D, Wolfson MR. The physiological effects of breathing fluorocarbon liquids at various temperatures. *Undersea Biomed Res.* 1984;11:287
59. Shaffer TH, Wolfson MR, Clark LC. State of the art review. Liquid ventilation. *Pediatr Pulmonol.* 1992;14:102
60. Sinderby C, Navalesi P, Beck J, et al Neural control of mechanical ventilation in respiratory failure. *Nat Med.* 1999;5:1433–1436
61. Smith TM, Steinhorn DM, Thusu K, et al A liquid perfluorochemical decreases the in vitro production of reactive oxygen species by alveolar macrophages. *Crit Care Med.* 1995;23:1533
62. Spragg R, Lewis J, Walmrath H, et al Effect of recombinant surfactant protein C based surfactant on patients with the acute respiratory distress syndrome. *N Engl J Med.* 2004;351:884–892
63. Veldhuizen R, Nag K, Orgeig S, et al The role of lipids in pulmonary surfactant. *Biochim Biophys Acta.* 1998;1408:90–108
64. Veldhuizen RA, Yao L, Lewis JF. An examination of the different variables affecting surfactant aggregate conversion in vitro. *Exp Lung Res.* 1999;25:127–141
65. Walmarth D, Grimminger F, Pappert D, et al Bronchoscopic administration of bovine natural surfactant in ARDS and septic shock; impact on gas exchange and haemodynamics. *Eur Respir J.* 2002;19:805–810
66. Whitsett JA. Surfactant proteins in innate host defense of the lung. *Biol Neonate.* 2005;88:175–180
67. Wolfson MR, Kechner NE, Rubenstein D, et al Perfluorochemical (PFC) uptake and biodistribution following liquid assisted ventilation in the immature lamb. *Pediatr Res.* 1994;35:A246
68. Yoshida S, Sekine Y, Shinozuka N, et al The efficacy of partial liquid ventilation in lung protection during hypotension and cardiac arrest: preliminary study of lung transplantation using non-heart-beating donors. *J Heart Lung Transplant.* 2005;24:723

69. Zapol WM, Snider MT, Hill JD, et al Extracorporeal membrane oxygenation in severe acute respiratory failure. A randomized prospective study. *JAMA*. 1979;242:2193
70. Zobel G, Dacar D, Rodl S. Proximal and tracheal airway pressure during different modes of mechanical ventilation: an animal model study. *Pediatr Pulmonol*. 1994;18:239

Chapter 18
Case Studies

The following modules represent some of the common situations that require troubleshooting on mechanically ventilated patients.

18.1 Case 1

Mr. A was ventilated 4 days ago for type-2 respiratory failure during a severe exacerbation of COPD. When recovering on the ventilator, he suddenly developed respiratory distress and tachycardia. SpO_2 which had hitherto been stable at 92% on an FIO_2 of 0.28, dropped to 69%. The peak airway pressure alarm became activated simultaneously with the onset of Mr. A's respiratory distress, and tidal volumes (set at 480 mL on the assist-control mode) became severely pressure limited and dropped substantially. Appropriate action at this stage would be:

(a) Disconnection from ventilator followed by bagging and suctioning the ET tube
(b) Chest X-ray
(c) ABG
(d) A careful physical examination

The correct answer is (a) since it permits immediate identification of whether the problem is with the machine or with the patient; it further enables diagnosis and treatment of an endotracheal tube block which is not only common, but must be urgently identified.

A. Hasan, *Understanding Mechanical Ventilation*,
DOI 10.1007/978-1-84882-869-8_18,

Mr. A was disconnected from the ventilator and manually ventilated with a bag and mask. The bag appeared stiff and substantial resistance to manual compression of the bag was encountered. A suction catheter passed down the endotracheal tube encountered significant resistance to its passage. After thorough suctioning, which resulted in the removal of sticky mucus, the suction catheter could now pass unimpeded down the endotracheal tube. Mr. A was reconnected to the ventilator and was now more comfortable; although the peak pressure was now lower, it was still high than before. Reasons for the persistently elevated peak pressure could include:

(a) A partial blockage of endotracheal tube
(b) Bronchospasm
(c) A small "occult" pneumothorax
(d) Any of the above

The correct answer is (d), since all three conditions can elevate the peak airway pressure.

Clinical examination did not reveal an overt bronchospasm, and a bedside chest film did not reveal a pneumothorax. The next logical option would be:

(a) Arterial blood gas analysis
(b) Change the endotracheal tube regardless of the fact that the suction catheter can be negotiated through it
(c) Chest physiotherapy
(d) Work up for pulmonary embolism

The correct answer is (b). Even slight narrowing of the lumen of the endotracheal tube can result in significant airflow obstruction. The endotracheal tube was, a short time ago, completely blocked, and it is likely that encrustations remain, causing partial blockage. Apart from the risk of reblockage, breathing through a narrowed endotracheal tube entails a high work of breathing and predisposes to respiratory muscle fatigue. When in doubt, the endotracheal tube should be changed.

On the evening of the next day, the low pressure and low minute ventilation alarms began to sound. Also, the inspired tidal volume exceeded the expired tidal volume. The potential problem could be any of the following *except*:

(a) ET obstruction
(b) ET cuff leak or rupture
(c) Air leak from temperature monitor port
(d) Leak from exhalation valve

The correct answer is (a). Note that this is an "except" question. Endotracheal tube obstruction leads to the activation of the high airway pressure alarm and not the low airway pressure alarm. The other three mentioned above can all lead to a fall in airway pressures.

Auscultation over the trachea revealed harsh breath sounds over the entire duration of the inspiratory phase. What should be done?

(a) Increase the minute volume
(b) Check and inflate pilot bulb to the required pressure
(c) Increase flow rate
(d) All of the above

The correct answer is (b). The presence of a hiss over the trachea during the ventilator delivered breath argues in favor of a cuff leak. The cuff should be reinflated by inflating the pilot bulb. If the pilot bulb fails to fill despite inflation with repeated boluses of air, a cuff rupture is likely and the ET should be replaced.
The ET was replaced, but with a much smaller sized endotracheal tube owing to some difficulty in reintubation. The inflation of the pilot bulb resulted in the disappearance of the inspiratory sound, but the pilot bulb pressure required to achieve this seal was 36 cm H_2O. The problem now was:

(a) Right main-stem intubation
(b) Size of ET too small for the patient's airway

(c) Defective pilot bulb
(d) All of the above

The correct answer is (b). Much more air needs to be introduced into the pilot bulb of an ETT which has a diameter that is small relative to the trachea, in order to ensure an effective seal.

18.2 Case 2

Mrs. B, aged 32 years was brought to the ICU after falling off the pillion of a motor-scooter half an hour ago. She had become unconscious after the fall and had not gained consciousness since. On arrival at the ICU, she had a BP of 140/90 and a heart rate of 108 beats/min. She had a single bruise on her occiput, and there were multiple lacerations on her chest and arms. Her lungs were clear to auscultation. Withdrawal response to painful stimuli was present and the pupils were equal and responsive. A CT scan of the brain showed an intracranial bleed. Mrs. B's chest film showed fractures of three ribs on her right side, as well as a small right sided pneumothorax. An intracranial probe revealed that the intracranial pressure was raised.

The indications for intubation in the case of Mrs. B would be:

(a) To protect the airway
(b) To ventilate with an intent to produce hypocapnia
(c) Both the above
(d) Nonc of the above

The correct answer is (c). In cases of neurological injury, mechanical ventilation with deliberate hyperventilation with the intent of producing hypocapnia is not resorted to unless the intracranial pressure is high. In cases of raised intracranial pressure, hypocapnia has been gainfully employed to quickly reduce the intracranial tension. In a patient with poor

airway defense mechanisms, intubation can protect the airway and prevent aspiration. Since even a small pneumothorax has the potential to transform itself into a tension pneumothorax on the ventilator, a chest drain was inserted into the right pleural cavity.

A while later, expiratory tidal volumes fell well below the inspiratory tidal volumes. A circuit check revealed no obvious leak in the system. The most likely cause of this phenomenon could be:

(a) Herniation of the endotracheal tube cuff
(b) Alveolar instability
(c) A large air leak through a bronchopleural fistula
(d) Any of the above

The correct answer is (c). Sustained bubbling from the underwater seal of the chest drain throughout the respiratory cycle was seen, which was surprising since the pneumothorax had been quite small. A large bronchopleural fistula was diagnosed.

Appropriate action should now include:

(a) Measures to reduce alveolar distension
(b) High frequency jet ventilation
(c) Sealing of the local bronchopulmonary segment by gelfoam or fibrin
(d) Laser coagulation of the leak

In theory, all these options have been attempted to treat bronchopleural fistulae. In practice, it is seldom necessary to do anything other than to limit the alveolar over-distension that often engenders them. Bronchopleural fistulae generally resolve parri-passu with improvement in the underlying lung pathology and in instances such as above where the minute ventilation is not compromised, a conservative line of management is often sufficient. Therefore, (a) is the correct answer.

18.3 Case 3

Mr. C, 56-years old, having chronic bronchitis, was admitted with an acute exacerbation of his condition, and in due course, had to be intubated and ventilated for hypercapnic respiratory failure which had progressed despite optional medical therapy.

On day 2 of ventilatio on the assist-control mode, Mr C's already elevated peak airway pressure suddenly rose further. Mr. C became tachypneic, began overbreathing the set respiratory rate, and looked distressed. A suction catheter passed down the endotracheal tube encountered no perceptible resistance and airway secretions were not much in evidence. Breath entry appeared markedly diminished on the left side. Diagnostic possibilities would include:

(a) Collapse of the left lung due to secretions
(b) Collapse of the left lung due to endotracheal tube migration into the right main-stem bronchus
(c) Left sided pneumothorax
(d) Any of the above

The correct answer is (d). Lack of aspirable secretions from the endotracheal tube cannot rule out mucus plugging more distally, and endotracheal tube migration into the right main bronchus can obstruct the orifice of the left main bronchus causing absorbtive atelectasis. Barotrauma in a patient on mechanical ventilation is also a possibility at any time and a high degree of suspicion for the same must be maintained.

An urgent bedside chest film revealed a collapsed left lung. The tip of the endotracheal tube was visualized well proximal to the carina and distal migration of the endotracheal tube was so ruled out. SpO_2 at this stage was 92% on a FIO_2 of 0.6.

Appropriate therapy at this stage would be:

(a) Chest physiotherapy
(b) Urgent bronchoscopic toilet

(c) Chest physiotherapy followed by bronchoscopic toilet, should the lung not expand with the former
(d) Deep suctioning

The correct answer is (c). Deep suctioning is not an option. In any case, a suction catheter would be liable to follow the path of least resistance and pass into the right main bronchus which is more aligned with the trachea and not the left main bronchus which is likely to be obstructed with a mucus plug or a blood clot. Chest therapy is a reasonable initial option since a saturation of 92% is for the time being satisfactory, but this should be followed up with a bronchoscopic toilet, should the lung not expand with chest physiotherapy alone.

18.4 Case 4

Mrs. D, aged 72 years was intubated and ventilated for type 1 respiratory failure secondary to cardiogenic pulmonary edema. Having improved, she was extubated after 48 h. Immediately post extubation, Mrs. D developed stridor and considerable respiratory difficulty. Diagnostic possibilities include:

(a) Laryngospasm
(b) Laryngeal edema
(c) Either a or b
(d) Tracheal stenosis.

The correct answer is (c). Since the stridor occurred within a short time of extubation, laryngeal edema (as a result of injury to the larynx during intubation) could be proposed as a likely cause of stridor. Laryngospasm is also possible; tracheal stenosis usually takes much longer to manifest.

Inspection of the larynx revealed laryngeal edema, but absence of other significant injury. At this stage, the initial treatment could include:

(a) Tracheostomy
(b) Corticosteroids

(c) Lidocaine
(d) Racemic epinephrine, followed by reintubation if required, with a smaller sized endotracheal tube

The correct answer is (d). Tracheostomy is not an option at this stage without allowing a little time for resolution of the laryngeal edema. Corticosteroids have not been convincingly demonstrated to be beneficial and although IV or tropical lidocaine has been used in cases of laryngospasm with some benefit, its role in laryngeal edema is unknown.

Mrs. D required reintubation, and a smaller sized endotracheal tube was used to negotiate the swollen larynx. She was extubated after another 48 h and made an uneventful recovery.

What parameter or test could have predicted the presence of laryngeal edema before extubation?

(a) SpO_2
(b) Tidal volume
(c) Spontaneous respiratory effort
(d) Cuff leak test

The correct answer is (d). Deflation of the ET cuff by evacuating the pilot bulb should result in an inspiration sound on auscultation over the trachea, as air leaks between the ET tube and the airway. Lack of such a sound would imply a snug fit between the ET and the airway, and the cause of this could possibly be laryngeal edema.

18.5 Case 5

On day 7 of ventilation for a neuromuscular problem, Ms. E, aged 22 years, suddenly developed ventilatory distress. She was removed from the ventilator and bagged. A suction catheter passed down the ET encountered no resistance, and on auscultation, the breath entry was normal and equal. The therapist then hooked her back onto the ventilator, and noticed that although the oxygen saturation had fallen, the lung compliance and resistance were unchanged. The possible problem could be:

(a) Pneumothorax
(b) Pulmonary embolism
(c) Lobar collapse
(d) Endotracheal tube obstruction

The correct answer is (b). Although it is possible for a small pneumothorax to go undetected on clinical examination, pneumothoraces in patients on mechanical ventilation often become tension pneumothoraces and become clinically obvious.

Endotracheal obstruction is virtually ruled out by the unhindered passage of a suction catheter down the breathing tube, and the absence of clinical wheeze or a rise in airway pressure can reasonably exclude bronchospasm. Likewise, the absence of a fall in pulmonary compliance and/or a rise in airway pressures argues against major lobar atelectasis. Pulmonary embolism is the correct answer since it *can* produce hypoxemia without a significant change in either compliance or resistance. An unchanged chest film in this case strengthened the suspicion of pulmonary embolism which was later confirmed.

18.6 Case 6

Mr. F, a 42-year-old persistent asthmatic was intubated and ventilated during an attack of acute severe asthma which failed to respond to conventional medical therapy. He was a hypertensive, well controlled on medication and was in the habit of taking 5 mg diazepam nocte for the last 10 years. Postintubation ventilator settings were: assist-control mode with a backup of 14 breaths/min, at 500 mL/breath, FIO_2 (which, a few minutes earlier had been 1.0) 0.6. After awakening from the sedation that he required at intubation, Mr. F became increasingly agitated and violent and had to be sedated and paralyzed. At this point, his pulse rate rose to 130 beats/min, respirations 36 breaths/min. SpO_2 was 98%. Possible causes of hiss restlessness could be:

(a) A blocked endotracheal tube
(b) Steroid psychosis
(c) Intrinsic PEEP
(d) Any of the above

The correct answer is (d). A blocked endotracheal tube is in many cases the cause of sudden restlessness and agitation in a ventilated patient. Tenacious secretions coat the luminal surface of the endotracheal tube and can progressively reduce the lumen of the endotracheal tube before a plug of inspissated mucus or clot of blood causes sudden total occlusion. The patient's distress may not immediately be accompanied by a fall in SpO_2, as a change in saturation usually takes time to register on the monitor. An acute rise in peak pressure is often the clue and resistance to the passage of a suction catheter down the endotracheal tube is virtually diagnostic of a tube block. Although ET blockage is unusual in a recently intubated patient, it should still be ruled out in such a situation. Sleep deprivation is also known to produce agitation and some patients on glucocorticoids develop steroid psychosis. The development of intrinsic-PEEP (auto-PEEP) can lead to considerable patient-ventilator asynchrony and this can manifest in the patient fighting the ventilator. In this instance, the cause of the patient's agitation proved to be a high intrinsic PEEP due to air-trapping and dynamic hyperinflation.

Appropriate corrective measures would include all, except:

(a) Bronchodilation
(b) Decreasing I:E ratio
(c) Increasing the duration of the inspiratory pause
(d) Adding a small amount of external PEEP (about 50–75% of the measured intrinsic-PEEP)

The correct answer is (c). Note that this is an "except" question. Decreasing inspiratory time leaves more time for expiration, and more complete lung emptying is possible, reducing dynamic hyperinflation, and thereby decreasing the auto-PEEP. The addition of a small amount of external PEEP reduces the gradient against which the patient must inspire, thus reducing the work of breathing.

Increasing the pause time, however, (note that the inspiratory pause is considered part of the inspiratory time) will actually leave *less* time for expiration and will actually worsen dynamic hyperinflation.

In Mr. F's case, despite the application of optimal ventilator strategies, peak and plateau pressures remained at unacceptable levels; the setting of maximal airway pressure at 45 cm H_2O resulted in termination of the inspiratory breath when 280 mL or so of the tidal volume had been delivered at each breath, and the hypoventilation resulted in a rise in the $PaCO_2$ to 72 mmHg. Appropriate strategies at this stage comprise all of the following except:

(a) Ventilation with helium–oxygen gas mixture
(b) Pressure control ventilation
(c) Permissive hypercapnia
(d) Raising the upper airway pressure limit

The correct answer is (d). Note that this is an "except" question. Since the set tidal volume is 500 mL and the breath is anyway being pressure limited to 280 mL, reduction in tidal volumes would serve no purpose. Since the low tidal volumes are now resulting in reduced minute ventilation, one way to allow delivery of the targeted tidal volumes would be to raise the upper airway pressure limit. This would, however, allow the upper airway pressure to rise and thereby unacceptably increase the risk of barotrauma.

The other strategies are all acceptable in this situation, though the usage of heliox is limited to a few centers and not yet in the realms of conventional ventilatory strategy.

18.7 Case 7

Mr. G, a 21-year-old man was admitted to the ICU, after a collision with a bus caused his vehicle to overturn. On examination, Mr. G was well oriented and alert but in considerable pain. His heart rate was 110 beats/min, respirations 22 breaths/min and BP 140/80. Breath entry was equal and satisfactory on both sides, but a flail segment of the sternum moved paradoxically with each breath.

The chest film confirmed the presence of multiple rib fractures bilaterally and some subcutaneous emphysema, but no obvious pneumothorax. The ABG on FIO_2 of 0.4 showed pH 7.36, $PaCO_2$ 38, and PaO_2 120 mmHg. Appropriate action now would be:

(a) Observation and adequate analgesia
(b) External stabilization of the chest by splints
(c) Internal stabilization of the chest by intubation ventilation and the application of PEEP
(d) Closed chest drainage

Mr. G's blood gases do not show the presence of respiratory failure, which is the indication for mechanical ventilation in flail chest. A $PaCO_2$ of 38 mmHg is reasonable: it certainly does not indicate hypoventilation. The respiratory rate is a bit high, which is understandable since the impaired mechanics of the chest wall do not allow complete excursions of the chest and Mr. G is fulfilling his minute volume requirements by raising his respiratory rate; the latter by itself, is not high enough to impose a significantly high work of breathing. In fact, noninvasive ventilation could be considered if the work of breathing were judged to be bordering on high. Subcutaneous emphysema does not always equate with pneumothorax, though the chest X-ray should be carefully scrutinized for a small inobvious pneumothorax; it is also mandatory in such cases to closely watch the patient for the subsequent development of a "late" pneumothorax. External splints are often not very effective. Analgesia plays an important role, facilitates bronchial toilet, and prevents chest infections. The correct answer therefore is (a).

Later on, Mr. G became increasingly tachypneic and distressed, and it was discovered that he did eventually develop a pneumothorax on the right. Closed chest drainage was performed, but during the while, Mr. G's saturations dropped and he had to be intubated and ventilated. A postintubation chest film showed that the pneumothorax had resolved, but the *left* lung had now collapsed. Diagnostic possibilities would include:

(a) Obstruction of the left main bronchus by clot
(b) Obstruction of the left main bronchus by a mucus plug
(c) Fracture of the left main bronchus
(d) Any of the above

The correct answer is (d). All three are possible in this setting. A diagnostic bronchoscopy discovered a mucus plug, the origin of which was uncertain, and the procedure proved to be of therapeutic benefit as well. Mr. G thereafter made an uneventful recovery.

18.8 Case 8

Mr. H, a 60-year-old diabetic, hypertensive, and smoker of thirty cigarettes per day for the last 40 years, was admitted with chest discomfort and difficulty in breathing since the last hour. On arrival, Mr. H was orthopneic, diaphoretic, and restless. His BP was recorded as 160/100, his heart rate 110 beats/min, and respirations 40 breaths/min. The JVP was raised, there was bilateral pedal edema, and profuse basal crepitations were heard in both lungs.

A chest film demonstrated cardiomegaly and bilateral symmetrical pulmonary parenchymal shadowing characteristic of cardiogenic pulmonary edema. The ECG showed evidence of evolving myocardial infarction. PaO_2 remained at 47 mmHg in spite of high flow oxygen, and there was lack of significant response to diuresis and other medication. Treatment options would include:

(a) Further observation and more diuresis
(b) NIPPV

(c) Intubation and ventilation
(d) All of the above

The correct answer is (c), since the patient already satisfies a number of criteria for intubation and ventilation viz., refractory hypoxemia, tachypnea, and increased work of breathing in the presence of cardiac ischemia, especially in the face of lack of response to medication. It is unlikely that NIPPV would be beneficial at this stage since it would likely be ineffective in supporting the patient at this stage.

The following is accepted as a conventional ventilatory strategy in CCF:

(a) High frequency jet ventilation
(b) Nitric oxide
(c) PEEP
(d) Heliox

The correct answer is (c). The benefits that occur due to the application of PEEP are due to its ability to reduce preload in a failing heart. Also, by decreasing transmural aortic pressure, PEEP improves cardiac output, and by increasing functional residual capacity, it improves oxygenation and compliance. Since the effect of PEEP in an individual patient is by and large unpredictable, the patient should be closely monitored.

18.9 Case 9

Mrs. J, a 28-year-old asthmatic was brought to the ICU in status asthmaticus. She was breathless and tachypneic, with a respiratory rate of 28 breaths/min. Auscultation revealed markedly diminished breath entry on both sides and her chest film showed hyperinflated lungs, but no obvious infiltrate. An ABG taken 2 h after the administration of IV steroid, O_2, and continuous nebulization showed pH 7.20, $PaCO_2$ 44, and PaO_2 75 mmHg on FIO_2 0.5. What should be the further course of action?

(a) Continue treatment with continuous nebulization
(b) Noninvasive positive pressure ventilation
(c) Addition of a diuretic
(d) Consider intubation and ventilation

The correct answer is (d). A patient in exacerbation of asthma should normally be hyperventilating and will therefore show a reduced $PaCO_2$. A normal $PaCO_2$ implies that the partial pressure of CO_2 is beginning to trend upward due to respiratory muscle exhaustion. In Mrs. J's case, the acidic pH testifies to this. At this juncture, it is very unlikely that NIPPV will provide enough support to the respiratory muscles to reverse the critical process. The choice in such a patient should be elective intubation and ventilation when it becomes obvious that the $PaCO_2$ is trending upward and the patient is fatiguing.

After the intubation and ventilation, Mrs. J was put on the assist-control mode. All of the following ventilator settings would be appropriate in her case except:

(a) Large tidal volumes to wash out the accumulating $PaCO_2$
(b) Titration down of the FIO_2 to keep PaO_2 above 60 mmHg
(c) See the upper airway pressure alarm at 40 cm H_20
(d) Low I:E ratio

The correct answer is (a). Note that this is an "except" question. Large tidal volumes in the setting of airway obstruction have the potential to exacerbate dynamic hyperinflation which is already a problem in such circumstances. A FIO_2 tailored to keep PaO_2 above 60 mmHg is sufficient, for at this PaO_2 the hemoglobin should be near-completely saturated with O_2. A low I:E ratio helps in that, with the shorter inspiration, a longer expiratory time is available to the overdistended lung to empty. A peak pressure of 40 and above has been linked to an increased risk of barotrauma, though it now appears that plateau pressures of more than 35 cm H_2O equally, if not more closely, correlate with pressure-induced pulmonary injury.

18.10 Case 10

Mr. K, a COPD patient was ventilated 2 days ago for type 2 respiratory failure. At this stage, his current ventilator settings were as follows: On the assist-control mode, the tidal volume was 550, the respiratory rate 15 breaths/min, FIO_2 0.28, inspiratory trigger –2 cm H_2O, and inspiratory flow rate 50 L/min.

Although the blood gases and vitals were acceptable, Mr. K evinced a sense of dyspnea. Which of the following changes in the ventilator settings would be likely to help?

(a) Increasing the tidal volume
(b) Increasing the respiratory rate
(c) Increasing the FIO_2
(d) Increasing the inspiratory flow rate

The correct answer is (d). Since the blood gases are acceptable the minute ventilation need not be changed. Similarly, if the PaO_2 is >60 mmHg on the present FIO_2 (0.28), no change in FIO_2 is required either. The inspiratory trigger is fairly low, so this should not impose a significant inspiratory load on Mr. K's respiratory muscles. It is important, however, to realize that many persons, particularly patients with normal respiratory drives, require high inspiratory flow rates to fulfill the demands of their respiratory centers. Increasing the inspiratory flows should help.

Later, Mr. K was put on SIMV (set rate 10 breaths/min) with a pressure support of 5 cm. The respiratory care practitioner noticed that Mr. K's spontaneous tidal volumes ranged between 130 and 210 mL. What could be done to increase the tidal volume of the spontaneous breaths:

(a) Increase the number of SIMV breaths
(b) Increase the level of pressure support
(c) Increase the tidal volume
(d) All of the above

The correct answer is (b). Increasing the level of pressure support can help increase the tidal volume of spontaneous breaths.

A few days later Mr. K seemed better; he was still being ventilated on the SIMV with PS mode, at a pressure support of 10 cm H_2O. Mr. K was then breathing at the SIMV backup rate of 9 breaths/min and taking an additional six breaths of his own at a tidal volume of 350–400 mL, through an endotracheal tube of size 7.5. In the morning, the ABG read as follows: pH 7.38, PCO_2 32 mmHg, and PaO_2 154 mmHg on 0.5 FIO_2. On switching to the pressure support mode (PSV of 10 mmHg), Mr. K's spontaneous tidal volumes fell to 250 mL and spontaneous respiratory frequency rose to 35 breaths/min, accompanied by subjective and objective signs of distress. The respiratory care practitioner reverted to the previous mode. Which of the following could make Mr. K wean successfully?

(a) Reduction in FIO_2
(b) Change in the endotracheal tube to a larger size
(c) Progressively raising the PCO_2 to approximately 50 mmHg before beginning the weaning process
(d) All of the above

The correct answer is (d). Theoretically, a reduction in FIO_2 to 0.28 or thereabouts would help boost the respiratory drive of the chronic lunger who is habitually accustomed to a high $PaCO_2$ though admittedly there appears nothing grossly wrong with Mr. K's respiratory drive at this moment. By the same token, the starting point for a spontaneous breathing trial for a COPD patient should ideally be at a $PaCO_2$ level that is at the patient's usual premorbid baseline, and so a $PaCO_2$ buildup to about 50 mmHg or even higher is considered appropriate in such cases before commencing the weaning trial. When weaning becomes difficult, a change in the endotracheal tube to as large a size as possible would help in substantially reducing the airway resistance and considerably help in the weaning process.

18.11 Case 11

Mr. L, a 72-year-old COPD patient was brought to the EMD. During transport, Mr. L had been given oxygen supplementation by a partial rebreathing mask at 12 L/min. At reception, Mr. L was drowsy and was breathing at only 5–6 breaths/min. An ABG performed on arrival showed pH 7.19, PaO_2 66 mmHg, $PaCO_2$ 92 mmHg.

Treatment options would include:

(a) Administering FIO_2 at 0.28 by ventimask
(b) Making the patient breathe room air
(c) Increasing FIO_2 by administering O_2 through a nonrebreathing mask
(d) Intubation and ventilation

The correct answer is (a). It is conceivable that the high flow oxygen administered to the patient during transport has suppressed his respiratory drive, compounding the hypercapnic respiratory failure. Reducing the FIO_2 to an acceptable level is logical, in that the patient would still be getting enough FIO_2 to maintain a reasonable O_2 saturation and the reduction in FIO_2 would also allow Mr. L's hypoxic respiratory drive to improve his ventilatory status.

Completely stopping supplemental oxygen is *not* an option. The PAO_2 (the partial pressure of oxygen in the alveolus) is determined by the following equation:

$$PAO_2 = [(\text{Atm pressure} - \text{Partial pressure of water vapour}) \times FIO_2] - [(PaCO_2 / \text{respiratory quotient})]$$

At sea level with a respiratory quotient of 0.8, assuming that 12 (LPM) by partial rebreathing mask corresponds to an FIO_2 of approximately 0.6,

$$PAO_2 = [(760 - 47) \times 0.6] - [(92/0.8)]$$
$$= 312.8 \text{ mm Hg}$$

If the supplemental O_2 were to be suddenly stopped, the patient would be breathing room air only (FIO_2>0.21) and with a PCO_2 of 92,

$$PAO_2 = [(760 - 47) \times 0.21] - [(92/8)]$$
$$= 34 \text{ mm Hg}$$

A low partial pressure of oxygen in the alveolus would mean that the arterial PaO_2 would be lower yet, and this could result in cerebral hypoxia. Supplemental oxygen should therefore never be completely removed.

Many physicians may feel that it would be hasty to intubate and ventilate the patient in a situation such as this, and would rather give the patient a chance to recover with a trial of initial conservative therapy. The role of NIPPV in this setting is unclear. Certainly, in a drowsy patient NIPPV is relatively contraindicated, (and here, there may be differences of opinion), but can be tried as the sensorium begins to improve. Bronchodilators, corticosteroids, antibiotics and respiratory stimulants may be used as the situation demands, with recourse to mechanical ventilation being taken if the PaO_2 is not sustainable at ≥60 mmHg with conservative therapy, or if there is a progressive rise in $PaCO_2$ with acidosis inspite of optimal treatment.

18.12 Case 12

Mrs. M aged 30 years, weighing 65 kg is being ventilated for severe ARDS. The mode of ventilation initially used is assist-control. Appropriate tidal volumes for this patient should be:

(a) 400 mL
(b) 600 mL
(c) 800 mL
(d) 1,000 mL

The correct answer is (a). Patients with severe ARDS have "baby lungs." This means that healthy alveoli comprise approximately a third of the lung volume; another third of the lung is represented by collapsed but recruitable alveoli, while the remaining third is composed of densely consolidated or collapsed alveoli. Ventilating such patients with large tidal volumes would cause overdistension of the healthy

and compliant alveoli, resulting in alveolar injury. Low tidal volumes coupled with enough PEEP to hold the unstable alveolar units open is the currently recommended strategy for ARDS. At approximately 6–7 mg/kg body weight, a 400 mL tidal volume would be appropriate for Mrs. M.
Mrs. M's set respiratory rate is 22 breaths/min, FIO_2 is 0.9 and PEEP is 5 cm H_2O. Her BP is 140/90 and her ABG is as follows: pH 7.39 $PaCO_2$ 43 mmHg and PaO_2 49 mmHg. An appropriate intervention to increase Mrs. R's oxygenation would be:

(a) Increase the FIO_2
(b) Increase the PEEP
(c) Increase the respiratory frequency
(d) Lower the tidal volume further

The correct answer is (b). The FIO_2 is already 0.9, which is too high to be safe and the physician should try to reduce the FIO_2 rather than increase it, in order to decrease the chances of oxygen-induced lung injury. Increasing the PEEP would be a good idea, since the blood pressure at this stage is well preserved.

During the incremental application of PEEP to 14 cm H_2O, monitoring of which one parameter is *particularly* relevant?

(a) Heart rate
(b) Blood pressure
(c) Urine output
(d) $EtCO_2$

The correct answer is (b). Increase in PEEP decreases the venous return to the thorax and can have an early impact upon the blood pressure which therefore should be closely monitored. Mrs. M tolerated a PEEP of 14 cm well, and her BP was steady at 130/80.
Over the next few days, Mrs. M's lung mechanics worsened further and she was switched to pressure control ventilation. Despite all attempts to decrease the FIO_2 to 0.6, it was not possible to do so and Mrs. M's PaO_2 was 50 on a FIO_2 of 1.0

and PEEP 16 cm H_2O. The next option to increase Mrs. M's oxygenation should be:

(a) Permissive hypercapnia
(b) Inverse ratio ventilation
(c) $ECCO_2R$
(d) ECMO

The correct answer is (b). PC-IRV (pressure control-inverse ratio ventilation) or VC-IRV (volume control-inverse ratio ventilation) should be the next option. Patients find the inversion of the respiratory time extremely uncomfortable and regularly require deep sedation with or without paralyzing agents. Placing the patient in a prone position too may help. The benefits conferred by extracorporeal life support are slender, though recent reports show better outcomes with LFPPV-$ECCO_2R$.

With the application of PC-IRV with a PCV level of 40 cm H_2O and an I:E ratio 1:1, a PEEP of 12 cm H_2O and an FIO_2 of 0.8, the PaO_2 was a bit better at 58 mmHg, but the $PaCO_2$ gradually climbed to 55 with a progressive fall in the tidal volume. Further attempts to increase the I:E ratio resulted in a fall in the patient's blood pressure. An appropriate option at this point of time would be:

(a) Permissive hypercapnia
(b) Increasing I:E ratio to 2:1
(c) High frequency jet ventilation
(d) Increasing the PEEP

The correct answer is (a). The problem now seems to be that the increasing airway pressure is limiting the tidal volumes causing the $PaCO_2$ to rise, and compromising the hemodynamics. In the end, it may be better to accept a moderate rise in CO_2 since the PaO_2 seems better than before.

Index

F

G

H

O

R

S

T